WEIGHT LOSS BY GINA

FALL 2022 PROGRAM

Posts and Guidelines

ISBN: 9798848959895

We are committed to making weight loss as easy as possible. In doing so, we have put together this booklet containing the instructional information which will be posted in the Fall 2022 Group week to week. Please keep in mind this booklet does NOT contain all of the information and posts, so you will still need to check into the Group day to day to review any newly added information and to watch the videos that go along with these posts.

At the end of this workbook you will find additional resources that may help with your journey. We have included 10 sample recipes that you can try. These are just to give you an idea of the types of foods you can have in the Program. We have also included a Science Guide, which contains additional articles that go more in depth into the science behind the Program. Lastly, you will also find some tracking sheets that you can use to track your progress. The tracking sheets will help you pick up on patterns of behaviour and how your body is responding to the changes you are making day to day.

I also want to acknowledge and thank Anna Blachuta, Sasha Spycher-Sulentic, Finn Sulentic, Krystyna Recoskie, Megan Corbett, Odette Ropchan, Kim Turnbull and Rebecca Ross-Zaiontz for contributing content that is included in this booklet. Special thanks also goes out to Terry-Ann Pighin, Kim Johnstone for their help in bringing it all together, and Chrissy Hobbs from Indie Publishing Group, who helped with all the editing and formatting. Thank you so much for all your efforts and this booklet wouldn't be possible without your help.

Disclaimer: These documents do not contain medical/health advice. The information is provided for general informational and educational purposes only and is not a substitute for professional advice. Please speak to your healthcare provider if you have any concerns before starting and/or during the Program.

CONTENTS

WELCOME TO GINA'S FALL 2022 WEIGHT LOSS PROGRAM

LET'S GET STARTED WITH PREP WEEK!

If you are new to the Program, Prep Week is all about reviewing the basics, like the Food Plan you are to follow, how the program works, as well as gather anything you might need and ask any questions you have. It's not about being perfect, it's about understanding the process and setting yourself up for success.

If you are a returning member, Prep Week is all about getting back at it and setting yourself up for success as you continue your weight loss journey on the road to finally & forever.

WHAT IS THE LIVY METHOD:

- The Livy Method is about losing weight in a way that is healthy for the body and mind so weight loss is easier to maintain.

- The approach is to systematically lower your setpoint by addressing weight loss from a variety of different angles, physically and mentally, week to week. Your setpoint is the weight your body is used to functioning at – also known as homeostasis – where all the regulatory systems in your body work together to maintain balance for the purpose of helping the body survive and work at its most optimal level.

- There is a basic Food Plan you will need to follow, where each week will have a different focus, so keep in mind what you eat and when you eat will change and evolve week to week.

HOW THE PROGRAM WORKS:

- The Program is broken down into a step-by-step process (The Livy Method) designed to systematically address why your body is feeling a need to store fat and help it focus on fat loss, so you can sustainably lose as much weight as you can in the time frame we have.

- What you eat and when you eat will change week to week as The Program progresses. Each week will have a different focus, although the kinds of foods you eat will stay the same (see Grocery List).

- The best way to approach the program is to check into the Facebook Group each day to watch the Daily Check In Video as well as any other added support videos/posts which will give a more detailed explanation of any changes you are advised to implement.

- The Facebook Support Group is also where you are to ask any questions if you have them.

- Each day, we will post a question board where you can ask any questions you have.

- Questions will be answered by Gina and her team of Program Specialists, as well as many previous group members. Group members' answers will always be confirmed by a member of our team. All of our Program Specialists will have a "moderator" badge beside their names to help identify them.

- Gina will be going Live Monday - Friday in the Group at 9AM and Saturday at 10 AM, all times in EST.

- The Live segments are not mandatory. All the info you need will be posted in the Group. The Live segments are saved in GUIDES to be viewed later. The lives will also be available on the Weigh In with Gina podcast found on all podcast platforms.

- This Program is very much designed to be followed day by day, week by week, for the full 12 weeks, regardless of how much weight you have to lose.

- With that said, it can also accommodate any time off or off day, and can be done on your own timeline.

- You can also use our new Livy Method app to journal and track your progress along the way.

DAILY CHECKLIST:

1. Read over the Weekly Basic Guidelines.
2. Check into the Support Group.
3. Watch the Daily Check In Video.
4. Ask your questions on the Daily Questions Post.
5. Watch/Review any additional Support Videos or Posts and click DONE to keep track of what you have read/watched.
6. Implement the changes you need to make.

7.   Watch/participate in the Facebook Lives and ask questions. *Suggested but not Required*

It's pretty simple so don't overthink it. No need to weigh or measure your food or count any calories... just have faith in the Process.

We will be posting a lot of information over the next few days. Take your time to review and let us know if you have any questions. Also, be sure to check out the Table of Contents to check out all the topics we will be discussing week to week.

3 WAYS TO GET YOUR QUESTIONS ASKED AND ANSWERED:

1.   On the Daily Questions Post. This is pinned to the top of the Facebook Support Group page and is where you can ask any questions you have day to day.

2.   Individual Posts. Each day we will be posting about a variety of different topics. Feel free to ask any questions you have about that topic on those posts.

3.   If you choose, you can also participate and ask your questions by way of the Facebook Lives 9AM Mon - Fri, and Saturday Mornings at 10AM EST.

PLEASE NOTE:

- Please avoid privately emailing your questions or sending DMs via social media, as our main focus while running the Group is to prioritize the questions being asked in it.

- You will find the Program is laid out and designed to cover just about any and every question someone would have about the Program and process, so there is a lot to cover in the first few weeks.

- Be sure to use the GUIDES to keep track of anything new being posted day to day and utilize the TOPICS section where you can also search specific topics that have been previously posted.

If you are feeling overwhelmed, trust we will be going over the info many times over and, as always, if you have questions let us know.

Please take the time to head over to the Facebook Group or the Livy Method App and watch the quick video that accompanies this post.

FAQS - ABOUT THE PROGRAM

Here are some of our most popular questions asked about The Program:

1. Is The Program low carb?

- No, although I do suggest taking out bread (except Ezekiel/Sprouted Grain and Ryvita/High Fiber crackers), all pasta, baked goods and obvious sugars. I have incorporated many nutrient rich and beneficial options for you to choose from.

2. Do we have to weigh, measure, or count calories?

- No. Stick to the scheduled plan and portions will adjust on their own. Right now, the key is to feel satisfied after each meal and snack. We will start to address portions in Weeks 3 and 4.

3. What kind of results can I expect?

- Although the goal is to take as much weight off as quickly as possible, there is a process to it.

- It is not unreasonable to expect upwards of a 60 lbs.+ loss for men and 40 lbs.+ loss for women, but that depends on the state of your body when you started, along with other variables.

- Remember that this is not a quick fix program and it is meant to be followed day by day for the entire 12 weeks, regardless of how quickly you reach your goal.

- Even if you have more weight to lose than possible in the time frame we have, the goal is to lose as much as possible and be well on your way to losing the rest once you complete the 12 weeks.

- Everyone's body will respond differently and at different rates, so please be mindful not to rush the process or compare what is happening with you to what is happening with someone else.

4.   What can I expect in the first week?

- In the first week you may notice an increase in energy, a decrease in bloating, and more intense hunger signals. You may also experience a natural decrease in portion sizes and more pronounced "full" signals from the body.

- Some of you will start dropping weight right away, while others may go into "repair and rebuild mode" in which case you might not see the scale move right away, but hang in there because it will…both are equally ideal.

- As your body goes into weight loss mode you may experience some "detox" symptoms like headaches, chills, flu-like symptoms, lack of energy, dry lips, loose bowel movements…to name a few. Be sure to check in with your healthcare provider if you experience any symptoms you are concerned about.

- While it is typical to start losing weight in the first week (again depending on the state you started, how quickly you implement the changes and how consistent you are with them), if you don't lose weight in the first 4 weeks there is nothing to be concerned about.

5. **What is "detox"?**

- "Detox" is a very loose term I use to describe when the body is specifically focused on fat loss or is in what I call "weight loss mode". Detox happens naturally in the body; therefore, it doesn't need any help. This is why I'm not a fan of detox kits, detox juice or juice cleanses. When it comes to detox and helping the body get the fat out, there is nothing you need to do other than follow The Program. The changes in food, the design of the food plan formula, and the process of releasing fat is what causes the body to react and go into detox. We will be discussing "detox" or "weight loss mode" in more detail later.

8. **Should I be concerned if my weight isn't moving?**

- No. This is a 12-week process systematically designed to address why the body is feeling a need to store fat and make it so you can lose weight in a sustainable way... and it's a process that works if you follow The Plan.

- Please try not to stress over the little ups and downs on the scale and if you are not losing right away. If you are doing everything you need to do, then it will all come together as we move forward.

9. **What about medications and health issues, how will they affect me and do I need to do anything special to compensate or adjust?**

- We will be talking more about this as we move forward but for now focus on the basics, regardless of health issues or medications. The suggestions I have made are beneficial to everyone, as they are safe and sound and designed to get your body functioning more optimally by giving it what it needs and being consistent long enough for it to make change. If you have concerns, be sure to check in and work with your healthcare provider along the way.

10. **Do I have to watch every Facebook Live video?**

- Although they are beneficial and informative, they are not a mandatory part of the process. You can choose to watch some, all, or none. They are posted in the Group under Guides so are always available for you to access. The lives will also be available on the Weigh In with Gina podcast found on all podcast platforms.

11. **What if you have a question about the program or plan?**

- The Support Group should be your first source for information. It is also the place where you are to ask any questions you have day to day.

THE FOOD PLAN

The Food Plan is designed to stimulate your digestive system, increase nutrient absorption, decrease insulin levels, and give the body the resources it needs to make change. The goal is to be as consistent as possible to allow the body to react and adjust to the Food Plan. You are to eat all meals and snacks, even if you are not hungry you still need to eat a small token amount. (A token amount is 4-5 bites with chewing in between)

You will be following the Food Plan for the next few weeks and as we progress, we will be making slight changes to it week to week. So, it's key to be as consistent as possible as soon as possible.

Although it's important to eat the suggested categories of food (protein, veg, fruit etc.) at meal and snack times, the variety and sources are up to you. Be sure to review the many examples given in the Grocery List and Meal ideas Post.

THE BASIC FOOD PLAN:

FIRST THING – Warm lemon water and/or apple cider vinegar (Wait 5-10 minutes to have coffee or tea or breakfast).

BREAKFAST – Protein is the focus.

SNACK #1 – Fruit on its own.

LUNCH – Vegetables are the focus with added protein, leafy greens, and healthy fats. Add in grains and heavier carbs when needed.

SNACK #2 – Raw veggies, can add dips, cheese or nut butters (can be cooked if needed).

SNACK #3 – Nuts and/or seeds on their own (see individual breakdown below for alternatives if needed).

DINNER – Protein heavy with added vegetables, leafy greens, and healthy fats.

The time between all meals and snacks should be anywhere from 30 mins to no more than 3.5 hours. It's important to keep the order of the food, but the timing between meals and snacks can change day to day.

Let's break it down and go into more detail...

LEMON/ACV WATER

Lemon Water = juice of half a lemon or 2 tbsp juice in as much warm water as you like.

ACV (apple cider vinegar containing "the mother") = 1 tablespoon in as much water as you need to get it down. If you are just starting out, you may want to start with 1 tsp and work your way up.

Why?

Warm lemon water first thing in the morning promotes hydration and helps to stimulate your digestive system. You can use fresh lemons or bottled lemon juice as long as it is all-natural.

Another option, or in addition to the lemon water, is Apple Cider Vinegar. If you suffer from acid reflux and other digestive issues, it can be very beneficial to add in. It's also beneficial for anyone who has had their gallbladder removed.

Both are beneficial in their own ways. You can take one or the other or both. This is not "make or break" but more of an added bonus, especially if you suffer from known digestive issues.

BREAKFAST - PROTEIN HEAVY

Breakfast is not the most important meal of the day; however, it can be greatly beneficial when trying to lose weight.

Why?

When you wake up, you are already full of energy from what you ate the day before. So, you don't need to eat breakfast to gain energy.

That's why you have the option of skipping it, carrying on with your day, then going to your morning fruit snack. With that said, there is absolutely a benefit to eating it. Starting your day with a high protein breakfast is a great way to "break the fast" and get your body working harder from the get-go.

It pains me to say it...but that means burning more calories throughout your day! (And NO, we still don't count calories!)

It's ideal to eat breakfast within 2.5 hours of waking. However, this is not a hard and fast rule. If you wake up at 5 am and you are not active or exercising you can still eat breakfast as late as 9 am and be fine. If you get up later, that gives you less time to have breakfast before your snack, so you might skip breakfast and go straight to snack.

We will be adding in bonus snacks to help fill in the blanks for those of you who are up early, are more active, or do shift work. For now, play around with the timing of your breakfast to figure out what's best for you.

SNACK #1: FRUIT ON ITS OWN.

Why fruit and why on its own?

Normally, it is a good idea to combine your carbs with a protein and fat which can help minimize the amount of insulin needed to convert the food you eat into energy.

Which may have you confused and wondering why we are eating the fruit on its own?!

Whether you have breakfast or not, by mid-morning, your glycogen (energy) reserves are starting to deplete. The goal is to replenish those energy stores before the body has to dip into, and utilize, your emergency fat reserves. When the body is forced to dip into its fat reserves, that sends a message to the body that you need to store fat. Which is something we are ultimately trying to avoid. So, by having fruit on its own, you are able to replenish those stores easily.

In the weeks to come, we will be making changes to your morning snack, but for now, you can have one or any combo of fruits. Fruit cups, frozen fruit, and applesauce are fine as long as they have no added sugar. Bananas are a little higher in sugar but are a great addition for anyone who is more active or in need of potassium due to leg cramps while sleeping.

LUNCH: VEG IS THE FOCUS (COOKED OR RAW) WITH PROTEIN, LEAFY GREENS (COOKED OR RAW), AND HEAVIER CARBS IF YOU FEEL THE NEED FOR THEM.

Why vegetable heavy?

Vegetables are carbohydrates, which are "energy foods". You want to eat those earlier in the day so your body has time to use them throughout the day.

If you feel you need a little more "oomph", this is also when you might want to add in some heavier carbs such as whole grains like rice or quinoa or carb-heavy veggies like squash or potatoes. These carbs are better eaten at lunch so your body has all day to use up the energy from them.

Side note: Leafy greens do not count as vegetables on this plan so if you are having a salad, be sure to load up on vegetables!

SNACK #2: RAW VEGGIES

Raw veggies can be very hard to digest, which makes them the perfect food for the first afternoon snack and after a bigger meal.

If you find you get bloated or have a hard time digesting raw veggies, that can be a sign you are low in digestive enzymes. If you need, you can cook or steam them but do so temporarily with the goal to work your way up to eventually eating them raw.

You can eat any raw veggies you like and do not need to worry about getting in a huge variety. You can stick to the ones you do like.

You can also add natural dressings or dips like hummus or guacamole. You can also add cheese or nut butter to make your veg snack more nutrient rich.

Pickles or fermented food like kimchi or sauerkraut also work! You could also do a salad and use leafy greens as long as it's loaded up with raw veg.

Keep in mind, even if you add raw veg to lunch, you will still need the afternoon snack.

SNACK #3: NUTS AND/OR SEEDS

Nuts and seeds ideally should have no added oil or salt.

Nuts and seeds are even harder to digest than raw veggies, which is why they make the perfect afternoon snack.

Try to keep the number of nuts you eat to a maximum of approximately 25 pieces and seeds to one shot glass full. You can have one or the other, or both. Remember that you are still eating to satisfaction. Note: Nuts and seeds can be very hard to digest, so eating too many can lead to digestive upset. This limit isn't suggested because of calories or fat.

Around 3-4pm, the body is naturally wired to take a dip in energy. What the body is really looking for is a nap. Other places in the world refer to this as a siesta and take time to snooze. Because most of us can't just take a nap during the day, this is where people go looking for sugar or caffeine as a pick-me-up.

By adding in the nuts and or seeds, you are keeping your digestive system stimulated and working hard, which helps to keep your energy up. The protein and fat from the nuts and seeds also helps to give you more sustaining energy, which will have you feeling more satisfied leading up to and going into dinner.

This helps keep your digestive system working hard to process and break down your larger meal and will also help prevent you from overeating your dinner.

You can also add nuts and or seeds to your meals. If you do, keep in mind you still need to eat your Nut & Seed Snack.

If you find them hard to digest, you can roast them or soak them. If you can't eat nuts due to allergies, you can stick to seeds. If you can't have either due to allergies or preparation for a procedure, the alternatives are dairy such as cheese or yogurt, olives and beans like chickpeas, edamame, black beans etc. Please Note: These alternatives are to be used as a last resort as nuts and/or seeds are the best choice.

BOTH SNACKS MUST BE EATEN IN THAT ORDER

DINNER: PROTEIN IS THE FOCUS WITH VEGETABLES (COOKED OR RAW), LEAFY GREENS (COOKED OR RAW), AND HEALTHY FATS.

Given that it's at the end of the day, try to think of dinner as more of a top-up rather than a need for fuel. Ideally, dinner "should" be the smallest meal of the day, especially if eating after dark when our bodies are naturally winding down to get ready for sleep. Most of us were raised in a culture where dinner was the biggest meal, and this habit is hard to break, but as you work through this Program, you will start to notice your appetite for a larger dinner will decrease.

Alternatively, there might be times where you won't be very hungry for dinner, but you still need to have a token amount. In this case, some protein with a bit of leafy greens would work.

You can add heavier carbs IF you feel you need them - like if you are being very active into the night.

Try to eat dinner as early as possible. Eating too late will prevent the body from following through on its wind down process, which will mess with your body's ability to get the deep REM and sleep it needs to make change.

After dinner snack: best if you can avoid it, but if you need a little something to take the edge off for now, you can have some air popped popcorn with butter and sea salt. We suggest eliminating this altogether by Week 2.

You can also have your favourite herbal teas in the evening that can help when breaking the nighttime snacking habit.

THE GOAL:

Keep things simple and routine. Don't overthink it, it is a process, and everything will come together in time.

I'm not concerned about portion sizes or weighing or measuring food. You are to eat to satisfaction. You will find as you go along, portions will adjust on their own and you will become very in tune with what your body needs.

This first week is all about taking the time to understand the process and making the changes you need to make. Be sure to ask any questions you have along the way!

For more information, be sure to check out the Food Plan FAQs.

Please take time to head over to the Facebook Group or the Livy Method App and watch the quick video that accompanies this post.

FAQS — THE FOOD PLAN

Here are some of our most popular questions asked about the Food Plan.

1. **Do I need to follow the plan exactly and do I need to eat all the meals and snacks even if I'm not hungry?**

   - Yes! This is super key! For best results do not deviate, improvise, or skip any meals or snacks. They are all equally important and for a rhyme and a reason. The only meal you don't need to eat is breakfast as outlined in the plan.

2. **How far apart should my meals and snacks be?**

   - Anywhere from 30 minutes to 3.5 hours is fine. The order of food is important, but the timing between meals and snacks can change day to day.

BREAKFAST

1. **Should I have both lemon water and apple cider vinegar?**

   You can have one or the other or both. You can also have them together as in your ACV in your lemon water.

2. **Can I use lime instead of lemon in my morning drink?**

   Yes, you can.

3. **Can I take ACV gummies?**

   Supplements in gummy form do not provide the same benefits as taking the real thing. We don't recommend them.

4. **Can I use bottled lemon juice for my morning lemon water?**

   Yes, you can, as long as it's made with all-natural ingredients.

5. **Can I drink coffee or tea?**

   Yes, coffee and tea are totally on plan.

6. **Does coffee and tea count towards water intake?**

   Yes, all beverages except for alcohol count towards water intake.

7. **Can I have cream and sugar in my coffee?**

   Yes, you can have cream or creamers as long as they contain all-natural ingredients and are not too high in sugar. Sugar is fine. Look for raw, or organic cane. You can also use honey or maple syrup. Keep sugar to a minimum.

8. **Can I have Stevia or Monk fruit sweetener?**

Although these are better quality sweeteners, it is best to use real sugar, honey, or maple syrup.

9. **Do I have to be consistent with eating or not eating breakfast?**

No, you can eat breakfast some days and not others.

10. **Can I have protein shakes?**

I am not a fan of liquid nutrients. Especially when trying to lose weight. You want your body to work hard to digest and process its food. Especially right now while we are preparing the body for weight loss. If you insist on keeping them in, be sure to use protein powder that contains all-natural ingredients and is low in sugar. Add little to no fruit and add in some healthy fat like avocado, nut butter, coconut oil etc.

LUNCH

1. **Do I have to have salad every day?**

Definitely not. You can have a vegetable heavy meal prepared any way you like. Soup, stir fry, roasted vegetables, raw vegetables etc. with added protein, healthy fats, and leafy greens.

2. **Can I add fruit at lunch?**

Yes, you can. Just keep it minimal.

3. **What if I'm on the road and have to stop at a fast-food restaurant?**

Most fast-food places these days have healthier options such as salads, soups, chilis, etc. These are your best bets. You can also have a sandwich or a wrap and just eat what's inside. It's okay to not be perfect every time. Sometimes life just happens so make the best choices with what you have.

4. **Can I use rice paper wrappers?**

You can, but keep in mind rice paper wrappers and rice noodles have the same effect on the body as pasta so best to avoid right now or keep to a minimum.

DINNER

1. **Can I use frozen vegetables?**

Yes, they are great for convenience. Canned ones are also fine.

2. **What about plant-based meat substitutes like Beyond Meat?**

You can, but keep it to a minimum. Many contain processed ingredients so look for quality ingredients.

3. **Can I cook with oil?**

Yes, you can use butter and oil. Choose higher quality oils such as olive oil, avocado oil, and coconut oil.

4. **Can I have potatoes or rice with dinner?**

You can, although these heavier carbs are best eaten at lunch.

5. **Can I have pasta made with Konjac, black beans, quinoa etc.**

Best to avoid any kind of pasta. Even when made with other ingredients it is still a processed product and not a whole food. No matter what the pasta is made from, it will still have your insulin levels up, which we are trying to avoid.

6. **Can I have breakfast foods for dinner?**

When it comes to eggs or things like tofu or beans then yes. But things like yogurt, cereals and oatmeal aren't the right kinds of protein for dinner at this time. There will come a time when you can have those at dinner.

7. **Can I have wine with dinner?**

Yes, alcohol is totally fine to have. You just want to drink extra water to compensate for dehydration (1 cup per drink).

8. **Can I use flour to thicken a sauce?**

Yes, small amounts of flour for thickening or breading are totally fine.

9. **Can I eat breaded meats, vegetables etc.?**

Yes, breading is totally fine.

10. **When is the best time to eat dinner?**

You want to eat dinner as early as possible and ideally before it starts getting dark.

11. **What if I'm not hungry for dinner?**

This will happen. You still want to have a token amount. In this case, some protein and leafy greens will do the trick. Further on in the process you will be able to skip dinner if you want to.

SNACKS

1. **Can I eat frozen or canned fruit for the fruit snack?**

Yes. Fresh is better but if you choose canned or frozen, look for all natural with no added sugar.

2. **If I have fruit with breakfast, do I still need to eat fruit for the morning snack?**

Yes. Fruit should be eaten on its own, mid-morning, regardless of whether or not you had some at breakfast.

3. **Can I have dried fruit for the fruit snack?**

It's not ideal but if you are in a pinch, such as on the road and stuck without any other option, it's fine once in a while.

4. **Can I have more than one type of fruit, like a fruit salad?**

Yes, any combination of fruit is fine as long as it's only fruit.

5. **Do I have to eat my veg snack if I'm still full from lunch?**

Yes, it is key to get in all meals and snacks. If you are not hungry, you still want to eat a token amount, a few bites, to stimulate digestion.

6. **Can I have a dip with my veggies?**

Yes, you can use dips or have with cheese, nut butter, olives or any type of healthy fat.

7. **Can I have sauerkraut or kimchi for the raw veg snack?**

Yes, fermented foods are excellent for gut health and considered a raw veg on plan.

8. **Can I have pickles for the raw veg snack?**

Yes, any kind of pickled vegetables work for veg snacks.

9. **What if I have problems digesting nuts and seeds?**

If you have trouble digesting nuts and seeds you can soak and/or roast them to make them easier to digest.

10. **What if I'm allergic to nuts?**

If you can't eat nuts due to allergies, you can stick to seeds. If you can't have either due to allergies or preparation for a procedure, the alternatives are: dairy, such as cheese or yogurt, olives, or beans like chickpeas, edamame, black beans etc. Please Note: these alternatives are to be used as a last resort as nuts and/or seeds are the best choice.

11. **Do I eat both nuts and seeds or just one?**

You can have one or the other or both.

12. **Can I switch out the snacks for other things or change the order?**

No. The snacks suggested are for a reason that goes far beyond just eating well. For optimal results, eat the suggested snacks at the suggested times.

LUNCH AND DINNER VISUAL GUIDELINE

Don't Take This Too Literally. I can't stress it enough. It's only meant as a visual guideline. We don't want you to start dividing up your plate.

Sometimes at lunch, your protein portion may be a bit bigger, or at dinner a bit smaller. Sometimes you may only have a pinch of greens added to a soup, or popped into your mouth, etc. As long as you just keep the focus on veg at lunch and protein at dinner you are totally fine. Even if it's totally off balance sometimes, it's no big deal! The point is to have you start thinking more about what you are eating and getting in some nicely balanced meals.

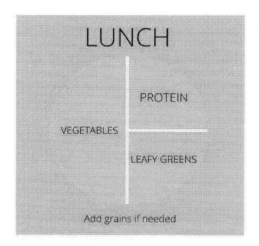
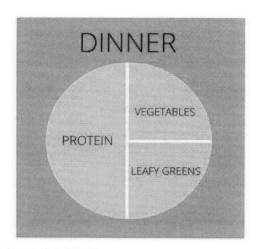

ADD HEALTHY FATS AT WILL

NOTHING NEEDS TO BE EXACT AND, WHATEVER YOU DO, DON'T MEASURE!

Sometimes you might be eating a chili, stew, soup or stir fry where the divided plate doesn't apply. As long as there is a good balance of veggies and protein you are good. When in doubt, toss in a bit of extra protein or veg if you feel the need. We just want you to start paying attention.

Portions - Eat to satisfaction. This looks different for everyone. We would rather you be overeating right now rather than undereating, so do not try to cut your portions. This will make more sense as we move forward.

Most importantly try not to overthink it. If your meals are slightly off balance, it's not going to affect your progress. If you are eating nutrient rich, whole foods, and following the guidelines, you are right on track!

Note About "Grains as Needed" - This will become easier to gauge as we move along, but basically if you are feeling you need a little more "oomph" to your meal, add them in. Like you are looking at your nice clean salad and thinking "I don't think this is going to satisfy me today" then add some grains or heavier carb veggies like potatoes etc.

LET'S TALK MEAL IDEAS

Following meal plans isn't really our thing. Although we are telling you what to eat and when, within certain categories, the choices within those categories are up to you.

As we move through the 12 weeks, the goal is to get you to a place where you are very in tune with your body's cues and signals – when to eat, what to eat, and how much.

As far as portions go, right now, the goal is to eat to satisfaction. That will be different for everyone. For example, some may need 3 eggs for breakfast and others one and that can change day to day. When it comes to portions, it's always about what you feel and not how big or small your portions look. Trust the process and follow as directed for best results. DO NOT purposefully try to reduce your portion sizes to try and speed up the process. This will backfire on you down the road.

BREAKFAST

Examples of higher protein breakfast (keep in mind these are not your only options, just some examples to get you started):

Eggs – Eggs are the best bang for your buck and by far the #1 recommendation for a high protein breakfast! Have them on their own, cooked any way you like, or with sautéed veggies, meat, cheese, a salad, small amounts of fruit, avocado etc.

Leftovers - Breakfast doesn't have to be breakfast-type food. You can also use leftovers you have in your fridge i.e., leftover meat or fish, a soup, stew, or chili. Some refried beans with avocado and salsa are some examples.

Tofu Or Tempeh – Baked, scrambled, omelets etc.

High Protein Cereal - Made with whole grains and seeds like Qia or Holy Crap brands.

Yogurt Or Cottage Cheese – Greek yogurt tends to be highest in protein. Avoid low or no fat. Add hemp hearts, nuts, nut butter and/or seeds to bump up the protein. A small amount of fruit is also okay. You can have plain or flavoured as long as it is made with natural ingredients. Added sugar is fine but watch the quantities as some brands are much higher in sugar. The higher the sugar, the higher the fat and protein content should be. Remember that we are trying to reduce insulin levels, so choosing lower to no sugar yogurts is ideal.

Chia Seed Pudding - With added hemp hearts, nuts, seeds etc. to bump up the protein.

Non-dairy Yogurt – The same as with regular yogurt, you want to add the extra toppings to bump up the protein. Coconut yogurt is low in protein so not the best option while on the program as a breakfast in itself but can be added to things like oatmeal.

Oatmeal - With added hemp hearts, nuts, nut butter and/or seeds for extra protein. You can also add high fat yogurt or other dairy/non-dairy milk or cream. Fruit and things like honey or maple syrup are fine in small amounts.

High Protein Pancakes are fine on occasion. But be mindful of what you are topping them with and be sure to add some hemp hearts or nuts/seeds.

A Note About Bread:

You can still lose weight while eating bread, but it can slow the process. If you choose to have it, look for Ezekiel bread in the freezer section at your grocery or health food store. If you can't find Ezekiel, look for other sprouted grain breads or darker denser breads that are high in protein and fiber and made with all-natural ingredients. Keep it to a minimum and have it at breakfast OR lunch. Not both.

LUNCH

Here are some examples for lunch. Keep in mind you want to have the main part of your lunch be vegetables. They can be cooked or raw and the same applies for greens.

You can also add in some heavier veggies or grains/rice if you feel the need for more oomph to your meal. Also, be sure to add in healthy fats.

Here are a few ideas to get you started.

Salad – Lunch doesn't always have to be salad, but it is a go-to for many and easy for packed lunches. Not all salads are made equal. For example, a piece of chicken on top of a Caesar salad isn't the best choice. Load up your salads with lots of veggies and things like avocado, olives, nuts, seeds, cheeses, meat, fish, beans, tofu etc. to bump up the nutrients. You can also add in grains or heavier carbs if you feel you need them.

Soup, Stew, Chili, Curry, Stir Fry – These one-pot wonders can be a life saver! You can make big batches and freeze for quick and easy meals. They can be with or without meat. Check the tips below for ideas of how to balance out the meal when necessary.

Lettuce Wraps – Use large lettuce leaves or other leafy greens to wrap up your fave sandwich fillings. Perfect for on the go!

Leftovers From Dinner – Use your leftovers for a quick and easy lunch.

Mix And Match – Lunch doesn't have to be a sit-down meal. You can toss some snack-like things into a container or onto a plate. Things like meats, cheese, boiled eggs, beans, olives, pickles, veggie sticks and dip (hummus adds protein). Add a few green leaves and you're all set!

Don't Like to Cook or Don't Have Time? – There are lots of prepared foods that fit into the plan. Check the ingredients list and look for quality. Avoid things like hydrogenated oil, MSG, artificial flavours and colours. Check the freezer section, the soup isle, the fresh made salads section etc.

DINNER

Eat dinner as early as possible to make sure your body is no longer focused on digesting food when it's winding down for sleep. There might be times you won't be very hungry for dinner, but for now, you still need to have a token amount. In this case, some protein with a bit of leafy greens would work.

There are countless possibilities for dinner but here are some ideas to get you started.

Meat, Poultry, Fish or Seafood – Grill it, bake it, bread it (yes you can use breading!), fry it (yes you can fry too!) Add your favourite veg on the side with some leafy greens (cooked or raw).

Tofu, Tempeh, Beans and Lentils – If you are looking for plant-based protein options, these are the best. Marinated tofu or tempeh, grilled, baked, or fried. Sauté some beans or lentils with veggies and seasoning or make a soup or chili.

Eggs – Eggs make a quick, light, and easy dinner. An omelet with spinach and mushrooms covers all the bases. Or eggs, any style, with some sautéed veg or a salad. Or make a Frittata and have it for breakfast, lunch, AND dinner!

Curry, Chili, Soup, Stew, Stir Fry – If you are used to having rice with your curries and stir fries, try using cauliflower rice instead.

Spaghetti Sauce – You can still make pasta for the family. Just have yours on top of zucchini noodles, cauliflower rice or cooked white beans instead!

Tacos – Put all your favourite taco fillings on a bed of leafy greens instead of in a shell or wrap.

Rotisserie Chicken – Pick up a rotisserie chicken (or 2!) from your grocery store. It's easy and convenient.

Don't Like to Cook or Don't Have Time? – There are lots of prepared foods that fit into the plan. Check the ingredients list and look for quality. Avoid things like hydrogenated oils, artificial flavours and colours. Check the freezer section, the soup aisle, the fresh made salads section etc.

TIPS TO BALANCE THINGS OUT
How To Add Extra Protein Without Using Meat:

- Hemp hearts
- Nuts and/or seeds or nut butter
- Beans such as Kidney or Chickpeas
- Lentils
- Tofu
- Nutritional Yeast

- Protein powder
- Cheese or other dairy such as yogurt or cream.
- Eggs – a boiled egg with a salad makes a perfect lunch!

HOW TO ADD LEAFY GREENS:

- Have a side salad.
- Add any leafy green to your bowl or plate and add the rest (such as a soup) on top.
- Add leafy greens to the recipe such as in a soup, stew, chili or stir fry that doesn't include it. A handful of baby spinach and you are done!
- Simply pop a handful into your mouth and away you go!
- Use them as a wrap.
- Sauté a big bunch of heartier greens such as kale, collard greens, Swiss chard, Bok Choy etc. with some butter and garlic and keep in the fridge to add to any meal.

HOW TO ADD IN HEALTHY FATS:

- Use natural oils and dressings.
- Add avocados, nuts, and seeds.
- Add quality cheeses.
- Add fish like salmon and fresh tuna twice a week.

GROCERY CHECKLIST

FRUIT

Any kind of fruit or combination of fruits you like. Literally ANY kind. Fresh fruit is best but frozen and canned are fine as well. Canned fruit should be without added sugar. Avoid dried fruits for this part of the program.

- Apples
- Apricots
- Bananas
- Berries (all)
- Cherries
- Cranberries (fresh)
- Dates (fresh & Medjool)
- Fresh figs
- Grapefruit
- Grapes
- Kiwi
- Lemons
- Limes
- Mango
- Melons (all)
- Nectarines
- Oranges (all types)
- Papaya
- Peaches
- Pears
- Pineapple
- Plums
- Pomelo
- Pomegranate
- _____
- _____
- _____

VEGETABLES

Any and all vegetables are on plan. Choose vegetables for both eating raw and cooked. Add your own to the list if some are missing

- Artichokes
- Asparagus
- Bell Peppers
- Beets
- Bok Choy (veg & leafy green)
- Broccoli
- Broccoli Rabe/ Rapini (veg & leafy green)
- Brussels sprouts (veg & leafy green)
- Cabbage (veg & leafy green)
- Carrots
- Cauliflower
- Celery
- Celeriac/Celery Root
- Corn
- Cucumber
- Edamame Beans
- Eggplant
- Fennel
- Fiddleheads (veg & leafy green)
- Green beans
- Green Peas (all types)
- Hearts of palm
- Hot Peppers (all)
- Jicama
- Kimchi (veg & leafy green)
- Kohlrabi
- Leeks/Scallions
- Mushrooms (all)
- Onions (all)
- Pickled Vegetables(all)
- Radishes
- Rhubarb
- Sauerkraut (veg & leafy green)
- Spaghetti squash
- Sprouts
- Tomatoes
- Turnip & Rutabaga
- Zucchini/summer squash
- Water Chestnuts

HEAVIER VEGETABLES (IDEALLY ADDED AT LUNCH WHEN NEEDED)

- Cassava
- Parsnips
- Plantain
- Potatoes
- Pumpkin
- Squash

- Sweet potatoes/Yams
- Yucca
- _____
- _____
- _____

PROTEIN

Protein is needed at breakfast, lunch and dinner so consider each meal when making your shopping list. Always look for quality products, "raised without hormones or antibiotics" "grass-fed" "all natural" "organic" etc. Quality is key!

Plant based proteins labeled as higher protein veg should not be used as a stand-alone protein source but are great when used in combination with other protein sources.

ANIMAL

- Eggs
- Chicken (all cuts, with or without skin)
- Turkey (all cuts, with or without skin)
- Beef (all cuts)
- Pork (all cuts)
- Game Meats
- Fish (all types)
- Seafood (all types)
- Canned meat/fish

PLANT BASED

- Tofu
- Tempeh
- Edamame Beans (higher protein veg)
- Sprouts (higher protein veg)
- Lentils
- Beans/Chickpeas
- Nutritional Yeast
- Hemp Hearts/Seeds
- Nuts (all)
- NutButters(all)

KEEP TO A MINIMUM

- Bacon
- Sausages (unless all natural/good quality)
- Deli Meats look for all natural

LEAFY GREENS

Leafy greens are added as roughage. Any leafy green works and can be eaten raw or cooked.

- Arugula
- Bok Choy (veg and leafy)
- Broccoli Rabe/Rapini (veg and leafy)
- Brussels Sprouts (veg and leafy)
- Cabbage (veg and leafy)
- Chinese Broccoli (veg and leafy)
- Collard Greens
- Endive
- Fiddleheads (veg and leafy)
- Iceberg lettuce
- Kale
- Leaf Lettuce
- Mustard Greens
- Radicchio
- Romaine lettuce
- Salad Mixes (all)
- Seaweed
- Spring Mix
- Spinach
- Swiss Chard
- Watercress

GRAINS

Whole Grains are best added to lunch if you feel the need to have a little more substance. You can have them at dinner too but keep the portion size small and try not to have it every day. Also, oats and high protein cereals are fine to have at breakfast with added hemp hearts, nuts and seeds or quality protein powder, to boost protein.

- Amaranth
- Barley
- Buckwheat
- Bulgur (cracked wheat)
- Farro
- Millet
- Oats Add extra protein when having for breakfast (See Meal Ideas Post for more details)
- Rice – black, red, wild, brown, white or brown basmati
- Quinoa
- Sorghum
- Teff

DAIRY

Avoid low or no-fat dairy products except for milk and cream, which can be any fat content. **Always avoid artificial flavors, colors, or artificial sweeteners.**

- Add hemp hearts, nuts and seeds, nut butter or quality protein powder to yogurt to bump up the protein.

- If eating non-dairy yogurt, nut and soy based are best. Coconut yogurt contains very little protein.

- Some sugar is okay in both yogurts and coffee creamers. Just keep to a minimum and with yogurt, add extra fat/protein.

- There are far too many cheeses to list them all here.

- All cheese is fine as long as it isn't processed or containing artificial colours or flavours.

- Although there is protein in dairy products, they are not a good stand-alone protein on program so should be used with an addition of extra protein such as nuts, seeds, hemp hearts etc.

- Greek yogurt -Ideally plain and unsweetened with 2% or higher MF. If sweetened, choose higher fat.
- Non-dairy yogurts
- Cottage Cheese
- Sour cream
- Milk (any fat %)
- Cream (any fat %)
- Non-dairy milk (all)
- Kefir
- Butter
- Havarti
- Swiss
- Gouda
- Provolone
- Mozzarella
- Parmesan
- Manchego
- Blue cheese
- Brie/camembert
- White cheddar
- Goat's cheese
- Cream cheese (no artificial flavours)
- Feta
- Bocconcini

FATS

Healthy fats are an important part of weight loss. Here are some examples of healthy fats to have on hand. Adding extra healthy fats to meals bumps up the nutrient value.

- Extra Virgin Olive Oil
- Avocado Oil
- Coconut Oil
- Cold pressed canola oil
- Ghee/Clarified Butter
- Butter
- Sesame Oil
- Nut Oils
- Flax Oil
- Hemp Oil
- Avocados
- Nuts (all types)
- Coconut
- Nut Butters (all natural)
- Seeds (all types)
- Olives

MISCELLANEOUS — OPTIONAL ITEMS

When looking for condiments, sauces, dressings, or pre-packaged food items, **avoid ingredients like artificial flavor, artificial colour, hydrogenated oils.** The organic and health food sections of your grocery store or your health food store are great places to look for quality prepackaged foods.

- Bottled lemon or lime juice (100% natural)
- High quality protein powder containing all-natural ingredients if using for oats or yogurt.
- Protein grain cereals such as Qia or Holy Crap
- Salad dressings
- Bottled sauces (BBQ, curry, stir fry etc.)
- Mayonnaise

- Ketchup/mustard & other condiments
- Dips for vegetables
- Premade soups, chilis, etc.
- Any herbs and spices
- Sugar - raw, organic cane, coconut, honey, maple syrup
- High fiber crackers such as Ryvita brand or equivalent
- Ezekiel bread (see Note)

A NOTE ABOUT BREAD

You can still lose weight while eating bread, but it can slow the process. If you choose to have it, look for Ezekiel bread in the freezer section at your grocery or health food store. If you can't find Ezekiel, look for other sprouted grain breads or darker denser breads that are high in protein and fiber and made with all-natural ingredients. Keep it to a minimum and have it at breakfast OR lunch. Not both.

LET'S TALK WATER

As you know, water and how much you need to drink is a hot topic when it comes to the Program. Increasing your water intake, in my experience, is one of the top things you can do to help maximize your efforts to drop fat.

Unlike traditional diets that force your body to burn fat by way of eating less or exercising more, my program uses the body's natural detox process to help the body release fat and water is key in helping that happen. The body releases fat when you pee, poo, breathe and sweat.

Lack of studies and a lot of misinformation about water and hydration has left people confused about how much they need to drink. The average person needs at least 2.7 - 3.5 litres of water for basic body functions like digestion, pumping blood through your veins, sweating, bowel movements etc. (Source: refer to original post in the group for source).

To help the body get into detox mode, you will need to drink above and beyond what it needs for basic body functions.

"Detox mode" is a loose term I use when referring to the body being specifically focused on releasing the fat. Although the body is capable of detoxing on its own, it will do so at a very slow and frustrating pace. This is why we have designed a program that will utilize and support that process.

Besides aiding in fat loss, being properly hydrated has many other health benefits such as:

- Increased energy and brain function
- Can help relieve constipation
- Increased cardiovascular health
- Increased function of muscles and joints
- Promotes healthy "glowing" skin
- Helps flush toxins from your organs
- Helps curb cravings, especially for sugar

SO HOW MUCH SHOULD I BE DRINKING?

This is a simple question with no easy answer.

Everyone requires different amounts, so you will have to play around with it to see what works for you, what helps to get you into detox and what helps keep you there. Your water intake can also change from day to day depending on many factors. Here's a list of things that can affect how much water you need above the 2.7- 3.5 litres.

YOU NEED EXTRA WATER WHEN:

- Your body is in detox
- You are fighting an illness
- You have your period
- You take medication that causes weight gain or dehydration
- You work or live in a dry environment
- You exercise or are active enough to sweat
- You drink alcohol
- You eat salty food
- You are taller than average (over 5'5" for women, 5'9" for men)
- You have weight to lose
- When the scale is bouncing between 2 numbers

Since you are all trying to get rid of fat, I suggest aiming for 3.5 litres to start. You can adjust from there depending on your height, weight and other factors listed above. Some of you might find this is enough and others might find they need more.

HOW DO I KNOW I'M DRINKING ENOUGH?

- You no longer feel thirsty.
- You no longer have dry mouth or lips.
- Your trips to the bathroom have decreased (they will increase until you are properly hydrated).

HOW MUCH IS TOO MUCH?

Overhydration and water intoxication happen when you drink more water than your kidneys can get rid of through urine. You have a greater risk of developing water intoxication if you drink a lot of water in a short period of time. When you drink too much too fast, your kidneys can't get rid of the excess water. Your kidneys can eliminate about 5 to 7 gallons (20-28 litres) of water a day, but they can't get rid of more than 27 - 33 ounces (0.8 - 1.0 litres) per hour.

Therefore, to avoid hyponatremia (low salt in blood) or overhydration from excess water, you should not drink more than 27 - 33 ounces (0.8 - 1.0 litres) of water per hour, on average and be mindful to include salt in your diet.

WHEN INCREASING WATER INTAKE:

- Increase slowly.

- Start early and spread your water drinking throughout the day. Don't chug a large amount at once.

- To prevent low sodium levels, add a pinch of pink Himalayan, Celtic or Sea salt to your warm water and lemon or ACV in the morning. This will add in minerals and electrolytes as well as support hormone and adrenal function. Or you can purchase trace minerals to add to your water.

- When it comes to water, it's not about drinking more and more. It's about drinking enough. Do what's right for you and always consult with your healthcare provider if you have any concerns.

TIPS TO GETTING IT IN:

- Make it fun! Make it a challenge!

- Start drinking early in your day. Most people find it easier to get the majority in the first half of the day.

- Sip, don't guzzle.

- Get a good water bottle or cup that you like to drink from.

- Track your water (and other fluids such as coffee, tea, bone broth) intake by using our Livy Method tracking app.

- Set reminders to drink.

- Add fresh or frozen fruit, cucumber slices, and/or fresh herbs or ginger.

- Stop drinking after dinner, so it doesn't mess with your sleep.

This can be the hardest part of the program but also the most important, so keep at it and do your best.

...it does get easier and if you make it a challenge it can be fun!

Once you have lost the weight, you can adjust and scale back on the amount you are drinking to maintain hydration without having to push more for the sake of weight loss.

On a final note: Tea, Coffee, soups, and essentially any other liquid (except alcohol) counts towards your water intake. Sparkling water is okay on occasion, but the majority of your water intake should be regular water.

Please take the time to head over to the Facebook Group or the Livy Method App and watch the quick video that accompanies this post. To read more about how water can support the weight loss process, head over to the Science Guide and read the articles on Detox, The Science of Fat and Fat Loss, and Maintenance and the Microbiome.

FAQS — WATER

Here are some of our most popular questions asked about water.

1. **Why so much water?**

   The average person needs 2.7 - 3.5 litres of water just for basic body functions like processing the food going in and going out. Because this program piggy-backs the body's natural detox response, you will need to drink above and beyond the minimum to get your body into detox mode (releasing fat).

2. **Can I drink too much?**

   You would really have to drink above and beyond the minimum recommended to an extreme, for there to be any detrimental side effects. However, although the kidneys can take in up to 20-28 litres of fluid per day, they cannot excrete more than 1 litre per hour. So, try not to drink more than 1 litre per hour and sip instead of guzzling.

   You also want to be mindful of low sodium. When increasing water intake, be mindful to add salt to meals or add in trace minerals to your water.

   Make sure you're drinking enough for your body's needs and not just drinking as much as possible.

3. **Does it matter when I drink the water?**

   Try to start early in the morning and spread it out throughout the day. Drinking into the later hours can cause disruption in your sleep so better if you can be done earlier rather than later.

4. **Will I always have to drink this much water?**

   The extra water is only necessary while you are trying to lose weight. When maintaining your weight, you can scale back to basic requirements. The amount of water you need will fluctuate from day to day both during and after weight loss.

5. **Can I add anything to my water?**

   You can add fresh or frozen fruit, fresh herbs etc. Anything that is all natural, with no sugar or sweeteners added. Naturally flavoured tea also counts towards water intake.

6. **How should I keep track of my water intake?**

   There are many methods, so experiment to find out what works best for you. It's a great idea to use the Livy Method App to record your water intake. Some people use elastic bands on a water bottle or glass to keep track or fill a large container and pour their glasses from that each day...More ideas will come up in the group discussions as we go.

7.   **Do other drinks count towards water intake?**

Yes, all drinks except alcohol count towards water intake.

8.   **Should I buy a water filter?**

This is a personal choice. Although it's always a good idea to make sure the water you are drinking is safe, it's up to you whether or not you want to use a filter.

9.   **Can I have carbonated or sparkling water?**

It is fine on occasion, but you want the majority of your water intake to be flat water.

10.   **I'm having trouble drinking so much water. Any tips?**

Start early in the day, set reminders on your phone with a goal of how much you want to drink each hour. Get a nice water bottle. Try using a straw. It will become easier as you go along.

11.   **Why do I have dry lips and a pasty mouth even though I'm drinking tons of water?**

These can be signs that you are still not fully hydrated and the body is asking for more water, or it can be a sign you are going into detox, so try increasing water slightly. Keep in mind this can also be due to medications or underlying health issues.

LET'S TALK LOW SODIUM

Sodium is the main component of salt and an essential electrolyte which helps with balancing water in the body, muscle function and nerve transmissions.

For years, health organizations have been warning people about the dangers of salt, linking too much sodium to high blood pressure and recommending people limit their intake. However, even though too much sodium causes problems, consuming too little can be just as unhealthy.

Insufficient sodium in your blood can occur when water and sodium are out of balance. In other words, there's either too much water or not enough sodium in your blood. Symptoms of low blood sodium can vary from person to person and can cause serious issues if not addressed.

Common symptoms of low blood sodium include:

- weakness
- fatigue or low energy
- headache
- nausea
- vomiting
- muscle cramps or spasms
- confusion
- irritability

**As you can see, some of the same symptoms of low sodium are also similar to detox, so keep that in mind. **

Although it's worth noting, low sodium levels are few and far between. Unless you are excessively drinking way more water than you need, sweating excessively, taking medication that can cause low sodium issues or avoiding salt, chances are there is nothing for you to be concerned about.

Many factors can cause low blood sodium. Your sodium levels may get too low if your body loses too much water and electrolytes but may also be caused by certain medical conditions.

Including:

- severe vomiting or diarrhea.
- taking certain medications, including antidepressants and pain medications.
- taking diuretics (water pills).
- drinking too much water during exercise (this is very rare).
- dehydration (please note low sodium can also be due to not enough water).

- kidney disease or kidney failure.

- liver disease.

- heart problems, including congestive heart failure.

- adrenal gland disorders such as Addison's disease, which affects your adrenal gland's ability to regulate the balance of sodium, potassium, and water in your body.

- hypothyroidism (underactive thyroid).

- primary polydipsia, a condition in which excess thirst makes you drink too much.

- using ecstasy or other hard-core drugs.

- syndrome of inappropriate antidiuretic hormone (SIADH), which makes your body retain water.

- diabetes insipidus, a rare condition in which the body doesn't make antidiuretic hormones.

- Cushing's syndrome, which causes high cortisol levels (this is rare).

(Sourced from Healthline)

WHO NEEDS TO BE MINDFUL OF LOW SODIUM?

- People who are older in age

- People who use diuretics

- If you use antidepressants

- If you are sweating a lot due to climate or exercise

- If eating a low-sodium diet

- If you have had heart failure, kidney disease, or other conditions

If you have any of these risk factors for low sodium, you may need to be more careful about your intake of water and be sure to add in salt or trace minerals as needed.

A blood test can help your healthcare provider check for low sodium levels.

TIPS FOR PREVENTING LOW SODIUM IN YOUR BLOOD:

- Keeping your water and electrolyte levels in balance can help prevent low blood sodium.

- Simply being sure to include sodium in your diet by salting foods with Pink Himalayan, Celtic or Sea salt, or adding in trace minerals to your water is not only healthy for you, but an easy way to ensure you are getting the sodium you need.

The moral of the story here:

- Be mindful of your water intake. Although water is key to the process, you want to be making sure you are drinking enough, and not just adding in more than you need. Be thoughtful when you are increasing water. If you are thirsty and in detox, listen to the body's cues and drink more when needed.

- You need salt in your diet, as much as you have been told it's bad for you...just like most things in the diet industry...that's a half truth. Be mindful of adding it in when following a healthy diet.

- If you have any concerns at all with your sodium levels, it is always recommended to get blood work done to confirm and to work with your health care professional.

Please take the time to head over to the Facebook Group or the Livy Method App and watch the quick video that accompanies this post.

LET'S TALK COFFEE

Coffee is totally fine to have on plan but here are a few things to note:

- You can drink as much coffee as you like but try to avoid drinking it later in the day if it messes with your sleep.

- Coffee counts towards your water intake, although it's not ideal so be sure not to use it as the main source.

- You can use any type of creamer you like, dairy or non-dairy, but we suggest you avoid any artificial flavour or colour. So, look for naturally flavoured and watch the amount of sugar added to some creamers.

- You can use real sugar, raw sugar or natural sweeteners like honey or maple syrup.

- I'm not a fan of agave. It is super sweet and high in fructose, which can feed into the need for something sweet and lead to insulin resistance, so best to avoid.

- And when it comes to artificial sweeteners, even though there are some better ones on the market like stevia and monk fruit, they can still lead to insulin resistance, so try to avoid it.

(Insulin resistance is when your body (pancreas) over produces insulin, something we will be focusing on further as we go...the goal is to decrease the amount your body needs to use.)

Please take the time to head over to the Facebook Group or the Livy Method App and watch the quick video that accompanies this post.

LET'S TALK ALCOHOL

This is a hot topic when it comes to weight loss, so let's discuss how alcohol fits into the plan.

When it comes to weight loss, I've never had a client or group member have to stop drinking alcohol in order to lose weight. Generally, that's because alcohol is not the reason your body is feeling a need to store fat. With that said, there are benefits to limiting your intake so still be mindful of what you are drinking when looking to lose weight.

If you like to enjoy a beverage every now and then, following these tips can help minimize the impact on your body and the scale.

- Most important tip is to get extra water in to compensate for dehydration that alcohol can cause. We recommend a minimum extra cup (250 ml/8 oz) of water per drink.

WINE

- Choose red wine over white. Although both are fine, red has more antioxidants and is slightly better for you. That isn't a reason to give up your white if that's what you prefer.

ROSE & CHAMPAGNES

- A little higher in sugar so don't be surprised if you wake up with a headache but also totally fine to have.

BEER/CIDERS

- Avoid "light" or "low-cal" beer. Light beer may have less calories but turns to sugar faster. That is an issue because we are not worried about calories, we are more concerned about how it breaks down in the body and affects your insulin levels and digestive system. Darker beers like Guinness are higher in nutrient value but any of your regular, all-natural ales, lagers, pilsners etc. are totally fine.

- When it comes to Ciders the same rules apply. Be mindful of added sugars and artificial ingredients.

- Non-alcoholic beer/cider is counted as an extra, just as juice would be. Be mindful of the ingredients and if there is a small alcohol percentage, you may want to add in some extra water.

HARD LIQUOR

- When it comes to the hard stuff, be mindful about what you are using as a mix. Try to avoid pop/soda, including diet and flavoured juice.

- Stick with carbonated water, mixed with a splash of natural juices, tomato juice or Clamato etc. If you enjoy something like rye and coke or gin and tonic once every now and then, it's no big deal.

The issue with alcohol is more the food you eat with it. If you are following the plan this is a non-issue but sometimes you might be at a party and be mindfully indulging. Here's a couple of things to keep in mind if you are.

- Drinking alcohol slows down the metabolism & your digestive system, so you want to avoid any heavy carbs like bread and pasta and stick to more protein, fats (like cheese and nuts) and veggies.

- Keep in mind alcohol can affect weight loss in other ways. For example, interrupting your sleep, messing with estrogen levels, causing dehydration, and causing you to crave both sugar and salt the next day. Alcohol increases the production of galanin, a neuropeptide in the brain, which causes you to crave greasy food. Pair that with the effects of dehydration that causes you to crave sugar and you are ready to eat your face off the next day!

- Bumping up good fats like oils, nuts, seeds, and avocados, increasing your water along with having a banana, which is high in potassium, first thing the next day will help the body metabolize the alcohol and reduce the galanin.

- Drinking can also affect the good bacteria in your digestive system, so if your stomach always feels off the next day, try adding in or doubling up on your probiotic. I will be talking more about probiotics and other supplements in the next few weeks.

MY FINAL TIP

The best thing you can do to offset negative effects of alcohol consumption is to add in that extra water of one cup per drink.

Besides that, enjoy your beverages!

Please take the time to head over to the Facebook Group or the Livy Method App and watch the quick video that accompanies this post.

LET'S TALK SHIFT WORK

How to manage the food plan with around the clock and off hours.

First, it's key to know that having a crazy or busy work schedule is not going to hinder your progress.

Working shift work can throw off your body's natural circadian rhythm, which in turn can cause you to be extra tired.

When tired, the body looks for pick-me-ups like carbs, caffeine, and sugar. This is generally a sign the body is asking for more water. Making water your focus will not only help with your energy levels but will also eliminate any cravings which will help you stay on track.

The more routine you can be with the food and water the better.

TIPS FOR WORKING OUT AN EATING SCHEDULE:

The basic rule for shift workers when it comes to the food plan is to start your day from when you wake up, regardless of what time of day that might be.

Even if it's 3pm or 9pm, wake up and have your warm lemon water or ACV and then your higher protein breakfast.

If you are eating breakfast at 9pm you may be more inclined to have something like fish or chicken and veg as opposed to more "breakfast-y" type foods, and that's ok.

If your day is broken up by taking naps, you can just insert the naps in your day and stick to your regular scheduled plan for food.

For example:

If you get up at 9am but then go back to bed at 12pm, you can have breakfast and then fruit... then nap. Or just breakfast then nap, then fruit when you wake up. When you wake up, continue with your day where you left off food wise, so in this case, go straight to lunch, if you had fruit before, or the fruit if you didn't, and then continue on with your day.

You also can extend your eating times by breaking your lunch and/or dinner portion into 2 servings. If you are working and awake for extended hours, it could look something like this:

- Breakfast
- Fruit
- 1/2 of lunch
- Other 1/2 of lunch
- Veg snack

- Nut/seeds snack
- 1/2 dinner
- Other 1/2 of dinner

This will have you eating 8 times a day so you can cover more hours.

Once we add in bonus snacks, they will also help with planning your day. For now, try to follow the food plan formula as much as possible. Bonus snacks are extra snacks you add to your day that can help fill in the gaps for those who get up extra early, those of you who are more active, and those of you who work shift work and will be awake sometimes for 24hrs.

As you become more in-tune with your hunger levels, you will notice some days you will feel hungrier than others. When working the night shift, for example, you may find your appetite is much lighter compared to the day, which is normal.

It might take you a while to find the right balance, don't stress. Play around with the timing until you find what works.

I will revisit this again when we introduce bonus snacks next week. Hope this helps!

Please take time to head over to the Facebook Group or the Livy Method App and watch the quick video that accompanies this post and if you need help with planning around your shifts, be sure to ask.

LET'S TALK THE SCALE

Let's take a moment and talk about the Scale.

I know many of you are not fans of stepping on the scale every day and for some of you it can be downright frustrating. Which is why it is ultimately up to you if you are going to use it while following the Program.

During weight loss the scale acts as a tool. Personally, I feel it can be very insightful, which is why I suggest you step on the scale every day during this process.

Trying to lose weight without using a scale is like trying to build a house without a hammer. It can be done…but it is so much easier when you use the right tools.

The scale can help indicate where your body is at in the process based on how it's responding in combination with the foods you are eating, the water you are drinking, and the supplements you are taking… along with how you are feeling from day to day.

HERE IS HOW TO USE IT SO YOU CAN LOSE IT!

What's happening on the scale can help you stay on top of the changes your body is making day to day. Noticing a pattern and using it as a tool can help you make the adjustments that help speed up the fat loss process and help the body focus on letting go of the fat.

When it comes to the scale, using The Livy Method, a drop is always a drop. When the scale moves down, you can count on it being because of actual fat loss and that is your new true weight. Whereas when the scale is up, it is always a superficial gain based on what you did or didn't eat or drink the day before.

So, when you say, "I gained weight last night" or "Why is my weight up even though I'm doing everything right?!" understand that it's the scale that is up and not your actual weight. It's impossible for your body to take the foods you eat and convert them into fat overnight. It's harder and takes longer than you think for your body to make fat.

Here are a couple guidelines about weight loss and weight gain that are helpful to understand before you let the scale freak you out or frustrate you:

- It is key to understand that weight loss is based on momentum, NOT on how you ate the day before.
- Meaning, weight loss happens after your body has geared up to go into "weight loss mode" which can be days or even a week.
- "Weight loss mode", or in "detox mode" are the loose and very general terms I use to describe when the body is specifically focused on fat loss.

THINGS TO KEEP IN MIND:

The scale is going to fluctuate. It will go up and down and you will have plateaus. Real weight loss is not a straight line down. Fluctuations are normal and expected.

- It is normal when you drop fat to have your weight go down on the scale & then back up again as fat cells retain water, getting ready to drop again, or before they have time to shrink… it does not mean you gained weight back.

- It's also normal to feel bloated and gross and have your weight up the day before it shows a drop on the scale…. this is not real weight gain, it's a sign to stay on plan because your weight is about to drop.

- It is also normal to feel like you have lost weight, but the scale is showing the same number or is up. This is usually a sign you are about to drop - it just hasn't translated on the scale yet.

- Drinking your water is so important! Water helps to get your body into detox, so it drops the fat in the first place. Not drinking enough water can slow the process of seeing the scale move.

- If the scale is bouncing up and down, it usually means your body needs more water because it is trying to get into detox.

OTHER THINGS TO KEEP IN MIND:

- Best time to weigh yourself is in the morning after you go to the bathroom. For shift workers, weigh yourself when you wake to start your day, after you go to the bathroom.

- A digital scale is ideal as you can see the small fluctuations, which can be helpful.

- The body doesn't care about how much you want the scale to move. It has no concept of time or your desire to lose weight as fast as possible.

- Your body also has no concept of any number you want to reach on the scale. Which is why going by how you feel can be just as important as stepping on the scale.

LET'S TALK ABOUT GOAL WEIGHT:

What is a good weight for you?

Without sounding cliché, I really do think it's when you feel comfortable in your skin. A good base line I use for clients is your lowest weight after the age of 21, that you were able to easily maintain.

That doesn't mean if you have always carried extra weight that you can't weigh less than you ever have, because you totally can. I always say weight loss is a side effect of being healthy. A properly functioning body has no need for excess fat, so given the opportunity and the time, it will be more than happy to get rid of it.

It is good to set a target weight as a goal, but I find most people underestimate their goals out of fear of failing. Group members are always setting new goals along the way and that's ok because it's a process.

On a final note, I have attached some photos (refer to the original group post) as a visual for you to see what weight loss really looks like on the scale. It is not the typical straight line down most believe it to be. It is very normal for weight to go up and down and up and down and be perceived to be all over the place when there actually is a pattern to it.

TO RECAP:

- As frustrating as it can be sometimes, the scale is a very helpful tool for weight loss and nothing to be feared.
- Best time to weigh yourself is first thing in the morning, ideally after going to the bathroom. Later in the day the scale will always read higher.
- Your weight being up does not mean you gained weight. It is normal for your weight to fluctuate whether you are losing weight or not, for a variety of reasons.
- A new low on the scale is always real weight loss and is your actual weight.
- It's also normal to feel bloated and gross and have your weight up the day before it shows a drop on scale.
- It's normal to "feel like" you have lost weight but have the scale up or the same. This also can be a sign you are about to drop.
- Weight loss is never a straight line down. The scale is going to go up and down whether you like it or not. It's a normal part of the process and is natural for the body even after you have finished losing weight.

I will be talking more in-depth about your body's response to the process and how to use the scale to your advantage as we move forward.

Please take the time to head over to the Facebook Group or the Livy Method App and watch the quick video that accompanies this post.

LET'S TALK TO THE MEN

It may seem like there are not a lot of men in the group but there are!

It's just that women tend to be more vocal about weight loss and the process.

Things to keep in mind for the guys:

- There is nothing men need to do differently.

- Follow the plan as designed and it will work wonders for both men & women.

- Eat all meals and snacks.

- Make your food as nutrient rich as possible and don't be afraid to add in the heavier carbs as needed.

- Eat to satisfaction and don't try to eat less.

- Get the water in!

Men tend to lose weight a lot faster than women, which can be an issue. With that said, it's a good issue to have, but one to be mindful of. Because the body can make change fast, it is a good idea to be checking in with your health care provider along the way. Especially if you have any health issues or are taking any medication.

As we progress, I will be addressing the men in the group specifically and will be sure to let you know if there are any tweaks or changes you need to make along the way.

Please take the time to head over to the Facebook Group or the Livy Method App and watch the quick video that accompanies this post.

LET'S TALK DETOX

How we use the body's natural detox process to lose weight.

"Detox" is a loose term I use to describe when the body is specifically focused on fat loss or in what I call "weight loss mode".

It is key to note the body doesn't need any help when it comes to detoxing naturally. This is why I'm not a fan of detox kits, detox juice, or juice cleanses. When it comes to detox and helping the body get the fat out, there is nothing you need to do other than follow the program.

The program is systematically designed to do all the work for you. There is nothing you need to do other than follow it exactly as designed.

Keep in mind not everyone will experience detox symptoms. If you don't experience symptoms that doesn't mean you aren't going into detox, everyone is different. You can be just as successful on plan without experiencing typical detox symptoms as someone who experiences strong detox symptoms.

Some typical "detox" symptoms include:

- feeling rundown
- flu-like symptoms
- runny nose
- dizzy as hormones balance
- headaches, chills, night sweats, aches and pains (nothing severe)
- feeling tired
- feeling bloated
- metallic taste in your mouth
- being thirsty and having dry lips even though you are drinking lots of water
- waking up around 3-4am to pee
- loose bowel movements and/or constipation
- Itchy skin or mild rashes (nothing severe)

Although some of you may experience strong detox symptoms, there is no need for concern. There is nothing you will do on this program that will cause, or lead to, any detrimental effects in the body.

**If you feel something is off, please make sure to always check in with your health care provider with any concerns. **

Keep in mind, all you are doing is eating healthy food and drinking enough water to be hydrated.

It's the changes in food, the design of the Food Plan formula, and the process of releasing the fat that causes the body to react. You can't expect your body to make life changing changes without noticing.

With that said, it's amazing what the body can do and how it will respond when you are giving it what it needs.

Please take time to head over to the Facebook Group or the Livy Method App and watch the quick video that accompanies this post. To learn more about the science behind our body's natural detox process please head to the Detox post in the Science Guide.

PROTEINS, CARBS, AND FATS

In my Program I talk a lot about the mix of protein, carbs, and fats that your body needs. And while this isn't something I need you to think too much about, here is a brief outline for those interested.

PLEASE NOTE: you do NOT need to worry about percentages or portions. Serving size and portion wise, all you need to do right now is follow the plan and eat to satisfaction.

This is just to give you examples of what foods fall under each category.

SOURCES OF CARBS (foods that break down into energy)

- Fruit
- Vegetables
- Heavier Root Veg like potatoes, squash, cassava, plantain
- Naturally occurring sugar found in things like beans and lentils and chickpeas
- Oatmeal and cereal like hemp hearts and buckwheat
- Rice and grains like black rice & quinoa, barley
- Ryvita crackers and Ezekiel bread

SOURCES OF PROTEIN (feeds the muscles helping to repair and rebuild along with maintain and build muscle mass)

- Fish
- Meat (Any Meat)
- Eggs
- Seafood
- Beans, lentils, legumes
- Nuts and Seeds
- Incomplete protein like oatmeal, quinoa and rice (not to be used as main source)
- Dairy - cheese, yogurt, milk products (not to be used as a main source)
- Tofu

PLANT PROTEIN

As you can see below, there is protein found in lots of things besides animal sources.

- Broccoli - 2.6g per 1 cup

- Asparagus - 2.4g per 1 cup
- Peas - 9g per 1 cup
- Cauliflower - 2g per 1 cup
- Brussels - 3g per 1 cup
- Bok choy - 1g per 1 cup
- Spinach, collard greens - 1g per 1 cup
- Mung bean sprouts - 2.5g per 1 cup
- Beans (kidney, pinto, black beans, chick peas etc.) - 7.5g per 1/2 cup
- Lentils - 9g per 1/2 cup
- Quinoa - 4g per 1/2 cup
- Tempeh - 11g per 1/2 cup
- Tofu - 7g per 1/2 cup
- Buckwheat - 6g per 1 cup
- Soy beans/Edamame - 10g per 1/2 cup
- Rice - 7g per 1cup
- Hemp seeds - 10g per 3 tbsp
- Pumpkin seeds - 5g per oz
- Chia - 4g per 2 tbsp
- Nut butter -15g per 2 tbsp
- Hummus - 7g per 2 tbsp
- Spirulina - 4g per 1 tbsp

Keep in mind you DO NOT need to worry about these measurements.

They are for reference only and to point out the fact that some proteins have carbs in them, some vegetables have protein in them, and that protein adds up.

As long as you are following the plan as outlined, you are getting enough and the right mix of everything you need.

SOURCES OF FATS (essential for cellular function, providing alternative energy and brain fuel)

- Fish/Fish oil
- Omega 3 and or 369

- Alternative oils like olive oil, coconut oil, avocado oil, grape seed oil, flax and hemp oil

- Salad dressings with good quality oils

- Olives

- Avocado

- Nuts

- Seeds

- Hemp hearts

- Dairy...like yogurt, cheese, butter

This is not a complete list, it is just to give you an idea of the kind of foods I'm suggesting when talking about incorporating proteins, carbs and fats to your meals.

Please take the time to head over to the Facebook Group or the Livy Method App and watch the quick video that accompanies this post.

LET'S TALK CONDIMENTS

This is a quick one, pretty much all condiments are fine to use. What you want to look for is quality ingredients, so nothing artificial.

Avoid:

- Artificial flavour
- Artificial colour
- Hydrogenated oil

Follow that rule and you should be fine.

This is for sauces and gravies and dips and all condiments in general. Use at will to flavour your foods.

Now, with that said some condiments can be super salty and may lead to the scale being up the next day...soy sauce is one of the main ones that has that effect. It is nothing to worry about and not a reason to not use it, as it's not real weight gain… just key to note when weighing yourself.

Please take the time to head over to the Facebook Group or the Livy Method App and watch the quick video that accompanies this post.

LET'S TALK DAIRY

Now if you are not into dairy, that's cool...you don't need to eat it or add it in. We get a lot of questions about dairy on plan so hopefully this post will help break things down for you!

FIRST LET'S TALK ABOUT CHEESE

When can I have it?

- With any of your meals AND it can also be added to your veg snack. With the veg snack just make sure raw veggies are the star of the show.

How much can I have?

- As with all meals and snacks on plan you are to eat to satisfaction...so add cheese to your meal and then eat said meal to satisfaction. See below regarding concerns about cholesterol.

What kinds of cheese can I have?

- Pretty much any kind is fine, avoid any processed cheese and of course any cheese with anything artificial in it including artificial colours.
- White cheeses are great, especially old white cheddar.
- Processed cheeses include things like Velveeta, Cheese Whiz, American Cheese, Kraft Cheese Slices, Cheese Strings, any cheese that comes in a tube or jar. Pre-shredded cheese has some questionable anti-caking agents so it is fine to have occasionally but keep it to a minimum.
- Always look for all natural ingredients.
- Avoid "light" or low-fat cheeses as they often contain additives to compensate for the fat removed.

What if I'm concerned about cholesterol?

- When it comes to avoiding high cholesterol, it's all about the kind of fats you are consuming.
- Cheese is a saturated fat and you do need to be mindful about how much saturated fat you consume.
- Saturated fat is a good fat, BUT the key is to make sure you are getting enough great fat like omega 3 and omega 6.
- If you are following the plan, this isn't something you need to worry about as the plan factors it in. Just be sure to be adding a mix of good fat to your meals.

To review a list of good fats, check out the post on Proteins, Carbs & Fats.

LET'S TALK ABOUT YOGURT

When can I have it?

For the first part of the program yogurt is eaten mostly at breakfast with added protein such as hemp hearts, nuts, seeds, nut butters and/or protein powder.

It can also be added to lunch and dinner as an added dip, dressing, sauce, or condiment to your meal. It can also be used as a dip with your afternoon veg. snack.

What kinds can I have?

Plain, Greek yogurt is the best option as it is higher in protein and lower in carbs. This is because of the straining process used to make it. By removing the excess liquid whey and lactose (natural sugars) a higher protein yogurt is created!

Avoid low or no-fat yogurts because they usually contain additives to compensate for the lack of fat that can jack up the carbs and sugars. There are some low & no-fat Greek yogurts that don't contain any additives, but we want the fat and protein for more sustaining energy, especially at breakfast.

Can I have flavoured or sweetened yogurt?

Yes, you can but make sure it has a higher fat content to neutralize the amount of insulin needed to break it down. Again, look for Greek yogurts higher in fat (4%+) and always bump it up even more with the above-mentioned proteins. The more sugar, the more fat and protein needed.

A better alternative to sweetened yogurt is to use plain and add a touch of honey or maple syrup instead. Or mix your favourite sweetened yogurt with plain yogurt. That way you have control over the amount of sugar added and can slowly reduce it as your taste buds adjust.

What about non-dairy or plant-based yogurts?

Same guidelines apply. Look for higher protein and fat without any artificial ingredients. Always add in extra protein as mentioned above.

LET'S TALK ABOUT MILK AND CREAM

When can I have it?

Milk and cream can be used at any time. You can have a glass of milk whenever you like, and it would count towards your water/fluid intake. Milk and cream can also be added to coffee, tea, high protein cereals, oatmeal, soups, sauces etc. at will.

What kinds can I have?

When it comes to milk and dairy you don't have to avoid low or no fat. The removal of fat here doesn't require additives to compensate for taste or texture. The fat is simply removed. So, you can enjoy anything from skim to full fat when it comes to milk and cream.

What about lactose free and plant-based milks and flavoured creamers?

Those are all fine to have on plan. When it comes to flavoured creamers, whether they are dairy or non-dairy, just make sure they are made with all natural ingredients, nothing artificial, and watch the amount of sugar added as some can be very high.

Keep in mind that although all dairy products have protein, they aren't a good "stand-alone" protein on program so should always be used in addition to other protein sources when eaten with meals. Check out the Grocery List for other protein sources.

Please take the time to head over to the Facebook Group or the Livy Method App and watch the quick video that accompanies this post.

LET'S TALK LEAFY GREENS

Leafy greens are an ideal addition to meals as they help to increase the Glucagon-like-Peptide-1 hormone that keeps blood sugar more stable and helps keep you more satisfied. They are also packed with tons of nutrients that are great for your health and cellular function and an excellent source of fiber which helps the body process food through your digestive system, which is needed for weight loss.

Plus, all of the changes you are making in your diet can affect your bowel movements. Leafy greens provide the roughage your body needs to keep you regular.

Leafy greens can be added to meals raw, like in a salad, but also cooked or sautéed and/or added to soups, stews & stir fries. Cabbage, Brussels sprouts, and bok choy, among others which are listed in the Grocery List, are also classified as veg and can be used as one or the other or both in your meals.

The general rule is…if it's green and leafy it works!

Getting your leafy greens in can be difficult especially in the colder months but cooking them and adding them to soups, stews, etc. is a great way to get them in when you're not feeling like having a salad.

If you are not a fan of eating your leafy greens, it is still key to get them in. You don't have to be fancy about it or get in a huge variety. It's also not a big deal if you are a bit hit and miss getting them in, as long as you are mindful to be as consistent as possible.

Although they are suggested at lunch and dinner, leafy greens can also be added to breakfast or to the raw veg snack.

** **Please note: Leafy greens are not considered a veg on plan.** **

Please take the time to head over to the Facebook Group or the Livy Method App and watch the quick video that accompanies this post.

LET'S TALK ABOUT GUM

Can you chew it on Plan?

It is not advised and here is why:

Digestion starts in the mouth, technically with smell first and then by chewing. Chewing gum artificially stimulates your digestive system, and without following through and eating food, that can be an issue. Especially if the gum you are chewing is artificially flavored and made with artificial sweetener.

Some sweeteners like sucralose, although low in sugar and calories, still causes a reaction in the body that secretes insulin (the chemical your body uses after it breaks down food to convert glucose into energy).

In small amounts it's a minimal concern, but if you chew a lot of gum it can lead to insulin resistance and higher insulin levels that can signal weight gain. We are trying to reduce the amount of insulin your body is used to using, which is why I suggest minimizing any gum chewing.

IF YOU NEED TO CHEW:

Try to chew natural gum which can be found online or at health food stores. Try to chew directly after a meal as opposed to in between.

Avoid using it to suppress your appetite. You want to be in-tune to your body's needs, not suppress them. In no way is chewing gum a benefit.

NOTE: MINTS HAVE THE SAME EFFECT

Please take time to head over to the Facebook Group or the Livy Method App and watch the quick video that accompanies this post. To read more about how chewing affects our digestive system head to the Science Guide and read The Basics of Digestion.

LET'S TALK CHOCOLATE

Dark chocolate can be a source of magnesium and, when it's good quality, it can be low in sugar. So, can you have it on plan?

I'm going to say NO and here's why:

You don't want to be using food for anything other than nutritional requirements right now. The goal is to get in tune to your body's needs and cut through your "wants". If you are craving sugar you want to ask yourself why? As every craving is a message from your body.

You don't want to be feeding into cravings or trying to manage or mask them. You want to address them, so you don't have them anymore. As always, when all is said and done, it's no big deal. It all depends on how much you want to get out of this process.

Down the road you will be able to add chocolate back in, but for now, if you are looking to maximize your results, I suggest keeping it out. If you are concerned about sugar cravings, then simply follow the plan, as the Program is designed to address them.

Eat all of your meals and snacks, make your food nutrient rich, eat to satisfaction, and drink your water. With that said, nothing is make or break and no one is expecting perfection. If you do end up eating some chocolate or indulging in any treats, all you need to do is keep moving forward and get back at it.

Please take the time to head over to the Facebook Group or the Livy Method App and watch the quick video that accompanies this post.

LET'S TALK ABOUT EXERCISE

How to incorporate it into the Program and tweak it so it is more conducive to fat loss.

As you move through The Program and focus more and more on giving the body what it needs, it will start to allow you more access to your energy reserves by maximizing your metabolism. Your metabolism is the rate at which your body functions day to day or to simplify, how much energy you use and calories you naturally burn on a daily basis.

When the body feels a need to store fat, it will keep you in "reserve mode" and limit the amount of energy you can use. This is why mentally you might be keen to exercise but energetically you might not feel so motivated.

As you move forward in this process and continue to put the time and energy into giving your body what it needs, your body is going to start giving you access to more energy. After a few weeks on the program, you may be surprised that you will want to move your body more and feel like being more active.

Although there are many beneficial reasons to exercise, it is not a mandatory requirement for weight loss on this program.

We will however be talking more about it as we move forward for those interested.

AMPLIFYING YOUR FITNESS FOR FAT LOSS:

Let's talk about the best way to implement exercises that will fall in line with your weight loss goals. If you are new to exercise, I suggest you start by simply being more active.

I know it sounds cliché, but things like taking the stairs and parking further away when getting groceries, going for walks or doing some push-ups or squats in your kitchen, can add up and have a big impact.

If you are looking for something more intense, there are a lot of great home workout options. It's best to start slow to minimize the stress on the body and build up to it. Whatever you choose to do, it should be something you enjoy so you make a positive association to exercise moving forward and it becomes something you look forward to doing.

**You also want to walk away from any exercise feeling good and energized, not tired, taxed or drained. **

You have to remember that you are working towards getting the body to focus on detox and fat loss. If you work out too hard and you create too much damage in the body, it will have no choice but to focus on repairing and rebuilding instead of detoxing and fat loss.

THIS BRINGS US TO THE TOPIC OF REST:

If you are going to work out to the point of being sore, you need to make sure you are giving your body adequate time to repair and rebuild, or you will run the risk of overtraining.

Overtraining happens when the body can't catch up to the damage that's been done, leaving your body feeling weak and in a deficit, which in turn can cause the body to feel the need to hold on to fat or store more fat for easy energy.

LET'S TALK CARDIO OR GETTING YOUR HEART RATE UP:

When it comes to exercise and weight loss, it's all about the message you are sending to the body. Your physical brain that runs your body doesn't see what you are doing for exercise, it only interprets what you are doing based on your movements and heart rate. This is where you can use the body's natural FIGHT or FLIGHT response to maximize your results.

Getting your heart rate up as high as you can for as long as you can, even if just for a few minutes, evokes the FIGHT or FLIGHT response in the body and immediately sends a message for the body to work to make you stronger.

The body's sole responsibility is to keep you alive, so if you repeatedly evoke the fight or flight response, your body will look to make you as strong and efficient as possible. In wanting to be as efficient as possible, your body will look to get rid of any extra fat that could be slowing you down. This makes cardio (exercise that gets your heart rate up) very effective for fat loss.

Cardio doesn't have to be running, it can be walking fast, skipping, swimming, dancing, lifting lighter weights with higher reps, sports activities, and anything else that helps get your heart rate up.

With cardio you are basically taking the muscle you already have in your body and using it to move your body, which will get your heart rate up without creating damage, making it a complement to the weight loss program.

LET'S TALK LIFTING WEIGHTS:

When it comes to lifting weights, things can get tricky because you are purposely creating damage in the body, so the body repairs the damage and makes the muscle stronger.

That is great for bone density, building muscle and shaping your body, but not great for fat loss. That doesn't mean you can't continue to lift weights, especially if that is something you enjoy. I would, however, suggest you lift a little lighter using higher repetitions, to use the muscle you do have to help to get your heart rate up with minimal damage.

During sleep is when the body detoxes and/or makes change, it doesn't do both at the same time. So, if your body is always sore, then your body is always focusing on repairing the damage that is making you sore. Leaving very little or no time left to focus on detox.

I know we have been taught to believe that exercise is how you lose weight, but that just isn't true. In fact, exercise is a really crappy weight loss tool and can actually work against you when it comes to the scale.

Now with that said, exercise is amazing for so many reasons, like stress release, heart health, and making your body stronger in general, so I'm not saying don't do it. I'm just saying be smart about it and understand the message that is being sent to the body when you do.

MY EXERCISE FAVES FOR FAT LOSS:

- Walking because it's also conducive to healing and the least stressful type of exercise you can do.
- Anything outside, because it stimulates the brain and works the body while communing with nature and relieving stress.
- Dance or Boxing/Martial arts type classes that move the body in different ways other than side to side and up and down, while evoking the fight response.
- Biking or spinning is great for getting your heart rate up and evoking the flight response.
- Exercises that use your own body weight as resistance.

Let me know if you have any questions and be sure to check with your healthcare provider before starting, or if for any reason you are feeling apprehensive about adding exercise into your routine.

Please take time to head over to the Facebook Group or the Livy Method App and watch the quick video that accompanies this post. For more information on exercise and weight loss check out The Science of Fat and Fat Loss in the Science Guide.

LET'S TALK BREAD, FLOURS, PASTA, AND CRACKERS

We're mindful of not giving people the impression that this program is low Carb...because it's not. It's more about the right carbs. On plan you are eating veggies and fruit, grains and legumes, with naturally occurring sugars...so the plan, if followed, is far from low carb.

We get asked a lot if it's okay to eat bread, pasta, crackers etc. on plan. The answer is yes, BUT…

By following the Food Plan you are trying to decrease the amount of insulin your body is used to using, which in turn will help you to feel more satisfied with smaller portions.

Bread, pasta, and flour in general, require a lot more insulin than whole foods when the body breaks them down, regardless of the type or source. So, when it comes to weight loss and this process, we consider bread and pasta to be processed foods. You can eat them, BUT it can slow down the process.

BREAD & CRACKERS

Although it is possible to lose weight on this program while continuing to eat bread, it can slow down the process. In the beginning we want you to have an easy transition into following the food plan so it's okay to keep bread in and keep it with breakfast or lunch, but not both.

It's also important the type of bread you choose. Best choice is Ezekiel Bread which is a high quality, sprouted grain bread that doesn't contain any flour. Because it is free from any preservatives and sugar, it is found in the fridge or freezer section in health food stores and many grocery stores.

Ezekiel Bread ingredient list: *Organic Sprouted Wheat, Filtered Water, Organic Sprouted Barley, Organic Sprouted Millet, Organic Malted Barley, Organic Sprouted Lentils, Organic Sprouted Soybeans, Organic Sprouted Spelt, Fresh Yeast, Organic Wheat Gluten, Sea Salt.*

If you can't find Ezekiel, and choose to keep bread in your diet, look for other sprouted grain breads that are dense, grainy, and seedy. Go for high fiber and quality ingredients. The less processed and shorter the ingredient list the better!

When it comes to crackers, we recommend high fibre crackers like Ryvita brand. Ryvita crackers have a short ingredient list, contain whole grains, and are high in fiber. If you can't find the Ryvita brand specifically, look for crackers with similar ingredients.

Ryvita Multi-Grain Crispbread Ingredients:

Whole grain rye flour, Toasted grains and seeds (buckwheat, soy meal, sesame seeds, flaxseed, kibbled rye), Rye bran, Salt.

Mary's Super Seed Crackers are a good gluten free alternative for those of you who can't digest gluten.

PASTA & FLOUR

We get asked a lot if it's okay to have pasta made with alternative flours such as chickpea, black bean or konjak. Although these pastas are a better choice than ones made with wheat flour, while trying to lose weight, it is recommended to leave them out.

It's not about what the pasta (or flour) is made from, it's about the process of making them that can still affect blood sugar levels. Right now, while trying to lose weight, we are working hard to decrease and balance out blood sugar levels so adding in pastas and larger quantities of flour is counterproductive.

Small amounts of flour used for breading or thickening a soup or sauce is totally fine as a small quantity won't have the same effect on your blood sugar levels.

As mentioned above, some people can continue to eat these things and still lose weight but if you are looking to maximize your efforts you might want to consider limiting or skipping them altogether. Remember it's not a "lifestyle" it's an effort to lose as much weight as possible in the time frame we have. Maybe you prefer to take a more relaxed approach and leave it in. That's also totally cool! The choice is yours based on how hard core you want to be about the process. If you find that your weight isn't moving and you've been adding it in, you may want to consider taking it out for now.

We understand that bread and pasta are convenient, easy, and taste great and we know you might miss having them ....but you won't miss the fat when it's gone and keeping them out can make that fat loss process happen a lot faster.

WEEK 1 GUIDELINES: IMPLEMENTING THE FOOD PLAN

The goal is to implement the changes with the food if you haven't yet. And if you have, continue with the food plan, focus on water, be as consistent as possible, and pay attention to how your body is responding to the changes you are making.

Any information not included in the Workbook, including all of the accompanying videos, you will find in the Facebook Support Group. Everything is posted in the GUIDES section, where the GUIDES are listed by the Week.

Another way to quickly find information in the Facebook Support Group is by using TOPICS, which is located on the same menu bar as GUIDES (mobile) or on the right-hand side of the page on a computer. You can also search for information by using the search feature located at the very top of the group page.

Each day, we post additional support info/videos to further explain the process and any changes you are to make. All of the information is posted in the Facebook Group so be sure to check there regularly.

THE GOAL FOR WEEK 1:

The goal for this first official week is to continue to implement the food plan, work on getting in the water, and be as consistent as possible. Also, if you need, take time to catch up on the information that has been posted and get yourself familiar with navigating the Group so you are up to date. We want to ensure you don't miss any need-to-know info moving forward.

MUST WATCH: If you have not seen them yet, please take the time to watch these videos (found in the Facebook Support Group and the Livy Method App) as they explain the basics of the program and the process.

- The Livy Method
- The Food Plan
- Detox

THE FOCUS FOR THIS WEEK:

- Continue to follow the Food Plan Formula.
- Eat ALL meals and snacks.
- Make food choices as nutrient rich as possible.
- Eat to satisfaction, meaning do NOT try to eat less.
- Continue to work on getting your water in.
- Even though these are healthy changes you are making, change is stressful on the body, so consistency is key as you give it time to adjust.

Keep in mind, how you eat in the beginning will change and evolve week by week, and each week leads into and sets up the following week.

YOUR DAILY CHECKLIST:

- Check into the Facebook Support Group daily.
- Watch the "Daily Check In" video.
- Watch or read any new support posts.
- Ask any questions you have on the Questions of the Day Post, so you are clear on the changes you are making week to week.
- Implement the changes you need to make.

FACEBOOK LIVES:

The live Q&A Facebook Times:

- Monday to Friday - 9 am EST
- Saturdays - 10 am EST

If you are having trouble finding the Lives, here are some tips:

- Once you see a live, be sure to set notifications. You will be prompted to do this while watching for the first time.
- Depending on what kind of device you are using, look for a menu option that is "Media" "Videos" or "Photos". Check in those menus after refreshing your page. Once you figure out the quickest way to find the video on the device you are using, this will be easy.

Please Note: Facebook Lives are NOT a mandatory part of the Program. You DO NOT need to watch them to be successful.

A LOOK AHEAD AT WEEK 2:

- The goal for Week 2 will be to fine tune and perfect the changes you have already made.
- We will also be introducing bonus snacks.
- We will also be talking about supplements and going over any that might be a benefit to the process moving forward.

Consistency is a super important part of this process as the first few weeks are all about giving the body what it needs so it no longer feels the need to store fat. The next step is to get the body to focus on detox and help it stay in detox long enough to drop the fat, so the more consistent you can be, the quicker you will start seeing results.

As you can see, it's a process. This may be a different process than you have experienced before but rest assured, it is a process that works and works well.

We are not concerned at all about anyone's ability to lose weight. The Program is all about following the plan, implementing the changes week to week, all while problem solving and moving forward.

Although this is a Weight Loss Program, the focus is NOT on the scale right now. It is NOT about how strong you start; it's about following through and finishing strong.

There will come a time where the scale will become the focus and main topic of conversation, but we are not there yet.

For now, focus on the basics and be as consistent as possible. It's the quickest way to get the scale moving and to keep it moving.

We have a long way to go, but there's no reason we can't have fun along the way. So, let's do this!

Please take the time to head over to the Facebook Group or the Livy Method App and watch the quick video that accompanies this post.

WEEK 1 GUIDELINES FAQS

1.   Is it normal for the scale to fluctuate?

Yes it's totally normal and to be expected. The scale can fluctuate for a number of reasons, none of which have anything to do with actual weight gain. Some reasons the scale can be up include your body reacting to a change in foods, your body being sore from a workout, poor quality sleep and medications, to name a few. Another reason the scale can be up is because your body is detoxing and your weight is about to drop. If the scale is fluctuating between a couple of numbers that is usually an indication that you need to add a bit more water as your body is looking to get into detox.

2.   Are bloating, constipation, and fullness signs of detox?

Yes, these are all typical signs of detox. Bloating and constipation are also normal as your body is adjusting to the Food Plan. Following the Program as designed and drinking enough water will help as everything comes together. If you are in detox, you'll want to support your body by being consistent with your water and getting in all of your meals and snacks, eating dinner early, getting a good night's sleep. If you're feeling full without much of an appetite leading up to a meal or snack, you'll still want to have a token amount to keep your digestive system working hard. A few token bites will do. For constipation, drinking plenty of water and adding leafy greens with your meals can help.

3.   I have esophageal reflux (GERD) and am concerned about taking lemon or apple cider vinegar (ACV). What do you suggest?

By following the Program and Food Plan, this can naturally help with your reflux. Adding in ACV can be very beneficial if you suffer from acid reflux. Feel free to dilute the lemon or ACV in as much water as you need to get it down. That said, it would be a great idea to speak with your healthcare practitioner if you have any concerns.

4.   What nuts are on plan?

Any type of nuts and seeds are great, preferably raw. It's best to avoid nuts and seeds that have oil or added salt, as they are usually made with poor quality oils and salt.

5.   Does skipping breakfast on some days and eating it on others have adverse effects? Should it be one or the other consistently?

Go by how you feel when it comes to breakfast. Skipping breakfast wouldn't have any adverse effects, and that is why you have the option to skip it, but there are definitely benefits to having a high protein breakfast in the morning. When you wake up in the morning, your body is already full of energy from what you ate the day before, so it doesn't need the energy from breakfast. However, having a high protein breakfast is a great way to "break the fast" and get your body working harder from the get-go.

6.   Can I have the ACV straight followed by a glass of water?

Yes, you are welcome to have ACV straight followed by water if this is the way you like it. You can also dilute the ACV in as much water as you need to get it down. There is some benefit to having your ACV in water as it is fairly acidic and some people find it can be gentler on their system.

7.   If something counts as a vegetable and a leafy green, does it cover both purposes in a meal?

Yes, if a vegetable also counts as a leafy green, it would count towards both your vegetable component and your leafy green component of your meal. Some great examples are cabbage, bok choy and brussel sprouts.

8.   If I am busy in the morning, is it better to skip breakfast and go straight to the fruit? Or eat breakfast late and schedule my other meals for later in the day?

It's always best to start your day with a high protein breakfast, and breakfast is ideally eaten within 2.5 hours of waking. However if you are up at 5am and not active or exercising you can still eat breakfast as late as 9am. If you get up later that gives you less time for both breakfast and fruit snack so you might skip breakfast and go straight to fruit snack. If you know you're going to have a busy day, it can be helpful to plan ahead by preparing some boiled eggs or overnight oats that you can quickly grab and go. Keep in mind you have between 30 min and 3.5 hours for your next meal or snack so you can still fit in all your meals and snacks into your day. Whether you have breakfast or not, you still want to have your fruit snack mid morning.

9.   Does it matter what time of day I have my coffee/tea?

You can have coffee and tea as you like at any time throughout the day. They would count towards your water intake. That said, if drinking coffee affects your ability to sleep at night, avoid drinking coffee too late into the evening.

10.   Are smoothies and/or shakes on plan?

At this point of the Program, while we are preparing our body for weight loss, we want our bodies to work hard to digest and process its food, which is why it's important to chew our food. There will come a time later in the program that you can add them in but for now it's best to follow the program as designed. If you do choose to keep them in, it's best to use a protein powder that contains all natural ingredients, without artificial sweeteners and low in sugar. Add little to no fruit and add in some healthy fat like avocados, nut butters and coconut oil, to name a few.

MUST WATCH VIDEOS (FACEBOOK GROUP AND THE LIVY METHOD APP)

Before you move ahead with the Program, you must watch these 3 videos, which are posted in the Facebook Group and the Livy Method App, if you have not yet watched them.

THE LIVY METHOD:

- I explain why The Livy Method is different from any other diet you have done. It is important you understand the method behind the process you will be following over the next 12 weeks.

THE FOOD PLAN:

- This is where I explain the rhyme and the reason behind what I'm asking you to eat and when, on the Food Plan. The sooner you start being consistent with the Food Plan, the sooner you will start and feel results.

DETOX VIDEO:

- This is where I explain how we use the body's natural detox process to help get fat out. It's key to understand how your body may or may not respond while following the Program.

As we go, I'll be talking more in depth about the Program and the Process. For now, focus on being consistent with the basics.

Please take the time to head over to the Facebook Group or the Livy Method App and watch the quick video that accompanies this post.

LET'S TALK BREAKFAST

If you need to eat it & how high protein it needs to be.

Breakfast is not the most important meal of the day; however, it can be very beneficial to your day and this process.

When you wake up, you are already full of energy, so you don't need to eat breakfast to get energy. That's why you have the option of skipping it, carrying on with your day, then going straight to your morning fruit snack. With that said though, there is absolutely a benefit to eating it.

Starting your day with a high protein breakfast is a great way to "break the fast" and get your body working harder from the get go. It pains me to say it, but that means burning more calories throughout your day! (And no, we still don't count calories.).

Going higher protein feeds the muscles without the need for as much insulin as carbs. High insulin levels signal weight gain in the body and we are trying to lower the amount of insulin your body uses on plan.

It's best to think about how you can maximize your meals and get the most bang for your buck portion wise, rather than trying to skew your meals to be something you enjoy. Meaning, be mindful not to be looking for variety, something to fit into your lifestyle ongoing, or to get excitement from your meals.

There will be lots of time for that later as we will be adding recipe share pages to the Facebook Group. For now, make sure to review the post on Meal Ideas in the Facebook Group where we break down some options for you.

The focus right now is to keep it simple and make sure to have the components you need at each meal and snack.

Ideally, you want to eat breakfast within 2.5 hours of waking. However, this is not a hard and fast rule. If you wake up at 5am and you are not active or exercising, you can still eat breakfast as late as 8-9 am and be fine. Some people are up earlier and some sleep later, and that might change day to day.

If you get up later, that gives you less time to eat breakfast before you need a snack, so you might skip breakfast and go straight to the fruit snack. We will be adding in bonus snacks to help fill in the blanks for those of you who are up early, are more active, or do shift work.

For now, play around with the timing of breakfast and then your fruit snack.

Please take time to head over to the Facebook Group or the Livy Method App and watch the quick video that accompanies this post. To read more about the benefits of a high protein breakfast check out the Hormones of Hunger and Satiety and Timing of Digestion post in the Science Guide.

LET'S TALK FRUIT SNACK

Why you need to have it and why you can't add anything with it.

Normally, it is a good idea to combine your carbs with a protein and fat, which can help neutralize the amount of insulin needed to break down your food.

Which may have you confused and wondering why are we eating the fruit on its own?! And why am I so adamant about that?

Regardless if you choose to skip breakfast or go higher protein...by mid-morning, your glycogen (energy) reserves are starting to deplete. The goal is to replenish those energy stores before the body has to dip into and utilize your emergency fat reserves.

Using your fat reserves sends a message to the body that you need your fat...so that is something we are ultimately trying to avoid.

When it comes to what fruit is best, that's up to you...no fruit is off limits, and you can choose to mix and match if you like.

Bananas, which we always get asked about, are a little higher in sugar but a great addition for anyone who may be more active or in need of potassium due to cramps while sleeping.

As with all meals and snacks, you are eating your fruit snack to satisfaction.

Please take the time to head over to the Facebook Group or the Livy Method App and watch the quick video that accompanies this post.

LET'S TALK LUNCH

Why it's not all about having salads every day.

Think of VEGGIES as being the star of the show and build your lunch around them, following the guidelines of vegetables, protein, healthy fats, greens and grains (if needed.)

It's not all about salads! If you do have them, be sure to load them up with veggies and make your lunch as nutrient rich as possible. Be sure to eat to satisfaction and be mindful that hunger levels change day to day. Lunch is the place to add in any heavier carbs like rice, quinoa, and potatoes to name a few, as needed.

Cheese, condiments, dressings, sauces, gravy and spices are all fine to use on plan. Best to leave out bread at lunch, especially if you had bread at breakfast, as well as any kind of pasta and noodles.

Please take the time to head over to the Facebook Group or the Livy Method App and watch the quick video that accompanies this post.

LET'S TALK VEG SNACK

Why, even though it tends to be the least appealing snack, it's important to get it in.

Raw veggies can be very hard to digest, which makes them the perfect food for signaling food in and food out. If you find you get bloated or have a hard time digesting raw veggies, then that can be a sign you are low in digestive enzymes.

Digestive enzymes build up in your digestive system by adding raw foods to your diet. They help the body process, digest and get maximum nutrients from the food you eat.

You can eat any raw veggies you like, and do not need to worry about getting in a huge variety. You can stick to the ones you like and you can mix and match.

You can also add natural dressings or dips like hummus or guacamole. You can also add cheese or nut butter.

Pickles or fermented food like cabbage also works.

You could also do a salad and use leafy greens as long as it's loaded up with raw veg. If you add raw veg to lunch you still need the afternoon snack.

If you do have a hard time digesting raw veggies, then you can cook or steam them, but do so temporarily with the goal to work your way up to eventually eating them raw.

The time between all meals and snacks should be 30 minutes - to not more than 3.5 hrs. between eating.

Please take the time to head over to the Facebook Group or the Livy Method App and watch the quick video that accompanies this post.

LET'S TALK NUTS AND SEEDS SNACK

Nuts and seeds can be very hard to digest, even harder than raw veggies...which is why they make the perfect afternoon snack.

Around 3-4pm the body is naturally wired to take a dip in energy. What the body is really looking for is a nap. Other places in the world refer to this as a siesta and take time to snooze.

Because most of us can't just take a nap during the day, this is where people go looking for sugar or caffeine as a pick-me-up. By adding in the nuts and or seeds, you are keeping your digestive system stimulated and working hard, which helps to keep your energy up.

The protein and fat from the nuts and seeds also helps to give you more sustaining energy, which will leave you feeling more satisfied leading up to and going into dinner. This helps keep your digestive system working hard to process and break down your larger meal, and will also help prevent you from over eating your dinner.

You can have Nuts or Seeds or a combination of both. You can use any Nuts or Seeds and ideally want to avoid oil or any salt added.

If you find them hard to digest, you can roast them or soak them.

The Nut & Seed Snack does not have an equal alternative so it is best to make a point of eating it unless you are allergic, in which case, you can *substitute with olives, beans or dairy.*

You can also add nuts and/or seeds to your meals - if you do, keep in mind you will still need to eat your Nut & Seed snack.

Please take the time to head over to the Facebook Group or the Livy Method App and watch the quick video that accompanies this post.

LET'S TALK DINNER

Given that it's at the end of the day, try to think of dinner as more of a top-up rather than a need for fuel.

(Read that again)

_With that said, if you are not hungry for dinner, it is still best to have a small portion of it. If you are hungry for dinner, be sure to eat to satisfaction. _

Either way, make your dinner nutrient rich and use the guideline of protein being the star of the show, with veg, healthy fats and leafy greens. You can also add heavier carbs IF you need, like root veg and/or grains.

Dinner can be in any combination like soup, stew, stir fry, chili, salad etc. When in doubt, go with protein and greens (cooked or raw).

Avoid using things like yogurts and oatmeal for dinner, or any kind of liquid nutrient (You can still use breakfast foods like eggs or sausage for dinner, but still incorporate the veg and greens).

There will come a time where you can have a greater variety of foods for dinner, but for now stick with the suggested components.

As with lunch, sauces, dressings, gravy, condiments, and spices can be used at will; just look for natural ingredients and avoid anything artificial.

You can also use flour in your recipes and use it for things like breading. Just do your best to avoid using excess amounts.

In terms of the timing of dinner, it is best to eat as early in your evening as possible.

Eating too late will prevent the body from following through on its wind down process, which can mess with your body's ability to get the deep and REM sleep it needs to make change.

Please take the time to head over to the Facebook Group or the Livy Method App and watch the quick video that accompanies this post.

LET'S TALK FRESH EYES

Fresh eyes are key for those of you who are redoing the program to continue to reach your goal.

First, it's important to note, redoing The Program is a **VERY EFFECTIVE** method for following through and finishing the process of helping your body release fat finally and forever.

The Program works **BETTER** each time around. Not only are you more in tune, but your body is also working for you more and more.

REASONS WHY PEOPLE MIGHT STRUGGLE WITH REPEATING THE PROCESS:

1. **You have done it before, and you know you can do it again.**

   - Sometimes rather than this being an advantage or a motivator, people use it as an excuse to allow in bites of bits that you didn't allow the first time.

   - Meaning, you know how to get back on track and you know what's to come so you give yourself more wiggle room to indulge. This is an issue because you end up spending more of the process getting back on track and never gain the momentum you need to see the results you expect.

2. **You know what's coming next and expect your body to respond the same way.**

   - This is an issue because you end up disappointed that your body doesn't respond the way it did the first time around.

   - You end up assuming the process isn't working simply because it's not working the same way as your last group, the way you want, or the way you expect. Your body is different this time around and you should expect and want it to respond differently.

   - What your body connected with the first time around will be different the second, third and fourth time around. By assuming how it will respond, you end up missing out on capitalizing on the areas that actually need work.

   - Meaning, you are getting in the way of your body making progress because you are trying to control what it is focusing on and how it responds.

3. **Your motivation has changed.**

   - This happens a lot when people try to use the motivation they had last time to lose weight this time.

   - Chances are what motivated you last time is not what is motivating you this time. Re-evaluating your "why" can make all the difference.

4. **You don't see an end-game.**

   - You need to see an end to the process. Leaving things open ended is not motivating and can keep you stuck in the cycle of trying to lose.

- Have a realistic time frame and plan of attack for crossing the finish line. Not only when, but also how that will feel and what it will look like.

5. **Completely missing the point that you have the advantage subsequent times around.**

   - If you are repeating the process then you should be all in, stepping up your game, and using your past knowledge to challenge yourself along the way and push yourself to the max.

   - You have no excuse, so perhaps that's what is holding you back, fear of being successful or fear of not following through.

   - Rather than being excited about what you can do this time around, you focus on what your body isn't doing in comparison to what it was doing last time. This robs you of the opportunity to capitalize in the moment and do the best you can day to day.

Regardless of your issue, re-doing the program is an ABSOLUTE advantage, so if you are struggling, chances are it's because you are getting in your own way.

So, take a step back and assess what you need to do to step up your game. Be all in and follow through and finish!

Please take the time to head over to the Facebook Group or the Livy Method App and watch the quick video that accompanies this post.

LET'S TALK SICKNESS

How to manage the plan while sick and still stay on track.

Being sick is never fun and it can be very discouraging when you are trying your best to follow the plan. Sickness always brings on detox so it can be used to your advantage so no need to worry about it setting you back.

WHAT TO DO WHEN YOU ARE SICK

1. **Drink extra water, especially if craving sugar and carbs.**

    - Resist the urge to go for crackers, white rice, bread products or sugar to settle your stomach. Sugar feeds a virus so sugar and carbs that break down into sugar are the last thing your body is looking for. Chances are what it really needs is an epic amount of water.

    - Water is essential for your body to detox out the virus, so drink as much as you can (within reason) and utilize teas and soup to get in even more liquid.

2. **Don't force the food.**

    - Chances are you won't be hungry when you are sick and that's for a reason.

    - The body is not interested in processing and digesting food, it would much rather stay focused on getting the virus out. This is a natural process that allows the body to divert all its resources into healing you.

    - The body stores a certain amount of fat for emergency purposes to use when you are sick. Your body using fat reserves for energy when you are sick is NOT the same as when you ignore hunger signals and purposely don't eat to force your body to burn fat.

    - Keep the food light and go for food that is easily digested, like soup. Be in the moment with your food choices and don't be afraid to keep it light. Once your appetite comes back, you can jump back on plan and force the formula.

    - Don't be surprised if you find your portions are naturally smaller when you resume eating. This is just your body resetting insulin sensitivity levels so go with it. It will help you fast track the process by putting you more in tune with your body's needs.

3. **Ignore the scale.**

    - Chances are your weight will be up while sick even if not eating, this is normal and happens because your body will retain the extra water it needs to get the virus out.

    - Antibiotics and medications can also have your weight up, it's not real weight gain so also not something to worry about.

    - Once your appetite comes back, your body will be looking to go into detox and that is where you will see the scale start to move.

4.   **Get lots of rest**

- You don't get points for powering through. Give your body the time it needs to recover and more importantly, to rest.

- Taking naps and going to bed early will have your body bouncing back sooner than later, whereas powering through can just end up prolonging the sickness.

5.   **Don't worry**

- Getting sick can feel like a major sidetrack, but it can work to your advantage. Your first priority is to feel better.

- Your body will look to rid you of the virus and make you stronger. This leads to your body working harder and fast tracking the repair and rebuild mode, which will only work to your advantage while working to lose weight.

- Once your appetite comes back, get back on track and re-establish the routine and then you can pick up where you left off and keep moving forward.

TO RECAP:

- Drink extra water.
- Keep the food light and easy to digest, don't force the formula.
- Avoid eating later in the evening which can mess with sleep.
- Have a hot epsom salt bath to help with detox.
- Take any medication needed to help.
- Get lots of rest.

Please take the time to head over to the Facebook Group or the Livy Method App and watch the quick video that accompanies this post.

LET'S TALK HOW TO MANAGE THE PLAN AS A DIABETIC

The program works well for all diabetics regardless of issues because the focus is on decreasing and regulating insulin while giving the body the resources & time it needs to become as healthy as possible.

It's a safe and effective program for not only weight loss but helping your body heal and address any and all health issues.

Although I have helped many people successfully lose weight who are diabetic and this program works well and can help with diabetes, this is not an issue I personally deal with, so I asked my former client and now Program Specialist, Kim Turnbull to share her firsthand experience. Please note, this is Kim's personal story. To make sure you're making the most of yours, be sure to check in with your healthcare provider along the way if you have any questions or concerns.

Hi all!

Thought I would share a bit about myself. I am type 1 diabetic been on insulin for 30 years and an insulin pump for 20 Years; in 2016 found out I had rheumatoid arthritis (RA).

I cannot imagine my life without Gina and The Livy Method, it has been a game changer. I wouldn't be where I am health wise without her plan and support.

Lowering the amount of insulin your body needs is the key with weight loss. The more sugar/carbs you put into your body the more your body needs insulin. The more insulin you need the more you crave sugar and the more weight you gain.

You do need carbs/sugar just not in the amount and type I was eating. I was gaining weight and my sugar levels were like a roller coaster some days.

Whether your body is making the insulin or you are giving insulin the response is the same. Before I started the program, I was taking upwards of 38-50 units a day and metformin as my body was becoming resistant to insulin, my A1C was 8.9.

Fast forward to today I am off the metformin and take 23-28 units of insulin today and my A1C is 6.5, however I have had it as low as 5.8 and I have lost weight!

My doctors could not believe the change in my weight, sugars and insulin levels. Not to mention how I feel everyday. More energy, more in tune with the foods my body is looking for, better sleep and the list goes on.

I still have carbs, just better ones, sweet potatoes, ryvita, fruits, vegetables, almond milk, Qi'a cereal etc. Just better food choices, more nutrient rich foods!

As soon as I add in something I shouldn't, I pay for it with how I feel, my weight is up, not to mention my sugar!

As for my RA, I have reduced my meds. I was on 14 pills a week now I take 3 a week. And again, if I go off with my food, I can feel it.

I was a huge Diet Coke drinker and I struggled to cut it out but as Gina says it can mess with your hunger signals which we want to get in tune with. As well we want to avoid artificial sweeteners and flavours as it can impact cravings and your metabolism.

Lowering the amount of insulin your body needs is real and has a direct impact on weight loss.

If you do take insulin or medication for diabetes, make sure you test your levels and if you are making adjustments, talk to your doctor along the way. Share this program with them so that they can support you along your journey.

I test a ton to know where I am sitting so I can minimize any high or low blood sugars.

At times I had to manage low blood sugars and dealt with them with Dex-4 tablets or some juice as advised by my doctor. Once I knew the cause of the low sugar or saw a pattern, I would make the changes in my daily insulin levels.

If my sugars runs high, I look at what I am eating and watch to make sure it wasn't a rebound from a low.

Being a diabetic sometimes it isn't always about the food impacting sugars it can be stress or illness but food choices have the biggest impact on insulin levels.

Week 3 – Consistency & Mindfulness is one of my favourite weeks, it allowed me to really focus on the choices I was making and being in tune with what my body was needing. For me being boring or predictable and consistent helped me adjust the insulin my body needed for the food I was taking in. For those that like to change things up you are going to love the Recipe Guide!

This program allowed me to lose 40lbs. I have had some ups and downs and right now I am up a bit but I know why and what I need to do to give my body what it needs to drop the weight.

It is a journey but one worth the effort and ride.

I would go weeks without my weight changing and then it would drop but even though the scale wasn't always moving, I could see the changes in my body. Remember everyone's journey is their own, I can't wait to hear about yours.

This is just my story and what has worked for me. Learn to love being bored - it works! — with love, Kim Turnbull

Please note: This inspirational post is not meant to replace your healthcare providers advice. If ever you have concerns about managing the plan, always check in with your healthcare provider.

To dig deeper into Insulin please visit the Science Guide and check out the Hormones Important to Weight Loss & Digestion Part 1: Insulin and Part 2: Hormones of Hunger and Satiety and Timing of Digestion.

LET'S TALK FERTILITY, PREGNANCY AND NURSING

The program has many benefits if you are looking to conceive, looking to lose while pregnant, looking to lose after, or while nursing.

WHAT YOU NEED TO KNOW:

Remember, this is not a diet, it's a method for helping the body focus on getting rid of fat that no longer serves a purpose. By giving the body what it needs, helping it to focus on fat loss and creating the environment for the body to follow through. All of which is done by making the body healthier in the process.

When following the Livy Method, you are helping the body decrease the weight it is used to function at as opposed to forcing the body to burn fat off by restricting calories and much needed nutrients.

The program has many benefits if you are looking to conceive, looking to lose while pregnant, or looking to lose after or while nursing.

WHEN PREGNANT:

The fat that makes you fat is not needed to grow a healthy baby, so there is no reason why you can't help the body get rid of fat that no longer serves a purpose while pregnant.

In fact, growing research suggests that losing some weight during pregnancy is not only possible, it can actually be beneficial for women who are overweight or obese.

Being overweight and pregnant can come with its own set of issues you need to be mindful of. Having excess weight can cause problems during pregnancy and can lead to:

- Premature birth
- Stillbirth
- Cesarean delivery
- Heart defects in baby
- Gestational diabetes in mother (and type 2 diabetes later in life)
- High blood pressure in mother
- Preeclampsia: severe form of high blood pressure that can also affect other organs like the kidneys
- Sleep apnea
- Blood clots (especially in your legs)
- Infections in mother

Not to seem extreme. This is just to put your mind at ease. If you are looking to lose while pregnant and feeling ways about it, know that contrary to popular belief, not only can it be beneficial to lose while pregnant, for some women it's essential.

Because the program is based on helping the body become as healthy as possible by increasing nutrient absorption and addressing the body's needs, there is nothing you really need to be concerned about.

Over the next few weeks, you will be focused on giving the body what it needs, which of course is only beneficial. However, as we move forward and start making changes to the food plan, I'm sure some of you might have concerns or wonder how you should proceed.

- Firstly, continue to check in with your doctor, or health care provider.
- Be sure to ask as many questions as you need day to day and along the way.
- Be in tune to your body's needs.
- Even when it comes to downsizing (Week 4), which is where you start to decrease portions, you will still be eating more than enough food (eating 6-8 times a day if using bonus snacks).
- Be sure to use bonus snacks (will be introducing bonus snacks at the end of the week) as needed.

WHEN LOOKING TO CONCEIVE:

If you are dealing with fertility issues, you will find a lot of what we do here on The Program falls in line with fertility protocols.

The Program allows for healing, repairing and rebuilding, and helps the body find internal balance.

If you have been advised to take additional supplements by your fertility expert or seeing an alternative medicine expert like a Chinese medical practitioner, just be sure to keep them in the loop with any supplements you add in on plan.

WHEN NURSING:

This program tends to be great for milk supply and after the initial changes you make with the food plan, you should find you are fairly consistent in food choices so any reaction to new foods should be minimal.

Even with downsizing (Week 4), which we will discuss when the time comes, you will still be eating more than enough food to feed both you and the baby.

All the supplements we will be introducing are safe, but for good measure, check in with your doctor as they may feel differently given your personal health history.

In fact, if you have any concerns along the way, be sure to check in with your doctor and make sure you are asking any questions you have day to day on the Questions Post.

Please take the time to head over to the Facebook Group or the Livy Method App and watch the quick video that accompanies this post.

LET'S TALK CRAVINGS

At this point, if you are following The Program, you should find any cravings you had or have are minimal. And if you do have them, they are nothing to be feared.

**Cravings are just simply a message from the body. They are the body's way of communicating it's needs by associating the foods that can help get it what it wants. **

If you are following the Food Plan and drinking the water, any cravings should be few and far between. And if they do pop up, it's usually just a matter of making a few tweaks.

LET'S TALK SUGAR:

The key to beating sugar cravings is to understand that it's not actually sugar people are addicted to; it's the high insulin levels needed to break it down that has you reaching for sweets.

Why?

- Insulin is the hormone that allows your body to use glucose for energy. Glucose is a type of sugar found in carbs like fruits, vegetables, and naturally occurring sugar that your body uses for energy. After you eat food and your digestive system breaks it down, your pancreas releases insulin to help regulate your blood sugar.

- When you reach for the sweets or foods with high sugar content, your body can flood with too much insulin, which causes your blood glucose levels to drop. This creates a dip in energy and a desire for even more sugar.

- This can create a vicious cycle that makes taking sugar and carbs out of your diet a challenge.

Why am I craving so much sugar in the first place?

Let's break it down:

1. **More is more:**
   - When you have sugar, your body will immediately want more sugar. These cravings can be so intense that if you create a habit of having sugar at the same time every day, your body will begin to crave and expect it at that same time daily. This is also the reason you end up eating that whole box of cookies in one sitting!

THE FIX:

- Add some protein and fat.
- Making sure to add in healthy fats to your meals along with protein, will help to prevent any cravings along the way.
- But if you do find yourself indulging, you can neutralize sugar cravings by having some

protein and fat with your sweet treat. For example, if you indulge in a cookie, you can cut the desire to eat another cookie by having a slice of cheese or a handful of nuts.

- The protein and fat will help neutralize the amount of insulin your body uses to break down the sugar and decrease your cravings, giving your will power a fighting chance to kick in and help.

2. **Dehydration is a factor:**

- When you are dehydrated and not picking up on the cues from your body to drink more, your body's next best bet is to crave foods with a high water content, like fruit. Fruits are also sweet, so you may mistake your body's cue to consume more water and instead find yourself reaching for processed carbs and sugar.

- This is why you may hear the advice to drink a glass of water before you eat to satisfy your appetite. It doesn't satisfy your appetite, but if it's water that you actually need, you may realize you are not really hungry after all.

THE FIX:

- Drink more water.
- Sip water throughout the day, aiming for a minimum of 3.5 litres a day and even more on days you exercise or are more active.

3. **You are tired:**

- When you are tired, your body goes looking for a pick-me-up, and you may find yourself reaching for something sweet.

- The same thing happens around 3 or 4 p.m. each afternoon when the body is wired to take a drop in energy and slows your circadian rhythm. What your body is really looking for is a nap. (There are places in the world that do just that: think of the siesta.)

- In our fast-paced, high-stress world, it's not always possible to take a nice afternoon nap, so the body goes looking for easy energy by way of higher sugar to pick it up and keep it going.

THE FIX:

- Make sure to eat all your meals and especially your snacks. This will help to avoid energy levels that dip when you go for long periods of time without eating.

- Your mid-morning snack of fresh fruit will top up your energy reserves in the morning and your raw veggies, nuts and seeds in the afternoon will keep your body working hard through-out the afternoon.

- These foods have a high nutrient value and are harder to digest, which will keep your digestion stimulated and your body awake and functioning when it's craving a nap.

- With a few adjustments, you can easily beat the need for sweets and stay on track to reach your goals and not be held captive by sugar cravings anymore!

LET'S TALK SALT:

When you crave sugar, it generally means that you need more water. When you crave salt, it generally means that the body is asking for more good fat. When you are stressed, your body is revving high, you burn lots of calories, your brain works really hard and your body quickly gets depleted of its nutrients.

Periods of high stress can rapidly deplete your vitamin and mineral reserves. So, when you are stressed, your body is looking for more sustaining energy by way of good fat.

You don't have to be stressed for the body to need more good fat. Fat is essential for cellular function as well as brain and heart health. It also works like a transport system for your body to process and digest carbs and protein.

Your body would rather get that fat from the foods you eat than to utilize its emergency reserve. Without enough good fat coming in, your body will be reluctant to let go of the fat that makes you fat. So, one way you can speed up that fat loss process is to make sure you are getting lots of good fats in your meals and adding in an omega 3 supplement, which we will be talking more about in Week 2.

LET'S TALK TUMMY RUMBLINGS & HUNGER PAINS:

We are taught to believe if your tummy rumbles you must be hungry, when in fact that's not what the noise and rumblings are about. It's actually your body's natural MMC or Migrating Motor Complex.

Your digestive system works like a self-cleaning oven where, in between processing and digesting food, it works to clear bacteria and food particles out of the small intestine.

Because we are eating so often during the day, the body is doing most of this work at night. As we move through the program, we will be phasing you into more natural patterns of eating which will be more in tune to your body's needs, which include the downtime it needs in between meals to self-regulate.

TO RECAP:

Cravings are nothing to stress about, though they can give you great insight into your body's needs. Usually, the smallest tweak or adjustments can make all the difference.

It's important to note it's not about controlling your cravings; it's about being in tune to them. As you progress through the program, you will become more in tune and able to differentiate between the body's needs and your wants.

You may also find yourself craving other kinds of foods and even specific foods. At the end of this process, your body will clearly let you know when it's hungry, what it's hungry for, and how much you need to eat.

Paying attention to those cravings can help you better meet your body's needs so that your body can focus on what you need…and get the fat out.

Please take time to head over to the Facebook Group or the Livy Method App and watch the quick video that accompanies this post.. To learn more about hunger and the science behind it, head to the Science Guide and have a look at The Migrating Motor Complex (MMC) and Hunger, and Hormones of Hunger and Satiety and Timing of Digestion.

NUTRIENT RICH MEALS

By now I'm sure you have heard us say "Make your meals nutrient rich". But do you know what that really means? I'm going to use a salad as an example, but the same idea can be applied to absolutely ANY meal.

LET'S BREAK IT DOWN...

- Spring Mix/Greens = leafy greens + roughage + vitamins + minerals + protein
- Variety of Vegetables = fiber + vitamins
- Avocado = healthy fat + potassium + fiber
- Feta cheese = healthy fat + protein
- Nuts and Seeds = healthy fat + protein
- An all-natural vinaigrette or dressing = healthy fat when made with good quality oils.

A simple, small salad loaded up with stuff, not only provides you with a variety of nutrients, but is also more sustaining!

**Look for quality over quantity and you will soon find that you don't need as much food to feel satisfied. **

Nutrient rich meals provide the most bang for your buck and give you longer lasting energy.

Even if you can just sneak in one or two extra things like a drizzle of olive oil, an extra veg, or a few nuts… it can make all the difference.

THINGS TO HAVE ON HAND THAT CAN QUICKLY BUMP UP YOUR MEALS:

Here are some great items to have on hand to quickly and easily level up your meals when something is lacking.

- A variety of nuts and seeds - good fat and protein and an excellent addition to yogurt or oats
- Olives - good fat
- Pickled and marinated veg like artichoke hearts, pickled beets, roasted red peppers, etc. - bump up your veggies.
- Good quality oils like extra virgin olive oil, nut oils, avocado and coconut oil. - good fats
- Coconut milk - a great healthy fat addition to things like your morning oatmeal or cereal.
- Salsa - extra veg
- Guacamole - good fat
- Hummus - good fat plus protein
- Tuna, sardines, smoked oysters - it's a great idea to keep these in the cupboard as a quick way to add protein to any meal.

Now go forth and eat RICH!

LET'S TALK WEIGHT LOSS

And get real about it.

Before talking about numbers on the scale, please make time to read the post about **THE SCALE**. There, I talk about the fact that the scale is going to **FLUCTUATE**.

I talk about what real weight loss looks like, the fact the scale goes up before it goes down, and that is not only NORMAL - in most cases, it's to be expected.

I also give a lot of reasons why the scale would be up, like water retention and dehydration, salty or hard to digest food, detox and hormone balancing… to name a few. None of which have anything to do with real weight gain. And most of which are a sign your body is about to start dropping fat.

The sooner you understand that the body is not trying to make you fat, the less stressed you are going to be throughout this process.

IT IS IMPORTANT TO UNDERSTAND:

- It is impossible to make fat overnight.
- It is impossible for the body to make fat over the weekend.
- And you would be hard-pressed to make fat over a week.
- Your body converting the food you eat into fat that makes you fat is a complicated and complex process and takes longer than you think.
- You have signed up for a weight loss program. A very effective one. You are going to lose weight.

THIS IS NOT ABOUT A QUICK FIX:

- We're into healthy, maintainable weight loss.
- Most of you are here because you know someone who has been successful in losing weight with the Program. You will be just as successful if you show up every day and do the work for as long as it takes to get the job done. Remember that might look different than the person who inspired you to join.
- We are not focused on numbers on the scale in the first few weeks. And you will find I'm not keen to even talk about it until we start to focus on it.
- If the scale moves in the first few weeks, great! And if it doesn't, I'm not worried. As frustrating as that is going to be for some of you, it's true.

Make no mistake, I am here to help you lose a lot of weight and make life changing changes, but that takes time and there is a process to it. Losing weight can be unnerving at times and can have you feeling overwhelmed and even hopeless, especially if you have a lot of weight to lose. The feelings and emotions you have about weight loss are very real and I want you to know that I take that seriously.

I want to make sure you are all clear and feeling confident about this process so please take time to head over to the Facebook Group or the Livy Method App and watch the quick video where I talk about expectations, what weight loss will look like, and things you need to keep in mind when it comes to the numbers on the scale.

For more information on weight loss head to the Science Guide and read The Science of Fat and Fat Loss.

WONDERING WHY YOUR WEIGHT IS UP?

While following the Plan, your weight might go up for various reasons, none of which will have anything to do with actual weight gain.

**Let me be clear...if following the Plan, eating all the meals and snacks, making foods nutrient rich and eating to satisfaction (or even overeating) you are NOT going to gain weight. **

The body is not inclined to want to store fat, in fact it's quite the opposite. The body wants your fat gone as much as you do! It's important to understand that throughout this Program, your weight is going to naturally fluctuate, no matter what you do.

Reasons your weight can be up:

- Stress
- Lack of sleep
- Salty food
- Hard to digest food (like red meat, although not a reason to not eat it)
- Dehydration
- Body fighting an illness
- Body sore from a workout
- Body reacting to change in routine
- Body reacting to change in food
- Body reacting to new medication or change in medications
- Body reacting to any new supplements or change in supplements
- Deficiencies like being low in iron
- Hormones balancing
- PMS
- Your scale needing new batteries
- And the last, and most important reason, is your body is detoxing and your weight is about to drop.

**If you haven't seen it yet, take time to review the Scale Post and watch the Video (posted in the Facebook Support Group) as it's important to understand what real weight loss looks like on the scale. **

If you stick around and keep showing up, you are going to be successful and lose your weight regardless of the little ups along the way. The ups are normal and to be expected. Although we do like to have fun around here, weight loss can have its frustrating moments so we don't want anyone stressing about the scale any more than they need to...or even at all!

Hope this helps. Embrace the little ups because they always lead to the big drops!

Please take the time to head over to the Facebook Group or the Livy Method App and watch the quick video that accompanies this post.

LET'S TALK WHAT TO DO IF YOU ARE NOT HUNGRY

With all the changes the body is making in the first few weeks, it's normal to feel hungrier.

However, it's also normal to not feel hungry.

Over the last few weeks, you have been working hard to give your body everything it needs so that it no longer feels the need to store fat. By being consistent and following the food plan, you are addressing your cravings and naturally helping the body reduce portion sizes without even trying.

This will lead to a change in your appetite as the body will be working hard to regulate your metabolism and blood sugar, as well as making internal and external changes and balancing hormones.

As your body works hard to make change and works hard to find balance, these changes will have your hunger levels changing day to day and week to week. Which is why it is normal to not feel hungry for meals and snacks. One day you might be hungry every 5 mins and then the next day, 5 hours can go by and you won't be hungry at all.

Which brings us to the question...why do you have to eat when you are not hungry?

- During the day, the routine is key. We are still in the early stages of making the body feel confident it is going to get what it needs so it doesn't feel the need to store fat. Therefore, you need to eat! Even if just a small token amount.

- Consistency helps to maintain and reinforce the routine of the Food Plan Formula. This will play a key role moving forward and with managing your weight loss.

- There are many benefits to eating a token amount of your meals and snacks even if you are not hungry. Having a small token amount of food signals food in and food out, which aids digestion and helps with processing food in and out.

- Being consistent helps to manage your hunger levels...since food takes time to digest you are being proactive in managing your appetite.

When it comes to dinner:

- There will come a time when you can skip dinner, but for now it's best you have something small.

- Stick with some leafy greens and protein if not hungry and just eat a token amount.

- Along with reinforcing the routine, it also helps to prevent the urge to snack later.

As we progress, we will be making changes to the Food Plan that will continually shake things up and in turn, have your appetite all over the place.

Next week, for example, we will be focused on being as consistent as possible. Consistent to the point of boredom which will help you work through any issues of utilizing food for anything other than nutritional needs.

You are going to notice that some days you will be hungrier than others, which is totally normal and why the focus right now is to eat all meals and snacks, make your food choices nutrient rich, and eat to satisfaction regardless of what that portion looks like.

Bottom line: if you are not hungry, then still eat a small token amount.

**Token amounts means just enough food to stimulate your digestive system so at least 4-5 bites of food with 4-5 chews each bite, give or take. **

Please take time to head over to the Facebook Group or the Livy Method App and watch the quick video that accompanies this post. To learn more about hunger, and the science behind it head to the Science Guide and read The Migrating Motor Complex (MMC) and Hunger and the Hormones of Hunger and Satiety and Timing of Digestion.

LET'S TALK ABOUT HUNGER

What it means to be hungry and the difference between true hunger vs. your body craving certain foods, your energy draining, hormones balancing, and detox.

As we work this week to fine tune and perfect the Plan, some of you will be introducing bonus snacks, which will be introduced shortly, as a way to manage hunger levels. I'm hoping this breakdown will give you more clarity as to if and when you need to add in the bonus snacks and when you can hold off till it's time to eat your regularly scheduled meals and snacks.

The most important things you need to understand about hunger:

- Hunger is the way your body checks in with you and lets you know where it's at and what it needs throughout the day.

- Hunger is just another way the body communicates its needs, a "heads up" kind of thing, and is not an immediate need for food.

- Hunger is nothing to be concerned about.

- The body knows that food can take hours to process and digest through your system. Therefore, it takes that into account when giving you a heads up on when you need to eat.

- Periodically throughout the day and into the evening your body will do a "systems check" and will let you know when it's time to start thinking about eating based on its current energy reserve.

It is normal for your hunger levels to be all over the place as your body adjusts to the food plan. Do the best you can to stay on track and you will notice that it gets better as you move along through the Program.

Please take time to head over to the Facebook Group or the Livy Method App and watch the quick video that accompanies this post. To learn more about hunger and the science behind it, head to the Science Guide and have a look at The Migrating Motor Complex (MMC) and Hunger, and Hormones of Hunger and Satiety and Timing of Digestion.

HOW TO ADVOCATE FOR YOURSELF

We want to help set you up for the best success moving forward. We have thrown a lot of information at you over the past few days and we understand that it's a lot to take in.

But remember... if you want to be successful you must read over the posts and watch the videos, to understand all the info. The videos expand on the written post so don't miss the extra tidbits provided within them. The information we provide in this Program is EVERYTHING. You must educate yourself so you can have a deeper understanding of how your body works. Then use it to GET THE FAT OUT!

Many other diets and weight loss programs out there are designed to spoon-feed and handhold. Telling you exactly what to eat, how much, on which days, and which meals etc. It has trained many of us to feel lost in thinking for ourselves when it comes to food, eating, and our bodies in general. We have become out of touch because of so much misinformation and old, archaic dieting bull-crap!

This Program takes you through a process that puts you back in tune with your body and teaches you how to think for yourself and listen to your body's cues...and that takes effort.

It is your "job" to read all the information and understand it as much as possible. Think of it as studying for an exam.

It might not make much sense right now but trust me, it all comes together in the end. It's a process and this Program is about so much more than weight loss. It's an epic course in getting to know YOU!

WHICH BRINGS ME TO THE QUESTIONS.

Although we are happy to answer all the questions you have, we are expecting those questions to be based on the information you have already read and listened to.

Given that this is the first week, and it's a lot of information, we understand that not everyone has had time to read everything over and watch the accompanying videos. Check into the Facebook Group and USE THOSE GUIDES to keep track of what you have read and/or watched.

Go back to Day 1 and work your way up to today. BE SURE YOU READ OVER EVERYTHING and watch the video content (found in the Facebook Group and the Livy Method App). We understand that many of you have very busy schedules and it can take some time to get to the info. So, of course, we are more than happy to answer your questions, but also keep in mind, if you want to be successful and lose weight, you need to also make the time. You do not have to watch the Facebook Lives, but if you can watch at least some of them, I can assure you, it will be very beneficial. Gina always goes into great detail to answer some of the questions asked during the Lives. Put your earbuds on and listen while you're cooking or cleaning the house, taking a walk...or relaxing in the bath! The lives will also be available on the Weigh In with Gina podcast found on all podcast platforms so you can listen to them whenever it is convenient for you.

Your job is to:

- Review the info in the Welcome, Food Plan and Prep Week Guides.
- Read all the posts and watch the informational videos.
- Take notes.
- Ask your questions AFTER reviewing the information.
- If you think of a new question, ask yourself if this has already been covered and go look for that post or posts, and read them over before asking your question. 9 times out of 10 the answer is there but it's been overlooked. Finding the answer yourself helps to better retain it.

You can't make epic changes without doing the work! We take weight loss seriously and we expect you will too! Make the time for yourself. You owe it to yourself. You deserve to be successful and feel amazing!

Now go start studying for this epic, life changing course so you can nail it!

5 PRO TIPS TO BE MORE PROACTIVE WITH THIS PROCESS

As we move forward, you are going to hear me talk a lot about being proactive with this process. So, I thought I would break it down and put together some tips for making the most of my Program from this point.

Proactive - adjective

pro·ac·tive (proh-ak-tiv)

"Definition of proactive 1 [pro- entry 2 + reactive]: acting in anticipation of future problems, needs, or changes"

1. **Make sure you are watching the videos that go along with the posts**

    -   The written information is only a short summary. In the videos, I go more in-depth and might also touch on other elements not listed.

    -   The more you understand the process, the more you will see it all coming together. When you can understand the process, it makes it so much easier to follow... which makes it so much more effective in the end.

2. **Be sure to keep up with the GUIDES**

    -   Guides are where all of the information is posted day to day. Not all of the information is included in the Workbook such as any videos, live content, share pages etc.

3. **Use TOPICS button and the SEARCH**

    -   You can use the Topics button or search using the magnifying glass at the top of the Group Page to quickly search & review any post or topic from past guides. Make sure you are searching in the group, not Facebook in general.

    -   Between all the Posts and all the questions and answers, the search bar can be quite handy.

    -   Using the Search bar literally searches every word posted in the group ...so if you search water, any post or conversation about water will pop up.

4. **From this point the program moves fast, so show up every day**

    -   Each week, the focus will change and you will be making changes to the Food Plan. The changes you make week to week become the jumping off point for the following week.

    -   Because there is no going back (and you don't want to keep looking back), the goal is to be all in and keep things moving forward.

    -   Set your intention in the morning and check in with yourself at the end of the day, taking note of where you excelled and any areas that could use more attention.

5.   Continue to ask questions

- Some weeks can be tricky, and some days are sure to be better than others. Because it can be easy to get sidetracked with this process for so many reasons, if you are ever unsure at any point on how to proceed, let us know.

- Don't spend time guessing or hoping you are doing the right thing. It's key to be clear on what you need to do each week so don't be shy about asking questions.

A BONUS TIP: Keep a journal and use our new app for tracking how your body is responding to the process. Journals (see Journaling Post) can help with any problem solving should it be needed along the way and give you great insight into how to make the most out of this process.

LET'S TALK KEEPING A JOURNAL/USING OUR NEW APP

Why it can be a great idea to be tracking your progress along the way.

BENEFITS OF JOURNALING

A journal can be a great tool to help give you insight into how your body is responding to the process.

It can help you pick up on patterns of behavior and responses, and give you a better idea of what weight loss looks like specifically to you.

It can help you pick up on any food sensitivities, especially if you have digestive issues. It can help you track bowel movements if you struggle in that department.

It can help you track your body's response to the supplements, or anything new you are adding in or taking out.

It can also help to track your mood and can be beneficial in helping you show up for yourself every day, by taking time to think about how you are managing your emotions and how you are feeling day to day.

THINGS TO TRACK

- Weight in the morning
- How you are feeling physically and mentally
- Food
- Water
- Extras (added food and drink on or not on plan)
- Bowel movements if they are an issue
- Notable responses from food
- Digestive upset
- Sleep
- Medications
- Supplements
- Notable wins not food related
- Energy day to day
- Changes taking place that aren't scale related

You can use good old pen and paper, your computer, or our new app. Whatever works best for you!

Not so much now, but as we progress, your journal can be a very helpful tool to problem solve in conjunction with the info being posted in the group.

The more tools the better!

Please take time to head over to the Facebook Group or the Livy Method App and watch the quick video that accompanies this post.

LET'S TALK ABOUT BONUS SNACKS

If you need them and when to add them in.

As we wind down this first official week of The Program, it's time to look ahead to Week 2, which will have you fine tuning and perfecting The Plan.

During the first week, you ate in a way that allows your body to adjust to lower insulin levels, which, in turn, will help to decrease the amount of food you will need to feel satisfied.

For Week 2, you are going to continue to follow the Food Plan but the focus will be on making adjustments day to day, so you feel more satisfied at the end of each day.

THIS IS WHERE BONUS SNACKS COME IN.

**Bonus snacks are extra snacks that can be used by those of you who are up super early, those of you who are more physical in your day (super active job), or for those long shift turnarounds where you are awake for 24hrs. **

First, it's key to note that Bonus Snacks are NOT meant to replace your regular snacks, so you will still need to eat them. And you cannot switch out your regularly scheduled snacks for bonus snacks.

Please note: If you are continually skipping breakfast and having to add in bonus snacks then you should be eating breakfast.

Bonus snacks are to be added **ONLY if needed** for nutritional requirements because you are feeling hungry...they do not need to be added in every day.

THE TIMING OF THE BONUS SNACKS IS VERY SPECIFIC:

1.   Can be added in between your morning fruit snack and lunch.

2.   Can be added between your lunch and raw veg snack.

For example:

- Protein for breakfast
- Fruit for morning snack
- BONUS SNACK
- Lunch
- BONUS SNACK
- Raw veg
- Nuts/seeds
- Dinner

The timing between these snacks and the rest is the same; 30 minutes to 3.5 hours.

WHAT YOU CAN HAVE FOR BONUS SNACKS:

MORNING BONUS SNACK:

- Yogurt or other dairy products, such as cottage cheese or other cheeses
- More fruit with nuts, seeds, nut butter, cheese or any protein and fat
- Vegetables raw or cooked and you can add dip or cheese
- Boiled egg or any other protein
- Half of your lunch eaten early
- Ryvita/high fiber cracker with spread (only if not used at breakfast)
- Shake with protein, veg or fruit and added fat (be mindful of portion size)

AFTERNOON BONUS SNACK:

- Can be any of the above except nuts & seeds.

Keep in mind, if you add in the bonus snacks and find yourself not hungry for your regular snacks, you still need to eat them even if you keep the portion small.

I recognize it may seem counterintuitive to eat more when trying to lose weight, but right now it is key to address why your body is feeling a need to store fat and to be more in tune with its needs.

This is the quickest and most effective way to get the body to focus on fat loss.

Some of you, depending on how early you get up or how active you are, may need to utilize the bonus snacks more often while others may not.

Please take the time to head over to the Facebook Group or the Livy Method App and watch the quick video that accompanies this post.

LET'S TALK WEEKENDS

Why they are nothing to worry about and how to make the most of them.

When it comes to weight loss, it can seem like there is always something getting in the way and throwing you off track; birthdays, holidays, vacation days, let alone just your average weekend.

Lack of routine, travel, eating off foods like salty food, hard to digest food, high sugar content foods, lack of water, and even lack of sleep can easily have your weight up.

Good thing it's not as easy as you think to gain weight, and it takes a lot longer than you think for your body to convert the food you eat into actual fat. So, when you find the scale creeping up after a little indulging, chances are it's not real weight gain.

Which is why I always say there is nothing you can do in a weekend or even a few weeks that can't be undone by getting back at it!

Having off weekends and going off Plan is going to happen, for the sake of weight loss, you want to keep those days to a minimum. But with that said, there is also nothing to stress about.

Staying as consistent as possible is key, but if you get off track just get right back on track, because as long as you stay in the game and keep showing up, you are going to get there.

Please take the time to head over to the Facebook Group or the Livy Method App and watch the quick video that accompanies this post.

LET'S TALK GOAL WEIGHT

People always ask me what's a good goal weight?

Without sounding cliché, I really do think it's when you feel comfortable in your own skin.

With that said though, a good baseline I use for clients is your lowest weight after the age of 21 that you were able to easily maintain.

That doesn't mean if you have always carried extra weight that you can't weigh less than you ever have… because you totally can. A lot of people have had weight issues from childhood but that doesn't mean you can't be successful at losing or losing a lot.

Once you address why your body is feeling the need to store fat (like we are doing in the first few weeks), the body will be happy to get rid of it, regardless of when you gained or how long you have carried the extra weight.

People think genetics plays a role, but it doesn't. People who have genetically more fat cells may have the capacity to gain more when they do gain, but that doesn't mean it's harder for them to lose.

I know that it's easier said than done but focusing on all the positive changes that come with weight loss can be more motivating than aiming for a certain number on the scale.

Also, when it comes to that number on the scale, I suggest you ditch the BMI charts and the old archaic means of measuring what your weight should be. There are so many variables that they don't account for. Instead, go by how you feel and aim to be as healthy as possible regardless of weight.

It can be good to set a target weight as a goal, but it can also just add more stress. Visualizing looking and feeling your best can be just as, if not more, effective.

When it comes down to numbers, I find most people underestimate out of fear of failing. Because with this Program, weight loss is such a process, it is normal to find yourself setting new goals along the way.

Please take the time to head over to the Facebook Group or the Livy Method App and watch the quick video that accompanies this post.

WEEK 1 RECAP AND A SNEAK PEEK INTO WEEK 2

As the first official week of the program comes to an end, I want to touch base and check in to see how you are doing!

LET'S TALK ABOUT MOTIVATION AND SUCCESS.

I recognize that for many of you the journey to lose weight thus far has been a frustrating one, having spent a lot of time, energy and money on diets. Because of that, please know that I am always super mindful about this program not being one more thing you have tried that didn't work.

I also understand that some of the things I am suggesting seem far removed from traditional diets, which I view as a good thing, since traditional diets don't work.

If you stick around, what you are learning and how your body is responding will start to come together and, not only will it make a lot of sense, but it will also help you lose a lot of weight.

Even if you feel like you have already messed up, are behind, or you are feeling apprehensive about moving forward, this program takes all those things into account.

Although I like to set the bar high, there is no such thing as "perfect" with this program because weight loss is a process. I always say, "there is never a good time to lose weight". There is always going to be something getting in the way, like holidays, birthdays, and times in life when the desire to lose weight may seem trivial in comparison to what you have going on.

Even though life keeps getting in the way, the desire to lose weight doesn't go away because I believe for most of you, this Process is not just about vanity and fitting into a pair of jeans. It's about being in tune with your body's needs and feeling comfortable in your skin as well as being as healthy and happy as you can possibly be.

As you move forward week to week, continue to check in each day, watch the Daily Check In Video and review all of the information. I am a big believer in having a deeper level of understanding, so if you have questions or need clarification, please never hesitate to ask!

My only concern, moving forward, is that you stay in the game, and you keep showing up, even on the days you want to give up. There absolutely WILL BE moments of frustration, but for the most part, we truly believe this process can be fun!

LOSING WEIGHT IS NOT A PUNISHMENT. IT'S A JOURNEY IN SELF LOVE AND LIVING YOUR BEST LIFE!

I have seen great things happen and amazing life changes take place when people put time and energy into giving their bodies what it needs to make lasting changes.

Chances are, you are here because somewhere along the way your body got the message it needed to store fat and that message has been reinforced time and time again over the years. This is why the first few weeks of The Program are all about giving the body what it needs.

Although many of you have already been experiencing fat loss, know that if you haven't, it's nothing to be concerned about. It might be frustrating, but it's also perfectly normal.

We have a long way to go, and everyone's body will respond differently. It isn't until Week 3/4 that we even start to focus on fat loss. If you have faith in The Process, take it day by day, and do the work, then you will be successful regardless of how quickly you start to lose.

A SNEAK PEEK AT WEEK 2

Week 2 is more of the same but with the focus on fine tuning and perfecting...as your body adjusts to the changes that you have already made.

In Week 2, you will continue to focus on giving your body what it needs so it no longer feels the need to store fat. The focus is all about making adjustments, so you are feeling satisfied at the end of the day.

In the first few weeks, by following the basic Food Plan, you are eating in a way that will allow your body to adjust to lower insulin levels, which will eventually lead to you naturally feeling more satisfied on smaller portions.

With that said though, you are not to try to eat less. Be open to your body's needs day to day and continue to eat to satisfaction. For example, one day you might need one egg to feel satisfied and then the next day you might need three.

The goal is to eat to satisfaction, not to TRY to eat less.

In fact, as you enter into Week 2, you may find your appetite has increased because of your increasing metabolism. So in order to satisfy this increased hunger, we have introduced Bonus Snacks. Be sure to read over the Bonus Snacks Post, watch the Video, and ask any questions you have.

At the beginning of Week 2, I will be introducing Supplements.

These can play a key role in this process and help the body drop fat. Supplements can help where the body is deficient, which can make all the difference when it comes to addressing the body's needs and speeding up the weight loss process.

WEEK 2 GUIDELINES: FINE TUNING AND PERFECTING

Week 2 has you fine tuning and perfecting the changes you made in Week 1, along with adding in Bonus Snacks and implementing the suggested supplements if needed.

Last week was all about implementing the changes you needed to make with the Food Plan and letting the body adjust.

This week is all about Fine Tuning & Perfecting the changes you have made so far.

THE GOAL FOR THIS WEEK:

- Eat all meals and snacks
- Make all food choices as nutrient rich as possible
- Eat to satisfaction
- Add in BONUS snacks IF needed
- Be as consistent as possible

The idea behind fine tuning and perfecting is making sure you feel satisfied at the end of the day.

So, if you are feeling full and stuffed at the end of the day, you want to pay extra attention to the portions the next day. And alternatively, if you are hungry at the end of the day, be sure to eat your meals and snacks (don't skip breakfast), make your foods as nutrient rich as possible, and use Bonus Snacks if needed.

Bonus snacks are extra snacks that you can add in if you find you are continuously feeling unsatisfied at the end of the day, or your appetite is increasing because your metabolism is increasing.

Bonus snacks are to be added ONLY if needed for nutritional requirements because you are feeling hungry not because you "feel like" a snack.

As a reminder, Bonus Snacks are NOT meant to replace your regular snacks so you will still need to keep those in.

Keep in mind, you can keep your food choices simple, or you can make them as fancy as you like if cooking is something you enjoy.

Even when keeping things simple, don't be afraid to add in and bump up your meals with a variety of nutrient rich ingredients.

It's not always about adding in more food, sometimes it's about eating the right food.

Along with veggies, cheese, dips and sauces, any of your favorite condiments or spices can be added as long as they are made with good quality ingredients. You can load up salads and make your soups, stews, and stir-fry with tons of fresh foods and flavours and if you prefer plain, then that's ok too!

Week 2 also has us introducing SUPPLEMENTS that can play a key role in this process.

Supplements can help where the body is deficient, which can make all the difference when it comes to addressing the body's needs and speeding up the weight loss process.

While working on fine tuning and perfecting the Food Plan, water intake & supplements this week, we will also be covering a variety of topics in the Group.

Be sure to check into the Facebook Group every day, utilize the GUIDES to see what is being posted day to day and, as always, if you have questions be sure to let us know.

Please take the time to head over to the Facebook Group or the Livy Method App and watch the quick video that accompanies this post.

WEEK 2 GUIDELINES FAQS

1.   I am still hungry at night, any tips?

It can be helpful to remember that hunger is not an immediate need for food, especially at night when your body is winding down and getting ready for sleep. Ways to help alleviate hunger at night are by starting your day with a high protein breakfast, eating all your meals and snacks to satisfaction, adding healthy fats to your meals and veg snacks and getting in your water throughout the day. Having herbal tea, taking a bath or going to bed earlier are some ways to help.

2.   What are some signs of reaching satisfaction?

Satisfaction signals will differ from person to person. As we continue to build our mind-body connection, these signals will become louder and clearer. It's a great idea to eat your meals and snacks without distractions to help you become more in tune to your satisfaction levels. Some people find they take a deep breath as soon as they are satisfied. Others may put their utensils down and pause. Once you slow down and tune in, your own satisfaction signals will become more and more apparent. This is something we will focus on over the coming weeks as recognizing your satisfaction levels is an important part of the Program.

3.   I feel bloated and my clothes are tight, any tips?

Feeling bloated is normal as your body is adjusting to the Food Plan. Follow the program as designed, get in your water and add in those leafy greens and everything will come together. You can also feel bloated when your body is retaining water and getting ready to go into detox. If you feel that there may be something else going on, best to check in with your healthcare provider.

4.   How important is the timing between my meals?

It's important to keep the order of food, but the timing between meals and snacks can change day to day. The time between all meals and snacks should be anywhere from 30 minutes to no more than 3.5 hours apart. We want to avoid our bodies needing to utilize its emergency fat reserves, which sends a message to the body that it needs to store fat.

5.   Do I still include the other snacks if adding in bonus snacks?

Bonus snacks are not meant to replace your regular snacks, so you cannot switch out your regularly scheduled snacks for bonus snacks. Bonus snacks are extra snacks that can be used by those who are up very early, are more physically active during the day, or those that have long shift turnarounds. Bonus snacks are to be added only if ned for nutritional requirements because you are feeling hungry. They do not need to be added every day.

6.   What foods can be used for the bonus snacks?

There are lots of options for bonus snacks for both the morning and afternoon. You can have yogurt or other dairy products such as cottage cheese or other cheeses. Fruit with nuts, seeds, nut butter, cheese or any protein and fat. Veggies raw or cooked with dip or cheese, boiled eggs or any other protein. Half of your lunch eaten early, ryvita cracker with spread (if not used at breakfast) or a shake with protein, veg or fruit and added fat (be mindful of portion size). Your afternoon bonus snack can be any of the above except for nuts and seeds.

7.   How can I stay consistent on the weekends?

Weekends can sometimes get you off routine. Birthdays, holidays, visits with friends and family can all lead to eating bits and bites, not keeping up with your water or even lack of sleep - All things that can have your scale up. What's important to remember is that this is not real weight gain and that it takes much longer than a weekend for your body to convert the food you eat into actual fat. Take a look at your social calendar and recognize where you can stay consistent with the food plan and when you have events that will have you indulging. Be sure to eat all your meals and snacks leading up to your event and don't worry if you indulge. The next day get right back at it, add in some extra water and leafy greens to help process the backlog.

8.   Is there an alternate option for leafy greens?

While there is no alternative to leafy greens, there are some vegetables that count as leafy greens. Vegetables like brussel sprouts, bok choy and cabbage all count towards your vegetable and leafy green component of your meals. Leafy greens are an important part of the Program and are full of vitamins, minerals, micronutrients and fibre that help give the body what it needs, supports the body in detox and helps with digestion. If you are having trouble getting them in you can also try sauteing, stewing or add them to soups, stews and stir frys.

9.   At what time should I finish drinking my water for the day?

This will vary from person to person. It's best to avoid drinking water late into the evening if it will affect your sleep and you find yourself waking to use the bathroom. The timing is something you can play around with based on your specific needs.

10.   What if I have a question about supplements?

You are welcome to ask questions regarding the suggested supplements and how they work with the Program and weight loss in the Facebook Group. That said, we cannot make suggestions on the timing and doses of supplements as we do not know your individual health history. For questions regarding supplements and your individual health needs, it's best to reach out to your pharmacist or healthcare provider.

LET'S TALK SUPPLEMENTS

The following are basic supplements that, over the years, I have found helpful to aid in deficiencies in the body that may affect your ability to drop weight and/or can help speed up the process. These supplements are suggested because in my experience they can help and work well with The Program and weight loss.

It's up to you to decide if you want to add them in. We aren't trying to push supplements on anyone and understand that some may not be able to take them or afford all of them.

We do not work with any supplement companies and do not make money from selling or promoting them. I will not ask you to buy any supplements from any specific company and if I do suggest a specific brand, it is because it is my personal preference or simply a good example. There are a ton of great brands at a variety of price points.

Please note that if you have any concerns with these supplements interacting with the current medications you are taking or for any other reason, consult your healthcare provider.

Before we get started:

- I'm not partial to any particular brands and even suggest switching up brands every now and then to find one that works best for you. I will often switch mine up based on what is on sale.

- I suggest getting to know the knowledgeable staff at your local health food store and/or pharmacy to help make the best choice for you.

- Take time to read over all of the information a few times and be sure to ask any questions you need to be clear on what to look for, or things to keep in mind when purchasing any products.

- The supplements I am about to suggest are, in my experience, beneficial to weight loss because when you are deficient in them, it can affect your ability to lose weight and achieve maximum results in the time frame we are working with.

- Although they are all beneficial to the human body and basic health in general, before you run out and buy them for the sake of weight loss, I want you to understand why they are a benefit and assess if they are right for you.

If you are unsure about any interaction with health issues you have or medication you take, be sure to check with your healthcare provider.

BASIC SUPPLEMENT LIST:

PROBIOTICS

A probiotic is good bacteria added to your digestive system that helps promote a healthy immune system, but more importantly for our purpose, helps with weight loss by improving digestion.

Digestion is important for weight loss because if your body is unable to process food properly and get the nutrients it needs, it will store fat to compensate or be reluctant to let it go.

- Probiotics come in pill, powdered, or liquid form.
- The probiotic added to foods like yogurt is usually not sufficient enough.
- I suggest looking for a "one a day" with higher potency. This helps minimize the number of pills you have to take each day. Probiotics come in a variety of different potencies and strains and also price ranges.

Look for a probiotic with a variety of strains, especially:

- L. acidophilus (Lactobacillus acidophilus)
- B. Longum (Bifidobacterium longum)
- B. bifidum (Bifidobacterium bifidum)
- L. rhamnosus (Lactobacillus rhamnosus)
- L. fermentum (Limosilactobacillus fermentum)

If you feel you have digestive issues, issues with bowel movements or suffer from chronic health issues and/or skin issues, we suggest investing in a higher quality probiotic, usually found in the refrigerated section. If you don't feel you have these issues, then you are just looking for one to cover the bases.

DOSE

5-10 billion CFUs is an average potency. Follow the recommended dosage on your product's label.

WHEN TO TAKE

Take either on an empty stomach 30 mins before breakfast or with breakfast. The advantage of taking with or without food is debatable. You can also take it before bed. Whichever time you choose, try to be consistent with it. Avoid taking after a meal.

PLEASE NOTE: If you're following SIBO or the FODMAP diet while also following the plan, you might be advised NOT to add in a probiotic. If unsure, always check in with your healthcare provider.

PROBIOTIC FOOD SOURCES

- Yogurt
- Kefir
- Buttermilk
- Some cheeses such as Gouda, Cheddar, Parmesan and Swiss
- Sauerkraut

- Kimchi
- Pickles that are naturally fermented like Strubbs. If they contain vinegar they aren't naturally fermented.
- Tempeh
- Miso
- Kombucha - be mindful of sugar content

VITAMIN D, D3:

Vitamin D is beneficial for weight loss because it tricks the body into thinking it is summer year-round, eliminating the need for the body to hold on to the extra fat it feels inclined to store over the winter months. It is also essential in supporting the body's metabolism.

Low levels of vitamin D are often found in people who have weight to lose because when someone is lacking Vit D, the hypothalamus (the very small part of your brain that regulates hormonal functions, amongst other things) senses low vitamin D levels and responds by increasing body weight.

- Vit D comes in drops or pills. I like drops but pills work.
- Vit D2 is the vegan form
- Vit D3 is the most effective for raising levels as it absorbs better.
- It is better absorbed if taken with a meal that contains fat.

DOSE

600-2000 IU/day is the recommended dose range. Follow package directions for dose.

WHEN TO TAKE

Take with breakfast or lunch because taking it too late in the day can interrupt the body's production of melatonin and mess with your sleep.

ALTERNATE SOURCES FOR VITAMIN D:

Very few foods contain any significant amounts of vitamin D so sun exposure is our best source if not supplementing.

According to the Vitamin D Council, a person with light skin needs approximately 15 minutes of sun exposure and a person with dark skin needs a couple of hours.

- Your skin produces more vitamin D from the sun during mid-day, when the sun is at its highest point.
- The more skin that is exposed the more vitamin D the body will make.

- Darker skin takes longer to make vitamin D than paler skin

OMEGA 3:

If your body is feeling a need to store fat, one way you can speed up the fat loss process is to add in more good fat. Without enough good fat coming in, the body will be reluctant to let go of the stored fat that it keeps around for emergency purposes.

30% of your diet should come from fat and ideally 10% of that should come from Omega 3. The primary source of Omega 3 is fish and unless you are eating a lot of it, it can be difficult for the body to get enough.

Best taken with food and ideally higher fat for best absorption. Because it can be hard to digest, you can divide the dose and take it at breakfast or lunch. Some find refrigerating or even freezing the capsules makes it easier to digest. Follow package directions for dose.

- Omega 3 comes in pill or liquid (oil). Both are equally good.
- If you don't like fish oil you can use vegan alternatives like a 3-6-9 combo.
- I would also look for a high potency one-a-day, again, to minimize the number of pills to take in a day.

DOSE

500-3000 mg per day is the recommended dose range. Follow the directions on your product's label.

WHEN TO TAKE

Avoid taking before bed or before exercise as the increased activity can cause heartburn or reflux.

PLEASE NOTE: *If you are on prescribed blood thinners, consult with a doctor before adding in.

OMEGA 3 FOOD SOURCES

Best fish Sources:

- Mackerel
- Salmon
- Seabass
- Oysters
- Sardines
- Shrimp
- Trout

Other Omega 3 Food Sources

- Seaweed and algae
- Chia seeds (ground or soaked for better absorption)
- Hemp Seeds
- Flax seeds (ground is best for absorption)
- Walnuts
- Edamame
- Kidney Beans

CALM MAGNESIUM (MAGNESIUM CITRATE):

Although magnesium is responsible for over 300 actions in the body, it is important to us because, it not only helps to convert your foods into usable energy, it also helps calm the nerves and balance out cortisol levels (caused by stress). This will help your body to relax, which can help with getting deep & REM sleep. Deep sleep is important because that is the kind of sleep you need for the body to best repair, rebuild, and detoxify.

- Calm Magnesium is also beneficial when it comes to addressing bowel movement issues, and in combination with omega 3 and a probiotic, can help make significant improvements.
- The most effective Calm Magnesium is in powdered form. The pill form doesn't have the same effect.
- It comes plain or flavoured. The flavoured ones have stevia added, but the benefit outweighs the effect of stevia if it keeps you taking it regularly.
- Make sure you are dissolving the Calm Magnesium in warm to hot water to activate the ingredients.

DOSE

1-2 tsp per day is recommended. Follow the directions on your product's label.

WHEN TO TAKE

Take at night as directed before bed. You might need to play around with the dose to find what works for you. Start with the recommended dose and increase in small increments to get the desired effect.

PLEASE NOTE: When it comes to magnesium, there are better sources than the one I suggest. However, for the purpose of weight loss, the magnesium citrate powder works best. Natural Calm Mag is a good brand but there are other mag. citrate powders available.

Also note: it is CALM Mag NOT CAL Mag.

MAGNESIUM FOOD SOURCES:

- Dark Leafy Greens - spinach, kale, collard greens, Swiss chard
- Pumpkin Seeds
- Nuts - especially almonds, cashews and Brazil nuts
- Tuna
- Avocados
- Bananas
- Legumes
- Whole grains

EXTRAS:

The following are a few extra add-ins that may be a benefit and worth considering.

DIGESTIVE BITTERS:

- Bitters are drops that you put into water in-between meals. Look for Canadian bitters, not Swedish. Swedish bitters can contain a mild laxative which is not recommended. Follow package directions for dose.
- If you have known digestive issues, or digestive issues that are as simple as getting bloated after eating raw veg or nuts and seeds, you may want to add in some digestive bitters.
- Digestive bitters help build up digestive enzymes that help with processing and getting nutrients from food.
- Bitters are better than taking digestive enzymes because they don't just help in the moment to process food, they also help to build up digestive enzymes that are normally created by eating raw foods.
- Bitters are also beneficial for anyone missing their gallbladder or suffering from acid reflux as they help to stimulate bile production.

DOSE

1-2 ml up to 3 times per day as directed on the label.

WHEN TO TAKE

Take between meals or 15 mins before meals.

PREBIOTIC WITH ADDED CLEAR FIBER:

- If you have inflammation, digestive, or bowel movement issues, you might want to pick up a prebiotic with added clear fiber.
- Prebiotic is food for the probiotic and together can help improve digestion and bowel movements.
- It is being used more and more in gut therapy to address things like bowel movement issues, leaky gut, high histamine levels, inflammation, insulin resistance, Crohns, and Colitis.

DOSE

Follow directions on your product's label.

WHEN TO TAKE

Prebiotic can be taken any time of day.

PREBIOTIC FOOD SOURCES

- Garlic (raw)
- Onions (raw or lightly cooked)
- Leeks
- Asparagus
- Radishes
- Bananas
- Apples
- Flaxseeds
- Cabbage
- Dandelion greens and root
- Shiitake mushrooms
- Oats, Bran, Barley
- Hemp seeds
- Unpasteurized apple cider vinegar

COLLAGEN:

- Taking collagen helps with tissue repair, improving the quality of hair and nails, but more importantly skin, which is important when it comes to weight loss.

- It's a non-essential protein naturally found in the body that depletes at a rate of 1% yearly after the age of 21.

- Because collagen is a non-essential protein it doesn't count towards protein in a meal.

- Collagen can also help with internal tissue repair and aid the body in making all the changes we are asking of it, as well as helping to maintain muscle mass.

- Most commonly sold in powder form and can be mixed into coffee, tea, water, oatmeal, yogurt etc.

- Collagen comes in either bovine sourced or marine sourced. Marine is better for skin and bovine is better for maintaining muscle mass, but both are effective. You can do your own research or speak to someone at your local health food store, to see which source and which brand is best for you.

- I personally use marine collagen. Specifically, the "Within Us TruMarine" brand and "Deep Marine" brand. But there are many quality brands to choose from.

DOSE

5-10g is the average dose recommendation. Follow the directions on your product's label.

WHEN TO TAKE

Collagen can be taken any time of day.

We will be posting a secondary supplement list in the weeks ahead with some examples of products that can amplify your results once your body is ready and you have laid a strong foundation.

Right now, you want to stick to the basics and be mindful about adding in too many things at once, which can just end up stressing the body and slowing the process.

When it comes to bowel movements specifically, we want to be mindful and allow the body to make new connections on its own without interfering too much. There is a separate post on Bowel Movements which lists supplements that can help specifically with bowel movement issues.

TO RECAP:

SUPPLEMENTS THAT ARE KEY RIGHT NOW ARE:
- Probiotic
- Vitamin D
- Omega 3 or 3-6-9 combo
- Calm magnesium

IF YOU HAVE DIGESTIVE ISSUES CONSIDER:

- Canadian Digestive bitters
- Prebiotic

SKIN, TISSUE REPAIR, AND MAINTAIN MUSCLE MASS:

- Collagen

WHEN IT COMES TO DOSES:

- Due to the many variables based on the large variety of products and individual needs, follow as directed on the package.

WHEN TO TAKE:

- Because everyone will have different needs and some of you are taking medications and other supplements, it's best to grab a pen and paper and make some notes on what times work best, given your individual needs and situation. Check in with your pharmacist or healthcare provider to inquire about any medications that could affect the timing of supplements.

We will be chatting about the supplements all week. Watch out for the post on FAQs.

There is no rush to add these in and you don't need to start taking them all at once. You can take your time adding them in, and they can be added in at any time.

If for any reason you feel uncomfortable taking these or cannot take them for whatever reason, please understand they are simply recommended, but not necessarily make or break when it comes to weight loss.

Please take the time to head over to the Facebook Group or the Livy Method App and watch the quick video that accompanies this post.

FAQS - ABOUT SUPPLEMENTS

Here's a list of frequently asked questions having to do with supplements.

1. **Where should I purchase the supplements?**

Shopping around can save you money so be sure to check different places if you can. Your local health food store or pharmacies are great if you want to talk to someone for recommendations. Here are a few good online shopping options as well:

- Bedrugsmart.ca (Canada & US)
- Well.ca (Canada)
- Vitamart.ca (Canada)
- Vitaminshoppe.com (US)
- Thrivemarket.com (US)
- Amazon.ca and .com (Canada & US)
- COSTCO (Canada & US) also has lots of supplements at great prices.

2. **If I'm taking my probiotic in the morning, should I take it before or after lemon water or acv?**

- You can take it before or after. Just wait about 10 minutes or so in between.

3. **Can I take magnesium citrate pills?**

- If the powder isn't available where you live then yes, take the capsules, but keep in mind they aren't as effective as the powder.

4. **Can we take supplements in gummy form?**

- The short answer is NO. Gummies are for kids and are not as effective. They also contain artificial colour and sweeteners.

5. **I take another magnesium supplement, Should I still take the calm mag?**

- Yes. There are hundreds of different magnesium supplements out there. The calm mag (or magnesium citrate powder) is suggested specifically to go with this program. You can continue taking your other magnesium, but we suggest you also take the Calm Mag. Be sure to speak with your pharmacist or health care provider if you have any concerns.

6. **Can collagen count as my protein for breakfast?**

- No, the protein in collagen is an incomplete protein. Plus, you can't drink your breakfast.

7. **When is the best time to take collagen?**

- Collagen can be taken any time of day, with or without food.

8. **I'm having acid reflux when taking the omega 3.**

- Try any or all of these things:

- Put the capsules in the fridge or freezer.

- Take just before a meal instead of after.

- Switch brands or try the oil if using capsules.

9. **I take a multivitamin. Can I take that instead?**

- You can continue to take any other supplements you were taking prior to the program but not in place of the ones recommended here.

10. **Is there a vegan form of collagen?**

- Collagen is animal-based, however, there are vegan collagen boosters that help your body make more of its own - check your local health food store as they would be able to guide you.

11. **Can you mix the collagen and Calm Mag and take them together?**

- You can mix these together and take at the same time. Be sure to activate the Calm separately in hot water and once it stops fizzing you can add the collagen and mix!

LET'S TALK BOWEL MOVEMENTS

If you have always suffered from bowel movement issues, then rest assured you will see significant improvement by following the program.

During this process, because we piggyback the body's natural detox response, your bowel movements will be all over the place, meaning every shape, size and consistency.

You may experience bouts of constipation, which are normal before detox or when the body is focused on making changes. You may also experience episodes of diarrhea or loose bowel movements, which are also a normal occurrence when the body is in active "detox" or eating any foods your body may be sensitive to.

Your digestive health is directly associated with, and affects your bowel movements. Food goes in and the byproduct eventually needs to make its way out. So, if you have experienced constipation issues in the past, this could have played a major role in your body feeling the need to store fat.

Here is what you can do, above and beyond following The Program, to help improve your bowel movements:

LET'S TALK CONSTIPATION:

THE BASICS:

- Drink lots of water
- Be sure to add leafy greens to meals
- Add in, and regularly take, the basic supplements: Omega 3, Vit D, Probiotic, and Calm magnesium.

In addition to what is listed above in regards to the basics, which all work together on Plan, we also suggest looking into adding:

1. **PREBIOTIC:**

- Prebiotic is food for your probiotic. Prebiotic does come in pill form but is best to get in a clear fiber.
- You can also increase your intake of prebiotic foods that help with digestion like: Onions, garlic, leeks, chickpeas, lentils, kidney beans, bananas, grapefruit, bran, barley, and oats.

2. **DIGESTIVE BITTERS:**

- Digestive bitters are herbs that support digestive function by stimulating bitter receptors on the tongue, stomach, gallbladder, and pancreas.

- They work to promote digestive juices such as stomach acid, bile, and enzymes, which help to break down food and assist in the absorption of nutrients.
- Look for Canadian Digestive Bitters that come in drops you add to water.
- Take bitters about 20 minutes before a meal to signal your body to produce more saliva, bile, and stomach acid.

3. **VITAMIN C:**
- When taking higher doses of vitamin C, the extra or unabsorbed vitamin C pulls water into your intestines, which can help soften your stool.
- Take 30 mins before food in the morning, dose is dependent on the individual and can range from 90-2000 mg.

4. **B COMPLEX:**
- B12, B1 & B5 deficiency can cause constipation. These can be found together in a B complex. If your constipation is caused by low levels of B's, increasing your daily intake of this nutrient may help ease your symptoms.
- B complex is part of the secondary supplements list I will be sending out in a few weeks.
- Not essential to weight loss, but B12 is key in supporting metabolic function, which can significantly help with weight loss, by helping to improve your energy.
- You may prefer to eat more foods rich in this vitamin rather than take a supplement.

EXAMPLES OF FOODS RICH IN B VITAMINS INCLUDE:
- Meat (red meat, poultry, fish)
- Beef
- Liver
- Trout
- Salmon
- Tuna fish
- Whole grains (brown rice, barley, millet)
- Eggs and dairy products (milk, cheese)
- Legumes (beans, lentils)
- Seeds and nuts (sunflower seeds, almonds)
- Dark, leafy vegetables (broccoli, spinach)
- Fruits (citrus fruits, avocados, bananas)

5. **TRIPHALA:**

- Used in Ayurvedic medicine for thousands of years, it is thought to support bowel health and aid digestion. As an antioxidant, it is also thought to detoxify the body and support the immune system.

- Triphala helps to keep the stomach, small intestine and large intestine healthy by flushing out toxins from the body.

- Triphala as a supplement, is available as a pill, and in powder form. The powder is meant to be dissolved in warm water and consumed as tea. It can taste bitter but can be mixed with honey or lemon without diminishing its effects.

- Triphala supplements have varying daily dosages based upon the manufacturer. It's important to follow package directions exactly.

- Triphala may be most effective when taken right before bed with a large glass of warm water.

- Some people prefer to take this supplement on an empty stomach, while others prefer to take it with food. Discuss these options with your healthcare provider.

6. **EXERCISE/MOVE YOUR BODY:**

- Exercise helps constipation by lowering the time it takes food to move through the large intestine. This limits the amount of water your body absorbs from the stool.

- Cardio exercise speeds up your breathing and heart rate, helping to stimulate the natural squeezing of muscles in your intestines which helps to move stool out quickly.

- Something as simple as going for a walk after dinner can make all the difference when it comes to improving digestion.

7. **TIME AND CONSISTENCY:**

- It is important to note that in most cases the body just needs time to rewire how it has come to function over the years.

- The foods you are eating, and the overall structure of The Program will help from a baseline level to address constipation issues.

- Try to keep things routine and be patient with the process, but also don't suffer. Sometimes you need to take something stronger like an over-the-counter laxative to help the body work through any backlog.

LET'S TALK LOOSE BOWEL MOVEMENTS:

Loose bowel movements can be unnerving but can also be a normal part of the process. All of the water you are drinking, leafy greens you are eating, and fiber rich foods like fruit and veggies all contribute to a natural daily detox.

In most cases, it's nothing to be concerned about. However, here are some things you can do to address them:

1. Continue to focus on digestive health. It can be a great idea to add in the prebiotic and bitters to help strengthen your digestive system.

2. Keep a journal and record how you are feeling after eating meals and snacks as sometimes food sensitivities can pop up that can cause loose BMs and discomfort.

3. Dairy and gluten are the most common sensitivities, but it can come down to specific food choices like a kind of fruit for example, or even spicy food.

4. Decrease calm magnesium. Although the calm mag is rarely the sole issue for loose BMs, decreasing it slightly may help.

5. If you are concerned about nutrient loss, rest assured, it's not a major concern when following the plan.

6. You can add trace minerals to your water or add in a pinch of pink rock salt or Celtic salt to your warm water and lemon in the morning and/or water throughout the day.

7. Add in Psyllium fiber. You never want to add in fiber while constipated as it can sometimes make the situation worse. It is however an excellent time to add in if experiencing loose bowel movements.

Psyllium is non-dependent and when added in, attaches itself to toxins stored in your fat cells and helps to draw them out. This can help make your bowel movements more binding and effective for fat loss.

*   The soluble fiber also helps lower blood cholesterol levels and control blood sugar levels. You can also get this type of fiber from oats, barley, oranges, dried beans and lentils.

*   Comes in pill or powder form. I personally like the pills.

*   Take before bed or in between meals.

TO RECAP:

The body will be working hard to address digestive and BM issues. Given enough time, your body will aim to make significant improvements.

Although usually nothing to be concerned about, when it comes to BM issues, it is always recommended to check in with your healthcare provider.

Some conditions including Crohn's disease, celiac disease, IBS, thyroid issues and medications can be the cause of loose BMs, but if your changes in BMs go hand in hand with following the program, chances are there is nothing to be concerned about and given the time, the body will sort out and address it on its own.

Please take the time to head over to the Facebook Group or the Livy Method App and watch the quick video that accompanies this post.

LET'S TALK NON-SCALE VICTORIES (NSVS) — ANOTHER MEASURE OF SUCCESS!

Our WLBG Maintenance and Mindfulness Group Manager, Odette Ropchan, who is now down 40lbs in her journey, put together this post in the hopes of providing insight into Non-Scale Victories that you may experience and may want to lean into during your weight loss journey.

Here you are. You've joined a weight loss program. You want to lose weight and you will! But let's talk for a minute of what you will gain. It is just as important and measurable but not on the scale! Those Non-Scale Victories are going to come, and often sooner than your scale victory will.

So, what is a Non-Scale Victory or a NSV as we like to call them around here? These are your measures of success that will not show up on that piece of metal on the floor. It could be a number like inches lost, it could be a feeling like more energy, or it could even be an emotion like pure pride! Some will present themselves easily and some you may have to look to find.

In the pursuit of weight loss, we have been conditioned to be hyper focused on the number on the scale and to only acknowledge and appreciate that. We only feel we are moving in the right direction to our finally and forever if the scale is moving in the perceived right direction. While doing the Livy Method, we want you to look beyond the scale, open your mind and expectations, and measure your success with those NSV's. They are there. We know losing weight can be frustrating and we can easily focus and be consumed with what *isn't* happening rather than what *is*. NSV's and the positive vibe they bring can have a big impact on your overall success! They will keep you determined to keep going even when the scale doesn't tell you what you want! They will help you trust the process and confirm that the time and work you put in has not been a lost cause!

We have put together a list of just some of the NSV's our members have reported. You will notice that some can be seen, and others have to be felt! We encourage you to make your own list or add to this one! Look for the positive changes that are happening as you are making change! Be sure to lean into those changes! These won't be on the scale, but they will in the mirror, and they will be inside of you!

NSV's that you can see:

- Body changes
- Increased Energy
- Clothing fits looser
- Tightening belt loops
- Tightening watch straps
- Wedding rings fitting again
- Improved complexion
- Not having to use ChapStick

- Seeing hip, cheek, and collarbones
- Towels feel bigger when wrapped around
- Ability to be on the floor playing with your kids/grandkids
- Lap for your kids to sit on
- Crossing your legs comfortably
- No longer snoring
- Lost inches when measuring
- Symptom management of chronic illness
- More regular bowel movements
- Less uncomfortable and strained bowel movements
- Easier time getting up in the morning
- Having coffee because you like it, not because you need it
- Wanting to drink water
- Decreased medications – blood pressure, cholesterol, blood sugar meds, antacids, etc.
- Improved Mobility
- Moved your car seat closer to the steering wheel
- Fitting in chairs, seats that you were previously uncomfortable in
- Being comfortable with doing simple activities
- Friends/family commenting that they are noticing positive change
- Inspiring kids/family/friends to change own poor diet habits
- New friends/relationships
- _____
- _____
- _____
- _____
- _____

NSV's that you feel:

- More in-tune with your body's needs
- Improved relationship with food
- Being hydrated
- Less brain fog

- More focus and concentration during the day
- Menopause and PMS symptoms improved
- Migraines diminishing or infrequent
- No more heartburn
- Less gas and less bloating
- Improved overall digestion
- Decreased pain
- Increased libido
- Better sleep
- Not needing an afternoon nap
- Feeling energized
- Less Inflammation
- Diminished cravings and snacking urges
- Don't get hangry
- Trying new foods and not being afraid of delicious food and fat
- Not being out of breath doing chores/daily activities
- Changing taste buds
- Appreciating how food smells
- Learning how to feed yourself
- Learning new information, understanding how your body works
- Recognizing feeling full doesn't feel good and is not what you need
- Knowing that certain foods don't make you feel good
- _____
- _____
- _____
- _____
- _____

We like to level up around here so let's take it one step further and talk about NSV's that have nothing to do with your body or a physical feeling. These are the ones that come from trusting you are doing something that is new, maybe hard at times, but is the most important and healthiest thing you can do to take care of yourself!

Intuition: "having the ability to understand or know something without any direct evidence or reasoning process" and ""using or based on what one feels to be true even without conscious reasoning; instinctive."

NSV's that are intuitive:

- Making yourself a priority
- More positive mood and attitude
- More focus
- Feeling confident
- Happier
- More patience
- Pride for being open to learning and doing this
- Pride of sticking to something
- Hope, not fear, that you can succeed
- Not wanting to quit when one day doesn't go your way
- Calmer about your choices knowing you will be ok
- Calm about grocery shopping. Buying real food and not diet food
- Recognizing stress and not running from it but understanding it
- Less anxiety around food and feeling deprived
- Being in-tune with how certain foods make you feel
- Knowing what you actually want to eat instead of just eating
- Developing positive eating habits and associations
- Not missing the types of food you thought you would because you don't feel deprived
- Realizing that you want to exercise not feel like you HAVE to exercise
- Not feeling shame and guilt and having food freedom
- Trusting you can do new things
- _____
- _____
- _____
- _____
- _____

We have a supportive community like no other! In this community our members share and encourage so everyone can get to their finally and forever. Have a look below at some real NSV's from our group!

- ☐ Best NSV is getting my mind and body to realize they're on the same team

- ☐ Putting myself first instead of everyone else and taking the time to know I deserve this

- ☐ Acknowledging and managing my stress much better

- ☐ My best NSV is not wanting to snack at night anymore

- ☐ Living each day with renewed energy

- ☐ Learning to love my body

- ☐ My NSV is last Saturday at the gym I noticed when doing a spin class that my knees and my stomach were no longer connecting

- ☐ Being scared but trusting the process and putting myself first!

- ☐ Able to do up buttons as my arthritis is better

- ☐ Eating the right amount of food for me, not what a tracker says or just because it's on my plate

- ☐ Today I had to move my car seat up. Suddenly I couldn't reach the pedals – sure sign my bum is getting smaller!

- ☐ After many years on my anxiety meds, I have finally been able to start dropping doses to get off them. This is such a huge non scale victory for me. My numbers on the scale may not always drop day to day, but my negative thoughts about myself do.

- ☐ What a wonderful non scale victory! Recognizing when I have eaten to satisfaction, so I don't have that feeling of having eaten too much and feel uncomfortable.

- ☐ Last week, a colleague said to me "you look really good these days" to which I replied, "Thanks, I feel really good." And in that moment, I realized that I meant it. I had been so focused on the scale that hadn't been moving that I wasn't paying attention to how all over awesome I have been feeling lately and all the little victories that have been piling up. Lesson learned – this program is also a wellness journey, not just a weight loss one.

Weight loss isn't always a smooth paved road to drive on. You will encounter speed bumps; pit stops and full-on roadblocks during your journey. None of these are a reason to stop from moving in the direction that will get you to your destination. When your scale is presenting that roadblock, embracing those NSV's becomes more important. Writing them down, reviewing them, and appreciating them will keep your determination strong and your goals in sight. You have got this!

LET'S TALK OILS

It's important to choose the right oil for the right job. Oils are used in all kinds of things from dressings to marinades, sautéing, searing, stir frying, roasting etc. But not all oils are created equal.

When it comes to cooking with oils, things can easily get complicated. Levels of saturation, smoke points, cold pressed, unrefined, hydrogenated. It's easy to go down a rabbit hole when it comes to oils, so let's try and simplify things a bit.

Let's break down some of those terms mentioned above so you know what to keep in mind when choosing your oils

SMOKE POINT:

The point at which an oil starts to smoke when heated is its smoke point. You want to avoid letting oils get to the smoke point because it indicates that the oil has been damaged and is releasing harmful chemicals into the air by way of smoke. If you accidentally bring oil to its smoking point, toss it out and start again at a lower temperature. PRO TIPS: Heat the pan first and then add your oil, let it heat for a few seconds then add your ingredients. This can prevent the oil from ever reaching its smoke point. In most cases for frying and sautéing high heat isn't necessary. Even for searing meats, a medium high heat works just great!

COMMON OILS WITH A HIGHER SMOKE POINT:

Refined olive, avocado, coconut, canola, grapeseed, peanut oil, sunflower, safflower and sesame.

REFINED VS UNREFINED:

Unrefined oils are only lightly filtered and have better flavour, colour, and fragrance than refined oils. The bottle will say "unrefined" or "cold pressed". They are more nutritious and are best used unheated as in a salad dressing or on very low heat for cooking. All the healthy stuff will disappear if heated too much.

COMMON UNREFINED OILS:

Extra virgin olive, avocado, coconut, nut oils such as walnut and almond, sesame oil. Extra virgin olive oil may not say "cold pressed" or "unrefined" because "extra virgin" means the same thing.

Naturally refined oils are more finely filtered with the use of a little heat. This can reduce the nutrient level and flavour but also makes them more resistant to smoking. They are not chemically refined like large crop oils (see below) Many common ones listed above under "Smoke Point".

WHAT ABOUT BUTTER?

Butter is great for cooking and has a medium smoke point so keep the heat to medium temperatures when using it for cooking. Ghee or clarified butter has a higher smoke point so can be used for higher temperature cooking.

Organic butter is always best, if your budget allows.

WHAT TO AVOID:

Unfortunately, many of the oils found on the shelves in the grocery store are chemically processed and are produced in large crops that are heavily sprayed with chemical pesticides. Oils like canola, safflower, soy, corn, palm, sunflower...as well as the generically labeled "vegetable oils" (which is just a combination of any of the above listed oils). These often contain trans fats as well. They are best to avoid or use sparingly.

HYDROGENATED OILS:

This is a highly chemical process that converts a naturally liquid oil into a solid oil. Best to avoid these or products containing these oils. Shortening and margarine are hydrogenated oils although there are now many non-hydrogenated margarines on the market so check those labels!

SO NOW WHAT?

When shopping for oils, look at the labels for words like "refined" "unrefined", "cold pressed", "extra virgin" and "organic".

LAST BUT NOT LEAST.... Nothing to worry or stress about from a weight loss perspective. You don't need to throw out any oils you don't think are good. We are just looking to provide you with some more information to continue making good choices when at the grocery store.

LET'S TALK DOUBLE DETOX & YOUR MENSTRUATION CYCLE

As much of a pain as it can be, your period is an awesome opportunity to capitalize on fat loss each month!

Because The Livy Method uses the same detox process that the body uses when you are sick (cold or flu), have food poisoning, or when you have your period, we can use those times to help with the weight loss process.

Which is where the concept of double detox comes from.

Your period each month is a time where the body looks to reset, to balance hormones, and to get rid of any fat it doesn't need.

When your **MENSTRUAL CYCLE** hits:

- Be consistent with supplements
- Increase the calm magnesium

Magnesium has many benefits like contributing to energy production, helping with digestion, and relieveing anxiety to name a few, but it can also help relieve PMS symptoms and keep your hormones more balanced. Taking magnesium daily has been proven effective in preventing menstrual migraines as your magnesium levels tend to be a lot lower on your period due to your hormones.

Magnesium is also effective in relaxing muscles, which can help with any cramping.

Magnesium can also help boost your mood by playing a role in serotonin production. Serotonin is a mood-boosting hormone. You can add an extra dose during the day or increase your dose at night. Taking during the day won't cause drowsiness as your body isn't producing Melatonin at that time.

Be mindful of iron issues. When blood is lost every month, the iron in red blood cells is also lost. If your monthly iron intake and absorption does not replace the iron lost during your period, you can end up with iron deficiency, which affects not only your energy, but your ability to lose weight.

**If you think you might be low in Iron, be sure to check in with your healthcare provider. **

Here are some tips to help support the body during Double Detox:

- Extra water
- Hit all meals and snacks
- Keep portions on the smaller side to allow the body to stay focused on the task at hand
- Lighter on the carbs and heavier on the leafy greens at lunch and dinner for increased roughage to help keep moving things in and out

- Eat as early as possible
- Go to bed earlier to help the body get extra rest
- Take warm epsom salt baths

The intention here is to help the body stay focused on the task at hand and capitalize on the natural detox process.

It's also key to note that this process allows the body the opportunity to balance hormones, which can lead to cycle syncing. Cycle syncing is the practice of eating, exercising, and aligning your lifestyle choices according to your menstrual cycle.

Cycle syncing is something that happens naturally while following the plan because of the holistic approach we are taking to lose weight.

This is why it's normal for your period to come early, late, or look and feel different than what you are used to while following the plan. Although this can be unnerving, rest assured your body is doing what's best to allow your body to work at optimal levels.

And as always, if ever you feel something is more off than it should be, always check in with your healthcare provider.

Please take time to head over to the Facebook Group or the Livy Method App and watch the quick video that accompanies this post. To learn more about the science behind our body's natural detox process please head to the Detox post in the Science Guide.

IS IT A FRUIT OR VEG?

This question gets asked a lot. Especially in relation to tomatoes and avocados. Because they are technically fruits, we get asked if they can be eaten at fruit snack, but on this program, we classify tomatoes as a veg and avocado as a healthy fat.

DID YOU KNOW….

A fruit develops from a flower and produces seeds or a pit. Like a tomato… and many other fruits we think of as vegetables inside and out of this program.

In the botanical world, the word "vegetable" doesn't even exist. What we call vegetables they refer to as leaves, stems, roots, flower buds etc. Like celery is a stem and radishes are roots.

The word "vegetable" is only a culinary term.

There are many foods on plan that are technically fruits, but we use them as veg. And there are some fruits that we categorize as healthy fats.

LET'S BREAK IT DOWN...

TECHNICALLY FRUITS BUT WE USE THEM AS VEGETABLES ON PLAN:

- Tomatoes
- Cucumbers
- Peppers
- Peas
- Green beans
- Eggplant
- Okra
- Corn
- Zucchini
- Pumpkin
- Squash

NOTE: Even though these are technically fruits, we use them as vegetables on plan. Then there are fruits (technically) that we use as fats on plan.

TECHNICALLY FRUITS BUT WE USE AS HEALTHY FATS ON PLAN:

- Avocado
- Nuts

- Olives
- Coconut (technically a fruit, a nut, and a seed!) But we use it as a healthy fat on plan.

Watermelon is both a fruit and a vegetable, but we use it as a fruit on plan and rhubarb is actually a vegetable. (Remember the stem example that was used with the celery above? Same, same).

Are you confused yet?!

We could go down a scientific rabbit hole with this subject but just wanted to provide some clarity as well as some fun facts!

LET'S TALK FALL: SEASONAL TRANSITION & TWEAKS

As you focus on being mindful this week when it comes to food portions, it's also a great time to work on being in tune to your food choices.

The fall can be the perfect time to lose weight, but you may find yourself struggling on Plan if you don't make the switch over to fall foods and help the body adjust to seasonal change.

In the summer, the body works like an air conditioner trying to keep you cool so you crave foods that cool you down when you eat them, like fresh fruit and salads. Eating fresh fruits and clean salads comes easy when the temperature rises; but when it starts to drop, your cravings change.

In the fall, the body is busy transitioning to keep us warm and working like a heater in the winter.

Sticking to your summer diet is a mistake many people make—they fight the urge to eat the heavier carbs and fatty meats they start craving, leaving the body no choice but to store fat to compensate.

The body not only craves - but needs seasonal foods like soups and stews, heartier root veggies like squash and potatoes, heavier carbs like rice and quinoa and grains & oatmeal for breakfast; foods that make the body work hard and create heat when you eat them.

The body is very in tune with seasonal changes and it's important to make the adjustments to maximize the food plan.

HERE ARE EXAMPLES OF 5 FALL FOODS:

Apples

Super high in weight loss-friendly fibre and polyphenols. Apples keep you feeling full and satisfied longer and they help to feed the good bacteria in your gut, which can also benefit metabolic health.

Pomegranates

High in vitamin C, folate, potassium and fibre, a cup of these delicious arils can help to lower blood pressure and cholesterol.

Pumpkin

Pumpkin is low in calories (not that we count) and high in fibre, which helps to regulate blood sugar—essential for weight loss. Nutrient-rich pumpkin seeds are also packed with fibre, plus essential fatty acids, vitamins and minerals, making them the perfect little snack to add to any weight loss program.

Brussels Sprouts

Rich in sulphur-containing-nutrients, which are essential for detoxing, these guys are high in vitamins and minerals and also high in protein.

Sweet potatoes

Naturally sweet, these potatoes have their share of carbs, but they also help to regulate blood sugar and have a relatively low glycemic rating, meaning they convert to sugar slower when you eat them. Nutrient-rich and high in water and fibre, sweet potatoes keep you satisfied longer.

Cranberries

Loaded with antioxidants and essential nutrients, these little berries pack a punch when it comes to vitamin C and fibre. Cranberries are well-known for helping prevent urinary tract infections and recent research suggests they may help prevent stomach ulcers too.

Along with switching up your diet, it's key to adjust your sleep.

Sleep is essential to any weight loss program because when you sleep is when the body makes change. The shorter days can have the sky turning dark well before we would even think about eating dinner in the summer, so it is important to adapt to the change.

When it starts to get dark outside, the body produces melatonin to help your body get ready for sleep. Eating after dark can interrupt this process and have your body gearing up instead of winding down and that can prevent you from getting the quality, deep REM sleep the body needs to make change.

It can get darker as much as three hours earlier in the fall and winter, so it is key to adjust your diet and sleep schedule.

The body is wired to be in tune with seasonal change, so choosing more seasonal foods, eating a bit earlier, and getting to bed sooner can make all the difference when it comes to weight loss.

Let's talk water:

Compared to the warmer months, as the temperature drops, the amount of water you need to stay hydrated decreases. So it's perfect timing to keep up your water drinking to promote a natural detox and get the fat out.

On the other hand, as it gets colder outside, we tend to turn up the heat inside which can be very dehydrating, so you may end up needing more.

If you are finding cold water is not appealing, then try drinking it at room temp or supplementing with tea.

So, although seasonal change is nothing to stress about and you don't need to be cross referencing seasonal foods, being in tune to your body's needs day to day can make all the difference when it comes to your body falling in line and focusing on fat loss.

WEEK 3 GUIDELINES: CONSISTENCY & MINDFULNESS

This week has us discussing issues and associations when it comes to food. The goal is to be as consistent as possible to allow the body time to calm down and get used to the changes you have already made. This is also where we start to address portions. How are your portions? How do you feel while eating? How do you know when you're full? What are your habits & hang-ups? How is your body responding?

LET'S TALK CONSISTENCY

I would love to tell you this is where things start to get exciting, but the goal of Week 3 is actually quite the opposite.

Week 2 had you working on fine tuning and perfecting the changes that you have made so far, as well as the addition of the bonus snacks and supplements.

Moving into Week 3, the goal is to be as consistent as possible to allow the body time to calm down and adjust from the changes you have made in the past few weeks. Follow the food plan, make nutrient rich choices, continue to eat to satisfaction, add in any supplements, and work the water.

If you are continually feeling unsatisfied at the end of the day, or hungry to the point where it's distracting during the day, be sure to add in the bonus snack/s when needed.

Consistency is key as we are still in the phase of making the body feel confident that it no longer needs the stored fat it has been hanging onto for whatever reason; high stress, lack of sleep, long periods of time without eating, just to name a few.

I recognize this is not the most exciting week, but it is a very important one. It is essential that you establish routine within the body to lay a strong foundation we can work with.

The first few weeks of the program were about giving the body what it needs so as you move forward, you can manipulate it into focusing more on what you want it to do, which is to drop fat.

If you are starting to feel bored with the routine or the foods you are eating, rest assured, that is normal for where we are in the process. Rather than looking for alternatives or swapping recipes to make things more exciting, I want you to indulge in the boredom.

If you are not bored, that is OK too, as some people enjoy the routine.

This week is key for these reasons:

- It is important to continue to allow the body to adjust to the changes you have made in the first few weeks so it can calm down internally and focus less on digestion and inflammation and more on making change.
- If you have ever used food for anything other than nutritional requirements, like eating out of boredom, distraction, stress, reward and so on, this stage will address that.
- This week helps you get more in tune with your body's needs over your wants.
- This week also allows the body time to adjust its hunger levels, which will have you feeling fuller faster as your portions naturally decrease.

At the end of this week, things will start to come together for you as your body starts to change, weight starts to drop, and you get to a place where you feel so good that the process becomes about maintaining that feeling and building on it as we move forward.

LET'S TALK MINDFULNESS

This is when we start to focus on fat loss by focusing on maximizing the food plan and being even more in tune to your portion sizes.

Because we don't weigh, measure or count anything when it comes to portions, the first step to adjusting them is to put some time into increasing the mind-body connection even further, by paying attention to how the body is responding to your meals and snacks.

It sounds a bit corny, but there is a reason why people always talk about the mind-body connection.

Most people, when asked what makes them stop eating or how they know when they are satisfied, will tell you it's when they are done eating everything on their plate or until they feel full. And because most people have been eating until they feel physically full, they end up eating way more food than they need. And then they get used to eating more than they need, which then becomes the norm.

The goal is to get to a place where your body tells you very clearly WHEN to eat, WHAT to eat, and HOW MUCH to eat.

The process of weighing and measuring foods, counting calories and macros is not a normal way to eat. Neither is this food plan formula of eating I currently have you following.

So, it's important to note, as we move forward in the program, we are going to transition into more of a natural way of eating. But first, we need to make sure you are completely in tune with where you are now. Which brings us to the purpose of mindfulness. This is where the focus is on addressing portions by being mindful about how your body is responding before, during, and after you eat.

HERE IS WHAT YOU ARE TO DO:
ASK YOURSELF THESE 4 QUESTIONS

1. **Before you eat, ask yourself if you are even hungry:**
   - The goal is to bring awareness to your changing hunger levels. For example, sometimes you are really hungry but then when you eat, you get full fast. Other times you are not hungry at all, but when you start to eat, you feel hungry. Both are normal and you are still to eat all meals and snacks regardless of hunger levels.

2. **When serving or portioning out your food and before you eat…ask yourself:**
   - How is this portion for me?
   - How would I feel if I ate all of this?
   - You may not get a really strong response or any answer from your body at first, but trust that after a few days of talking to yourself, your body will start to talk back.

3. **While eating your food, pay attention to how you feel and ask yourself:**
   - Are you getting full, is this food satisfying you?
   - How would you feel if you took a few more bites?
   - How would you feel if you stop eating now?
   - Do you feel any physical effects of eating?

4. **When you are done eating, ask yourself how you feel:**
   - Do you feel full and if so, what is your definition of full?
   - How do you know when you have eaten enough?

- How do you feel physically? Meaning, is it a physically full belly feeling or is it more of a tired feeling? Or is it that you just eat everything on your plate because it's there - kind of thing? Or maybe you feel like you could eat more?

I know some of you may be inclined to start cutting and decreasing portions thinking it's going to get you ahead. I promise you it won't. It will only lead to confusion down the road if you miss this very important step.

If you follow these simple steps, your portions will naturally decrease on their own. For now, focus on eating enough food so that when you are done and walk away from your food, you don't feel any physical effects. Meaning, when you walk away from your food you shouldn't physically feel like you ate. If you do, chances are you have eaten too much.

With that said...You are NOT TRYING to decrease portions sizes based on counting, weighing, measuring, or what they look like.

This is about being in tune to them. Your hunger levels will change day to day so **it's about what the portions FEEL like... not what they LOOK like**, so each day might look different, portion size wise. If you decrease portions by too much too soon, you will have a hard time moving forward in the Program.

This week is about being more in tune with your body's needs so when we do start to address portions, you will know what to do. Although you may notice your portions are naturally getting smaller, make sure to still eat to satisfaction regardless of what that portion looks like day to day.

TO RECAP:

Your task for this week is a very simple but important one: to be as consistent as possible and to take time to connect with your body and get in the habit of being mindful of hunger levels and portions.

Ask yourself the 4 Questions. Try to eat without distractions so you can focus on your body's signals.

As we move forward in the coming weeks, you will need to have a clear understanding of when you are hungry, what you are hungry for, and how much.

As a look ahead into Week 4, we will start to reduce portion sizes - so it is very important that it comes off the heels of your body feeling satisfied and confident that it no longer needs the fat it has been storing and holding on to.

CONSISTENCY REMAINS KEY.

This is a very exciting time. You have patiently been putting in the time and work to lay a super strong foundation that will not only lead to weight loss success but will set you up to move forward from this process to live a normal life when it comes to food.

The goal is to not only lose weight and lose it in a way that is sustainable, but also to move on from the fight of constantly trying to lose. To let go of the "diet talk", the counting, weighing, measuring and stress from trying to lose over the years.

Let's work on changing that internal dialogue this week while also being mindful of your portions and maximizing your efforts each day.

Please take the time to head over to the Facebook Group or the Livy Method App and watch the quick video that accompanies this post.

WEEK 3 GUIDELINES FAQS

1.   I am struggling to overcome the habit of eating all of the food on my plate, any tips?

When serving your portions ensure you are asking yourself the 4 mindfulness questions, especially "How is this portion for me?". It is a good way to start thinking about what the portion feels like, as opposed to what it looks like. If throwing out the uneaten portion feels uncomfortable for you, save the remaining portion for another meal, or another day. Over time, these new habits will become wired in your brain, especially as you start to feel better about yourself and more in tune with your body's hunger and satiety signals.

2.   Any other tips to strengthen the mind-body connection?

What makes The Livy Method different from all the other diets out there, is that apart from the Food Plan, another main focus is on developing a mind-body connection. Keep following the food plan as many of these strategies are built into the weekly tweaks as we progress through the Program. Asking yourself the four mindfulness questions with every meal and snack will really help you to develop this connection. Practice, repetition and consistency will help to strengthen this connection. Over time you will find the more you get in tune with your body the clearer your body will communicate its needs.

3.   Is it ok to graze while eating your meals?

It is totally fine to take your time while eating your meals. Just be sure that you are eating to your hunger levels and staying in tune with your body. Ask yourself the four mindfulness questions with every meal and snack and keep in mind that your hunger levels will change day to day. Once you have finished your meal or snack, be sure to allow at least 30 min and up to 3.5 hours to have the next one.

4.   How do I know the difference between my hunger and migrating motor complex?

Hunger is just another way the body communicates its needs, a "heads up" kind of thing that lets you know where it's at and what it needs throughout the day. Once you have eaten to satisfaction the hunger feeling subsides. The migrating motor complex (MMC) is the digestive system's self-cleaning oven, signified by the "grumblings" and "churning" of the stomach, as your digestive system works to clear bacteria and food particles out of the small intestine. This takes place in between processing and digesting food. Because we are eating so often during the day, the body is doing most of this work at night. As we move through the program and phase you into more natural patterns of eating, this will also include the downtime your body needs in between meals to self regulate.

5.   I eat until I am satisfied but am hungry not long after, any tips?

If you are finding yourself hungry after eating, be sure you are making your meals nutrient rich and adding in good fats to help with sustaining energy, and eat to satisfaction. If you find you need more added oomph you can add some heavy veg or grains to your meal. If 10-15min after eating you still find you are hungry, you can always go back for more. Keep in mind the timing of eating, anywhere from 30 minutes to 3.5 hours so you can always move on to your next meal or snack.

6.   Should I be reducing my portion sizes?

It is recommended to not be decreasing portions intentionally at this point. You still want to be eating to satisfaction, asking those 4 mindfulness questions and giving your body what it needs so it no longer feels the need to hold on to your fat. As you continue to focus on your hunger levels and how you are feeling at each meal and snack you may notice that your portions will naturally start to decrease. Be open to your changing hunger levels, as portions are about what they feel like and not what they look like.

7.   I can't make the connection on the purpose of why I'm asking these four questions. Any tips?

The practice of asking the four questions is to bring awareness to how your body is responding to the food plan and the portions you are consuming now. By continually asking those four questions for each meal and snack, you are bringing awareness to how you are feeling in the moment and this will help differentiate between your body's actual needs over your wants. By slowing down, minimizing any distractions, asking yourself those 4 questions, and paying attention to how you are feeling as you eat your portion, you will begin to start making those associations. This is something that will take practice. Be gentle with yourself and day by day you will notice it all coming together.

8.   If meal prepping, should I pack extra and eat to satisfaction, or pack exactly what I think I'll need?

Hunger levels will vary from day to day and from meal to meal and you want to ensure that you are eating to satisfaction. Packing extra can help for when you find yourself extra hungry and in need of more than what you felt when packaging up your foods. Continue to ask those four questions when it comes time to eat and continue to eat to satisfaction for each meal and snack.

9.   What does Gina mean when she talks about consistency?

Consistency is when you are following the Program as it is laid out the best you can each day. You are eating all of the nutrient rich meals and snacks to satisfaction, within the designated time frames. You also want to be "consistent" with your hydration, getting good quality sleep, managing stress, getting in your supplements and following the Food Plan as designed.

WHY MINDFULNESS IS KEY

I know a lot of you have probably read over the Week 3 Guidelines and are left thinking "what the heck?!" You might be also thinking "I'm not really into all this mindfulness and meditation hullabaloo so this just isn't really for me". I get that but let me explain why, especially when it comes to weight loss; it's super important and you don't want to just blow it off.

When it comes to weight loss, there is never enough emphasis put on the mind-body connection. Especially in Western societies where large (HUGE!) portions have become the norm. Many of us were brought up being taught to not waste food and finish everything on the plate, sometimes not even being allowed to leave the table until everything was finished. "After all there are starving children in Africa!" How many of you heard that growing up?

This idea that you must clean your plate goes way back in history and has to do with food shortages beginning in World War I. It has become totally normal for parents to urge their kids to finish everything on their plates, regardless of how they feel. So, at a very young age we start learning how NOT to listen to our bodies. We have literally been trained to be mindless eaters, blindly shoveling food in until the plate is clean and that "oh-so-glorious" feeling that comes from overeating. Anything sounding familiar?

So that brings us to why this week is so important. We need to take the time to unlearn all of that training and start to feel and understand what our bodies are telling us. It's not going to be easy. For many, you have been taught your entire life not to listen. It's not easy or quick to unlearn and retrain this way of thinking...or not thinking in this case.

Start slow and don't expect to get it right away. You may not have any answers to those questions when you first start and that's okay. You might say "I never feel hungry." That's probably because you have spent years going very long periods of time without eating. Keep asking and you will begin to have answers. It will take time and lots and lots of practice. Just like learning a new skill, you need repetition, and it will slowly become more natural. This isn't a week you are trying to nail as it is not as straightforward as just following the Food Plan. We are asking you to dig a bit deeper here.

Take the time to:

- Focus
- Slow down
- Pay attention

Learning to listen to your body's cues, especially when it comes to portion sizes, is THE MOST IMPORTANT PART OF THIS PROGRAM. It's the thing that will keep that weight off. For good! You will always be in tune and very aware when you've let yourself go off track and your body will let you know.... if you are listening.

TOP TIPS FOR NAVIGATING MINDFULNESS:

Try Not To Eat While Distracted

Watching television, your phone, driving etc. can take the focus away from connecting with your body signals so try to eat in a calm state away from rushing and distractions where you can slow down and pay attention. If you are eating with a distraction, be extra diligent about checking in with yourself periodically about how you are feeling.

Eat What's Most Appealing on Your Plate

You still want to prepare your meals using the guidelines of more veg at lunch and more protein at dinner but don't put too much focus on that while eating and being mindful. Instead, eat what's most appealing to you in the moment (more mindfulness) and don't worry if you think you had more protein at lunch or less at dinner.

Am I Still Hungry?

"Eating to satisfaction" can be a hard concept to grasp at first, so try rewording it into something else. "Am I still hungry?" or "Is it my body wanting more or is it my mind or my taste buds wanting more?". If you need, come up with your own question that makes it easier for you to connect.

Wait A Few Minutes

If you decide you are satisfied but just can't believe all the food left on your plate, wait 10 minutes or so and if you decide you need a few more bites then have them. You will often find that you don't.

Try Not to Be "Afraid"

It's normal to feel anxious about being hungry later because you think you didn't eat enough. Remember that the next snack or meal is right around the corner and you can also add in bonus snacks if you need them.

Save Food for Later

Remember that when you don't finish what's on your plate you can always save it for later.

For more information on how mindfulness can benefit your digestion and weight loss please head to the Science Guide and read The Migrating Motor Complex (MMC) and Hunger.

LET'S TALK GROUP CHECKLIST

As we move forward the conversation is going to be more forward moving...it's a good time to make sure you are up to speed on the basics.

Even though we switch up the Food Formula as we go through the 12 weeks, nailing the basics sooner than later is key, so that as we move forward, you are ready for each new week.

Be sure to review the basics so your path moving forward is as clear and calm as possible.

Here are some tips on how to navigate and keep up with the information in the Group:

1. **EMAILS**

   - Please note, we are not emailing out any information as everything is posted in the Facebook Support Group and can be found in Guides and Topics.

2. **CHECK INTO THE SUPPORT GROUP DAILY**

   - Be sure to use the GUIDES section to keep track of anything new being posted each day.

   - Most of the information in this Workbook has an accompanying video posted in the Group. Be sure to check into the group and watch all the videos as they can provide additional information and clarity.

   - Be sure to use the Topics in the Weight Loss Group option to review any previous posts.

   - And be sure to use the magnifying glass search at the top to search all posts on any topic. Make sure you are searching in the Group and not all of Facebook.

3. **WATCH THE DAILY CHECK IN VIDEO**

   - This is a short daily video where I check in and let you know what you need to know or focus on each day.

   - These are key as I talk in more detail on what you need to know each day and will become more instructional as we go.

4. **ASK YOUR QUESTIONS ON THE DAILY QUESTIONS POST**

   - The questions post is always pinned to the top of the page.

   - This is where you are to ask any questions you have. Ask as many as you need to be clear about the process.

   - Keep in mind, we are asking you to base those questions on the information you have already reviewed.

5. **WE KINDLY ASK YOU REFRAIN FROM SENDING US PERSONAL DM'S AND EMAILS**

    - Once the group is up and running, it is our primary focus. Asking questions in the group is the quickest way to get an answer.

    - You signed up to participate in the group format, so questions are to be asked in the group.

6. **WATCH ANY ADDITIONAL SUPPORT VIDEOS**

    - Each day, I will be posting info relevant to The Process that you will need to know. We are expecting people to keep up with new information. The videos are just as important as the written posts, so be sure to read the post as well as watch the video.

    - We are mindful of your time, but also mindful of the info you need to be successful.

7. **WATCH FACEBOOK LIVE**

    - Weekdays at 9 AM and Saturday at 10 AM EST, unless otherwise noted.

    - This is a live Q and A format. Gina answers as many questions as possible in the hour.

    - Although this is suggested, watching the Lives is not required...they can be of great value, help give greater insight into the process, as well as hearing input from previous members.

    - If you don't have time to watch them live, you can always listen to them as they are now available on the Weigh In with Gina podcast found on all podcast platforms.

If you have not watched them yet, please take time to check out these 5 videos found in the Facebook Group:

1. THE LIVY METHOD
2. THE FOOD PLAN
3. DETOX
4. THE SCALE
5. WEIGHT LOSS

THE FOUR MINDFULNESS QUESTIONS

WLBG's Learning and Training Assistant, Rebecca Ross-Zaiontz, who is down over 90lbs in her own journey, put this post together to help provide even further insight and some tips on how to practice the 4 Mindfulness Questions.

Asking yourself the Four Mindfulness Questions is an important aspect of learning to become in tune with your body and its needs.

Since we don't count, weigh or measure our food, asking these questions is what we use to guide us if we are feeling hungry or not, when we know we have eaten enough and if we know we are satisfied after finishing eating our meals and snacks. These questions are key to knowing when you have had enough food to support your body's changing hunger levels and needs.

LET'S DO A QUICK REVIEW OF THE FOUR MINDFULNESS QUESTIONS:

1. Before you eat, ask yourself are you hungry? Could you eat? Should you eat?

2. When serving or portioning out your food and before you eat...ask yourself, how much food do I feel I need to be satisfied? Is this portion enough for me? Would I feel satisfied if I ate it?

3. While eating your food, pay attention to how you feel and ask yourself are you getting full? How would you feel if you took a few bites more? How would you feel if you stopped eating?

4. When you are done eating, ask yourself how you feel? Do you feel full and if so, what is your definition of full? How do you feel physically?

Though these questions may seem very simple, and can sometimes be brushed off in importance, the thinking involved when asking them is more complex. These questions are the bridge to your mind-body connection. They move you from focusing on what you want to eat, to focusing on what your body needs to eat, to provide you with appropriate nourishment and ultimately lose weight through this process.

PAY ATTENTION TO PHYSICAL CUES

When asking yourself the four mindfulness questions, it is important to "get out of your head and mouth" and into your stomach. What we see and want, and what tastes good, is different from what we actually feel in our physical body. It is a shift of focus that will help support laying the foundation of giving our body what it requires.

Sometimes your body may give you a particular cue, sign or tell you that you have finished your meal. Some of those cues may be:

- Moving food around on your plate;

- Burping;

- Sighing;

- Sitting back in your seat; and

- Change of breathing patterns (e.g. it may slow as you come closer to being finished), etc.

For some, your body may provide you with a sign to help you know you are done, as mentioned above. For others, there will not be anything specific that stands out. Either way, it is important to really assess how your body is feeling physically, and zero in on your stomach to gauge your satisfaction while finishing your meal. It is not easy, and takes practice, so be kind to yourself as you navigate these questions.

PROGRESS OVER PERFECTION

For those of you that have always eaten until you have cleared your plate, or have used other dieting habits to structure knowing when you have had enough, the process of asking the four mindfulness questions will require lots of patience. It may take many tries to slowly figure out how you know you are done and satisfied. Make "progress over perfection" your focus in this process. It is okay to not get it right every single time, but it is also important to keep trying. At some point, it will become second nature that you will no longer have to formally ask the questions, and you will intuitively know what to do in portioning and preparing your food, and in knowing when you are satisfied with your meal and snack choices.

Asking the four mindfulness questions is an important aspect of this program to lose weight, and for continued success in maintenance, finally and forever.

Check out the accompanying video in the Facebook Group or the Livy Method App to watch how Rebecca walks through the Four Mindfulness Questions as she eats her lunch.

LET'S TALK STRESS & SLEEP

Because managing your stress and getting enough sleep can make all the difference when it comes to getting and keeping the scale moving.

Just by following the Food Plan, you are helping the body manage stress because this process helps to provide an environment where the body can focus on making change and addressing issues. It also helps to calm down the body internally with the routine and structure of how everything works together.

Although the basics of the Program; the food, the water and the supplements suggested all help with both stress & sleep...there are quite a few things above and beyond that you can focus on to help with this process.

Although the basics of The Program; the food, the water and the supplements suggested all help with both stress & sleep...there are quite a few things above and beyond that you can focus on to help with this process.

Keep in mind the goal isn't to make stress go away, it's more to recognize it, and help the body manage it, so you can capitalize on it.

TIPS FOR MANAGING STRESS:

1. Be consistent with the basics of the program; the food, water & supplements.

2. Practice deep breathing exercises.

3. Get outside and commune with nature.

4. Move your body more. Go for walks, dance, stretch, find activities you enjoy doing like sports and other leisure activities.

5. Get better sleep:

    • The body needs deep and REM sleep to repair, rebuild and detox. You will find that following The Program will help with your overall sleep, but there are things you can do now to help make a difference when it comes to the scale.

    • Take naps when you feel the need. Naps are not advised in general when trying to improve sleep patterns, but when it comes to this Process, the body is working so hard on making change so it needs all the sleep it can get.

    • Turn lights down low in the evening.

    • Use blue light glasses.

    • Stay off of screens or get off them earlier.

    • Take the calm magnesium before bed and adjust the dose as needed. It will work well with your natural melatonin production.

- Eat as early in the evening as possible.

- Keep a journal and glass of water beside the bed.

6.   Have a warm epsom salt bath before bed.

7.   Keep up with health issues. Seeing a Naturopathic doctor, Chiropractor, Acupuncturist, Massage Therapist and other health care providers can be helpful.

8.   Add in helpful supplements like Omega 3, and add good fats to your meals along with being consistent with magnesium and any stress tonics or immune boosters you have added in.

9.   Check your attitude and be self-aware of where you are at and what you are struggling with.

10. Look for things that bring you joy. Look to have fun with this process. Don't underestimate the power of having a good conversation with a friend or spending time with a loved one. Some good laughs over a glass of wine can do wonders for relieving stress.

Getting enough sleep, getting a handle on your stress and helping the body manage it, can help you to use your stress as an advantage in this process.

Stress will challenge your body and with your body working for you, it will rise to the occasion; which can lead to your body wanting to be stronger and healthier, which helps put a greater focus on fat loss.

Please take the time to head over to the Facebook Group or the Livy Method App and watch the quick video that accompanies this post..

LET'S TALK MAXIMIZING AND 20 QUESTIONS YOU CAN ASK YOURSELF

Are you trying to figure out why you might not be losing as much or as fast as you like...then this post is for you!

Even though it is still WAY too early in The Program to be concerned about the scale, as you move forward you may find yourself wondering or questioning if you are doing everything right or if there is anything more you can do to help the process.

These are some of the questions that I will ask you...if you ask me why things are not working the way you think they should. I suggest you grab some paper and a pen and go through it making notes on the areas that need your attention.

20 QUESTIONS TO ASK YOURSELF:

1. **Are you doing everything you can to create the ideal environment for your body to focus on fat loss?**

   - Are you following the program 100% day in and day out? Like actually, because there is a difference between trying and doing.

   - Are you being as consistent as possible, day in and day out?

   - Have you watched these videos that break down the rhyme & reason behind the order of the meals and snacks? 1. The Livy Method 2. The Food Plan 3. Let's Talk Detox 4. Let's Talk The Scale5. Let's Talk Weight Loss.

   - Are you making all the necessary tweaks and changes along the way?

   - We are not talking about kind of, or sort of doing, we are talking about maximizing what you are doing to your full potential. Literally doing all of the things you can and need to do to be as successful as possible!

2. **Has your body had time to consistently focus on fat loss?**

   - Meaning has your body had days and weeks of working the plan where nothing trumps the body from focusing on fat loss? Day in and day out? Or have you had some off days and/or off weekends?

     Be real about the time your body has had to focus on fat loss. Have you been hit or miss with following the food plan, sick or stressed out, or are there things you are dealing with physically or mentally that need to be taken into account?

3. **Have you had the flu or a cold or any other sickness that your body is dealing with, or had to deal with and focus on?**

   - Is your body more focused on healing right now?

- Are you taking antibiotics or meds that might mess with digestion or make you dehydrated that you need to address?

- Are you following the Sickness Protocol?

  Are you following the sickness protocol and helping the body heal so it can better focus on fat loss when the time comes?

4. **Are you managing your stress levels?**

- Are you meditating, deep breathing, stretching, moving your body, going for walks, taking epsom salt baths and so on...and if so for how long and how often?

- Have you read the post on managing stress?

  Are you really doing all you can do to help the body manage your stress? Stress can play a major role in preventing the body from focusing on fat loss. Managing your stress can go a long way in getting the scale to move.

5. **Are you getting lots of deep & REM sleep?**

- Are you helping your body prepare for sleep by eating earlier in the evening, going to bed earlier, keeping lights low and avoiding stimulants like TV and phone, taking a relaxing bath, keeping a journal by your bed?

- Have you read the post on Sleep?

  Are you actually making changes? Or still staying up late?

6. **Are you drinking enough water?**

- Not just a set amount, but adjusting it according to the body's demands? (Not just "more than before" or "lots" ...are you drinking enough, spreading it out and sipping on it for maximum absorption & utilization?)

- Are you adding in salt or trace minerals?

- Have you read all of the posts on water?

7. **Are you making your food as nutrient rich as possible?**

- Are you adding different elements to your meals? Veg, protein, greens, healthy fats? (Not just grabbing what's convenient or easy or what you like or love...think most bang for your buck and maximum value).

- Have you read the Making Your Meals Nutrient Rich Post?

8. **Are you exercising? Are you moving your body?**

- If so, what are you doing and how often? Are you getting your heart rate up?

- Are you making an effort to be more active?

- Are you taking the stairs, parking further away, participating and not just sitting on the sidelines?

- Are you factoring in time for the body to repair and rebuild any damage from your workouts?

- Have you read the post on exercise?

- Are you being mindful to move?

9. **Are you helping the body while in detox?**

- Watching portions, keeping food light, drinking lots of water, eating early at night and getting lots of sleep and maximizing everything else you can and need to do?

- Have you watched the Detox Video? Have you made an effort to really understand and help the body maximize when it's in detox?

10. **Are you taking medications or have health issues that need to be factored in?**

- You can lose weight regardless of your health issues but they will impact your journey, so if there are things you can do to help the body adjust to medications and help to address or heal the issue ...it will help when it comes to the scale.

- Have you looked into other ways you can help your body heal or deal with your health issues?

11. **Are you missing any organs?**

- Are you helping the body compensate for missing organs like adding in the bile salts or digestive bitters if missing your gallbladder?

- Are you going the extra mile to help your body manage any deficiencies?

12. **Do you have hormone issues you need to address? Or that needs to be factored in?**

- Are you seeing a specialist or adding in supplements that can help?

- Have you looked into addressing hormonal issues you may be dealing with?

13. **Have you had your blood work done?**

- Do you have any deficiencies that could be affecting your body's ability to function properly?

- Have you seen or checked in with your doctor recently?

- Have you had a physical done?

- Are you keeping up with appointments like your Chiropractor or Therapist?

14. **Are you taking all the supplements and taking them consistently?**

- They all work together and are all key in weight loss. Are you maximizing your efforts by adding them in?

- Are you consistent with taking them?

- Have you read all the posts on supplements?

15. **Is your body changing? Has your body been focusing on repairing and rebuilding and making change?**

   - What changes have you seen that can't be seen on the scale and is your body changing shape and size?

   - What are the non-scale victories you are experiencing?

Pay attention to what your body is focused on and when, the non-scale victories can be just as key because your body is always working and it can't all be about weight loss.

16. **Are you eating a lot of red meat and meat in general or are you switching between veg proteins, seafood, fish, and meat?**

   - Be mindful about those quality protein choices.

   - Are you making an effort to maximize your food choices?

   - Are you choosing the best options or are you stuck on eating what you like and love?

17. **Do you have any digestive issues?**

   - Have you added in the supplements to help?

   - Are you maximizing your food choices to help your body better digest and process your food?

   - Are you eating things you are sensitive to like dairy or gluten?

   - Are you keeping a journal and taking notes on how your body is responding to your food choices?

18. **Do you have issues with bowel movements and if so, what are you doing to address them?**

   - Have you added in the supplements to help and are you maximizing your food choices?

   - Are you making the best choices possible?

   - Are you adding leafy greens to your meals and mindful to add in fiber rich foods?

19. **Are you sabotaging yourself?**

   - Do you continue to get in your own way of reaching your goals?

   - Are you making choices that take you further away, not closer to, your goals?

   - Are you indulging in your frustration?

   - Are you having real conversations with yourself?

20. **Do you genuinely believe you have what it takes to follow through and finish?**

   - Do you have faith that you can lose the weight?

   - What is your WHY? What is motivating you to keep showing up and following through till the end?

   - Do you truly see yourself still here at the end?

HOW TO USE THE 20 QUESTIONS AS A TOOL:

These are the questions I ask people when they say things are not working or they ask me why or what else they can do to speed things up. I suggest you take these 20 questions and give yourself a grade or a mark out of 10.

For example, when it comes to water, how are you doing on a scale of 1-10?

Or, when it comes to trying to get a better sleep, how are you doing on a scale of 1-10? Or, on a scale of 1-10, how are you doing with being consistent?

You get the idea!

Give yourself a score out of 10 and if you don't score a 10, make a list of the things that you can do that can help you address those areas and maximize your efforts.

That way you can easily see the areas that need your attention and better focus on the things you need to step up your game.

PLEASE NOTE:

If you are struggling and wondering if you are missing something along the way, these questions will help you get to the bottom of it and figure it out.

With that said, sometimes you CAN be doing everything right and all the body needs is time...but this is a good checklist to make sure.

As we continue to move forward in the program and the focus becomes more about getting the body to focus specifically on fat loss, it is key that you maximize your efforts far beyond the food, water and supplements.

As you can see, there are a variety of factors that may be affecting how your body is responding along the way.

Being realistic about those factors will help you make the adjustments you need to keep moving forward so you can successfully lose as much weight as possible in the time frame we have.

If you would like to dig deeper into the psychology of maximizing your efforts, please head to the Science Guide and read The Psychology of Effort.

TROUBLESHOOTING: MAXIMIZING AND 20 QUESTIONS CHECKLIST

This checklist is designed to help you look for areas of opportunity and for the things you may not be doing but can still do! It is time to assess your situation, get real with yourself and assess where you are at!

Be sure to go through the Let's Talk Maximizing and 20 Questions post and review the information thoroughly. Once you have read that post, pull out this checklist and work one by one through each point giving yourself a checkmark on all the points that you are maximizing your efforts on. You can leave points that don't apply to you blank, or if they apply to you but you haven't implemented them yet. You can highlight areas of opportunity for you to reflect on and implement. Be sure to utilize the blank spaces for your own unique points you are hitting the mark on!

This checklist is meant to be used as a tool to help you work on areas that need your attention. You can revisit this checklist daily, weekly, or whenever you are feeling like there is more you can be doing! It is time to put your best foot forward, be all in, do all the things to set yourself up for success.

** Please note, some posts listed in the checklist will be coming out in the coming weeks. As you move through the Program week to week, you may want to revisit this checklist to see if there is any area that you can level up!

1. **Are you doing everything you can to create the ideal environment for your body to focus on fat loss?**

   - Are you hitting all meals and snacks?
   - Are you having token amounts of meals/snacks when you're not hungry?
   - Are you following the order of the food plan?
   - Are you eating your meals/snacks 30 mins - 3.5 hours apart?
   - Are you checking into the Facebook support group daily?
   - Are you reviewing the information repeatedly until you are super clear on it?
   - Are you asking yourself the 4 Mindfulness Questions before each meal/snack?
   - Are you open to your hunger levels changing day in and day out and adjusting portions accordingly?
   - Are you setting/hitting your water target daily & adjusting as needed?
   - Are you weighing and recording every day to track your body's natural fluctuations and patterns?
   - Are you having your morning lemon/ACV water?
   - Is the majority of your fluid intake flat water?

- Have you watched the 6 key videos that break down the rhyme & reason behind the order of the meals/snacks:
- The Livy Method
- The Food Plan
- Let's Talk Detox
- Let's Talk about the Scale
- Let's Talk Weight loss
- Let's Talk Hunger
- _____
- _____
- _____

2. **Has your body had time to consistently focus on fat loss?**
   - Are you consistently following the program day to day, week to week?
   - Are you consistently taking your supplements (if you have added them in)?
   - Are you consistently hitting your water target?
   - Is the majority of your fluid intake flat water?
   - Are you setting intentions in the morning?
   - Are you checking in mid-day?
   - Are you reflecting at night?
   - Are you consistently hitting all meals and snacks?
   - Are you making sure to have the "stars" at each meal/snack?
   - Are you having token amounts when you're not hungry?
   - Are you hit or miss with the food plan/water or all you in?
   - Are you making all meals and snacks nutrient-rich?
   - Are you managing your stress?
   - Are you getting quality sleep?
   - _____
   - _____
   - _____

3. **Have you had the flu or a cold or any other sickness that your body is dealing with, or had to deal with and focus on?**

- Are you on antibiotics or any medications that might mess with digestion/ make you dehydrated?

- Have you adjusted your water intake to help your body detox out the virus/process any medications you may be on?

- Are you working hand in hand with your Health Care Provider?

- Have you visited the Let's Talk Sickness post?

- Are you following the sickness protocol to allow your body the time to heal?

- Are you getting enough rest to allow your body the time it needs to recover?

- If you are sick, are you taking into consideration that the scale may be up simply because you are sick?

- Are you managing your stress?

- _____

- _____

- _____

4. **Are you managing your stress levels?**

- Are you allocating time for breath work?

- Are you stretching?

- Have you added in movement?

- Are you communing with nature?

- Are you having Epsom salt baths?

- Have you added in meditation?

- Are you being consistent with the basics of the program?

- Have you revisited the Let's Talk Stress & Sleep post?

- Have you revisited the Meditation and Stress Management Share page?

- Are you taking the time to journal to process and work through all the feels/associations that may come up during this process?

- Are you eating as early into the evening as possible?

- Have you added in the suggested supplements that can help aid in stress relief?

- Are you redirecting your thoughts?

- Are you looking for things that bring you joy?

- Are you keeping up with health issues and seeing health care providers?

- _____

- _____
- _____

5.   **Are you getting lots of deep & REM sleep?**

- Are you fostering good sleep hygiene?
- Are you avoiding blue light at night?
- Are you staying off screens/getting off them earlier?
- Are you diming/adjusting your lighting in the evening?
- Do you have a nighttime routine?
- Are you taking naps when needed?
- If you are having sleep issues (i.e., snoring, gasping) have you reached out to a sleep specialist?
- Are you reducing your caffeine intake if it is affecting your sleep?
- Have you added in the suggested supplements that can help aid in sleep?
- Have you visited the Let's Talk Stress and Sleep post?
- Are you keeping a journal beside your bed?

- _____
- _____
- _____

6.   **Are you drinking enough water?**

- Are you consistently hitting your water goal day in and day out?
- Is the majority of your fluid intake flat water?
- Are you adjusting your water intake according to your body's needs?
- Are you starting early in the day?
- Are you spreading it out, sipping and avoiding guzzling for maximum absorption and utilization?
- Do you have a good water bottle or cup you are drinking out of?
- Are you setting timers/reminders?
- Have you visited the Let's Talk Water post?
- Have you visited the Low Sodium post?
- Have you watched the Let's Talk Water with Dr. Andrew Feifer, MD video?
- Have you watched the segment with Dr. Andrew Feifer?
- Are you adding in Trace Minerals/ good quality salts to your water to avoid low sodium levels?

- Are you drinking the minimum amounts of water required for basic body functioning 2.7-3.5 L and adjusting according to your body's needs?

- Are you looking out for signs to know you have reached your optimal amount (You are no longer thirsty, lips/mouth no longer dry, bathroom trips have decreased)?

- Are you tracking your water?

- Have you measured the cup or vessel that you drink your water from to be sure of your intake?

- If your water is not appealing, are you adding in fresh fruit or lemon/lime juice?

- If drinking alcohol, are you adding in one extra cup of water per drink?

- _____

- _____

- _____

7. **Are you making your food as nutrient rich as possible?**

- Are you adding in healthy fats to your meals and snacks? (Avocados, nuts, seeds, olives, cheeses, good quality oils etc.)

- Have you visited the Nutrient Rich post?

- Have you visited the Let's Talk Oils post?

- Have you visited the Proteins, Carbs, and Fats post?

- Are you consistent with making sure you are getting each component of each meal/snack by adding different elements to your meals?

- Are you going for foods that are more bang for your buck and avoiding grabbing what is convenient?

- Have you eliminated breads?

- Have you eliminated crackers?

- Have you eliminated popcorn?

- Are you having protein-rich breakfast?

- Are you switching up your proteins?

- Are you switching up your fats?

- Are you being mindful of your sugar intake?

- Are you avoiding artificial flavours/colours/sweeteners?

- Are you avoiding low fat/no fat dairy products?

- Are you avoiding processed foods?

- _____

- _____
- _____

8. **Are you exercising? Are you moving your body?**

- Are you being more active?
- Are you taking the stairs instead of the elevator/escalator?
- Are you parking further away when buying groceries?
- Are you going for walks?
- Are you doing light movements throughout the day?
- Are you walking away from exercise feeling good and energized, not tired, taxed or drained?
- Are you choosing exercises that you enjoy and have a positive association towards?
- If you are lifting weights, are you lifting lighter and using higher repetitions?
- Are you giving your body adequate time to rest to repair and rebuild?
- Are you getting your heart rate up as high as you can for as long as you can even just for a few minutes to evoke your fight or flight response?
- Have you visited the Let's Talk Exercise post?
- _____
- _____
- _____

9. **Are you helping the body while in detox?**

- Are you consistent with your supplements?
- Are you consistent with hitting all meals and snacks?
- Are you eating those token amounts if not hungry?
- Have you visited the Let's Talk Detox post?
- Have you visited the Supporting the Body in Detox post?
- Have you visited the Let's Talk Double Detox post?
- Are you keeping portions on the smaller side to allow the body to stay focused on detox?
- Are you choosing easier to digest proteins?
- Are you keeping your heavier grains on the lighter side?
- Are you keeping leafy greens on the heavier side?
- Are you going to bed earlier?
- Are you taking Epsom salt baths?

- Are you getting in extra water?
- Are you lightly moving your body?
- If you are double detoxing, have you increased your calm magnesium?
- _____
- _____
- _____

10. **Are you taking medications or have health issues that need to be factored in?**

- Are you working hand in hand with your doctor, pharmacist, or health practitioner when it comes to your specific medical conditions/medications?
- Have you gotten your blood work done?
- Have you sought out a specialist/expert to address any health issues above and beyond what we are doing on the program?
- Have you adjusted your water intake to help your body process medications/health issues?
- Have you watched the Dr. Paul Hrkal expert chats for need-to-know information on all the other things you can do to help your body while dealing with health issues?
- Have you introduced (after speaking with your pharmacist/health care provider) any supplements that may help aid in inflammation?
- Have you visited the 4 Reasons Why your Scale May Be Slow to Move post?
- _____
- _____
- _____

11. **Are you missing any organs?**

- Are you working hand in hand with your doctor, pharmacist, or health practitioner when it comes to your specific medical conditions/medications?
- Are you helping the body compensate for missing organs by adding in supplements that may help? (Example: Bile salts/digestive bitters if you are missing your gallbladder)
- Are you going the extra mile to help your body manage any deficiencies?
- Are you supporting your body by getting quality sleep?
- Are you getting adequate hydration?
- Are you managing your stress?
- _____
- _____

- _____

12.   **Do you have hormone issues you need to address? Or that needs to be factored in?**

- Have you sought out a specialist/expert to address any health issues above and beyond what we are doing on the program?
- Are you moving your body?
- Are you managing your stress?
- Are you getting good quality sleep?
- Are your meals truly nutrient-rich?
- Have you added in breakfast?
- Is your breakfast truly protein-rich?
- Have you considered decreasing or eliminating your consumption of alcohol?
- _____
- _____
- _____

13.   **Have you had your blood work done?**

- Have you read the article on getting a blood test?
- Have you asked for further blood work testing?
- Are you working with your health care provider to interpret your results?
- Do you have any deficiencies that could be affecting your body's ability to function properly?
- Have you added in supplements that address any deficiencies?
- Have you had a physical done recently?
- Have you seen a naturopath?
- Have you seen a chiropractor?
- Have you seen a physiotherapist?
- Have you seen an acupuncturist?
- _____
- _____
- _____

14.   **Are you taking all the supplements and taking them consistently?**

- Have you visited and reviewed the Let's Talk Supplements post?
- Have you visited the Supplements FAQ post?

- Have you considered all the suggested supplements and added them in?
- Are you consistently taking them day in and day out?
- Have you given your body enough time to adjust to and adapt to the supplements you have added in?
- Have you watched the live segments with Naturopath Dr. Paul Hrkal?
- Have you booked a consultation with your pharmacist to discuss the suggested supplements?
- Have you created a personalized supplements schedule?
- _____
- _____
- _____

15. **Is your body changing? Has your body been focusing on repair and rebuild and making change?**
- Are your clothes looser?
- Do you have increased energy?
- Are your measurements changing?
- Are your rings looser?
- Has your complexion improved?
- Have you been taking photos each week to track your physical changes?
- Have you visited the Let's Talk Non-Scale Victories (NSVs) – Another Measure of Success post?
- Have you visited the Let's Talk Non-Scale Victories post from Week 6?
- _____
- _____
- _____

16. **Are you eating a lot of red meat and meat in general or are you switching between veg proteins, seafood, fish, and meat?**
- Are you maximizing your food choices?
- Are you having a good balance of plant-based proteins and animal-based protein?
- Are you being in tune and adjusting your proteins when you are in active detox? (Keeping harder to digest proteins to a minimum)
- Are you going for the most bang for your buck or are you going for what you like and love?
- Have you visited the Grocery List for a breakdown on the variety of protein on plan?

- Have you visited the proteins, carbs and fats post?
- Have you visited the Vegan Meal Share page?
- _____
- _____
- _____

17. Do you have any digestive issues?

- Have you seen your doctor regarding your digestive issues?
- Have you followed up with a naturopath?
- Have you visited the Let's Talk Supplements post?
- Have you visited the Let's Talk Bowel Movements post?
- Have you added in the suggested supplements that help aid in digestion?
- Are you maximizing your food choice to help your body better digest and process your food?
- Are you consistently adding in leafy greens?
- Are you journaling to track, and isolate any potential food allergies/sensitivities?
- Have you watched the segments with Naturopathic Dr. Paul Hrkal?
- _____
- _____
- _____

18. Do you have issues with bowel movements and if so, what are you doing to address them?

- Have you seen your doctor regarding your bowel movement issues?
- Have you followed up with a naturopath?
- Have you visited the Let's Talk Supplements post?
- Have you visited the Let's Talk Bowel Movements post?
- Have you added in the suggested supplements that help aid in constipation/loose bowel movements?
- Are you consistent with your water intake and adjusting it according to your body's needs?
- Are you adding in leafy greens to your meals?
- Are you being mindful to add in fiber rich foods?
- Are you moving your body?
- Are you being consistent with the food plan/water and allowing your body the time to adjust and adapt to the changes you have made?

- Have you added in Trace Minerals/good quality salts to your water?
- Have you been journaling your foods to track and isolate potential sensitives or triggers?
- _____
- _____
- _____

19. **Are you sabotaging yourself?**
- Have you identified your WHY?
- Are you making a list of positive affirmations/self-talk and revisit them often?
- Have you made a list of all the things you can turn to besides food?
- Have you identified your triggers/what you're afraid of?
- Have you visited the Self-Sabotage post?
- Are you journaling?
- Have you made a list of non-negotiables?
- Are you putting in effort to make life changing change or are you looking for a quick fix?
- Are you setting realistic goals?
- Are you being patient with the process?
- Are you taking responsibility?
- Are you avoiding accountability?
- Are you trying to rush results?
- Are you comparing your journey to someone else's?
- Are you future tripping (anxious for what the future holds)?
- _____
- _____
- _____

20. **Do you genuinely believe you have what it takes to follow through and finish?**
- Do you have faith that you can lose the weight?
- Have you established and solidified your WHY?
- Are you setting your intentions?
- Have you visualized yourself at your finally and forever?
- Do you see yourself at the end?
- _____

- _____
- _____

Now that you have reached the bottom of the checklist, take a moment to reflect. Look at all that you have accomplished!

If there are still boxes left unchecked that you need to revisit, try not to get caught up in the feels. Get excited! This means that there are more things you can be doing! Time to take action and continue working towards becoming the best you!

Finally and forever here we come!

MAXIMIZING YOUR FOOD CHOICES

In the first few weeks of The Program, we really want the focus to be on settling into the routine. We want you to nail the Basic Food Formula so moving forward you are super clear, since it is the basis of the whole Program. Now is the time where you can start leveling up your efforts by maximizing everything you are doing, including your food choices.

Here are some things to think about tweaking as we move along. Keep in mind these are things that some people never have issues with and can continue to see results without having to think about, reduce, or eliminate. You have to decide for yourself how relaxed or hard core you want to be.

This is also a post you might decide to revisit down the road, after we start focusing on fat loss, if the scale seems to be stuck or moving slowly. Sometimes the smallest tweaks can make all the difference.

If you want to be really all in or hard core here are some things to keep in mind around your food choices. Remember it's also okay to decide you want to take a more relaxed approach and aren't in that much of a hurry. But for those of you who want to see that scale move as much as possible in the time that we have, then Maximizing is what you want to be doing.

Here are some questions to ask yourself. They will help find areas where you might be able to make some tweaks and move on to the next phase of leveling up and maximizing your efforts.

1.   Are You Still Eating Bread?

When asked if you can have bread, I always say you "can", but will also always follow it up with "but it can slow down the process".

Here's the thing about bread...by following this plan we are trying to decrease the amount of insulin your body is using which will eventually help you feel more satisfied with smaller portions. Things like bread and pasta require a lot of insulin to break down, no matter what it's made of. It's the process of making it that has it turn to sugar too quickly which can affect blood sugar levels. What about crackers? Crackers are the same as bread. There is nothing in them that your body needs. They, like bread, are just a transport vessel, or a way to add some crunch. So, if you really want to maximize, best to skip the crackers.

2.   Are You Eating Popcorn or Snacking At Night?

We know it can take some of you a bit longer to make the changes you need to make to address your cravings, and no doubt many of you are still working on that. Popcorn was added in the beginning to help with that transition. Since then, we have talked about hunger and how to address it. Be sure to watch the Hunger Video if you haven't already. We have also talked about how the body doesn't need food after dark and how eating and snacking can mess with your sleep and prevent your body from doing the work it needs to do during sleep. So now that you understand that, it's time to cut the popcorn or any night time snacking. It absolutely will slow down the process if you continue to snack at night.

3. Are You Still Having Heavier Carbs At Dinner?

I know we all love our potatoes and rice at dinner time, but the body absolutely does not need these heavier carbs (energy foods) at night. Unless you do heavy workouts or play sports at night you should seriously think about cutting out those heavier carbs at dinner. Add them to your lunch instead, when you feel you need them.

4. Are You Eating Breakfast?

Or have you been purposefully skipping it because you are thinking less food (or calories) is going to get you ahead? Or maybe you just aren't making an effort to be organized and have something easy to grab if you are busy. Make no mistake, having a protein packed breakfast will absolutely help with the weight loss process. Although it is fine to skip it, and sometimes it's just going to happen, it will help with the process if you have it. Even if it's just one egg or a couple bites of chicken or a few spoonfuls of yogurt with hemp hearts.

5. Is Your Breakfast Truly Protein Rich?

When eating oatmeal, cereals, or yogurt with added sugar and/or fruit for breakfast are you making sure that protein is the star of the show? The more sugar and carbs in your breakfast the more protein and fat you need to counteract that. Be sure you are bumping up the protein as much as you can. Remember to choose foods that give you the most bang for your buck.

6. How's Your Sugar Adding Up?

Let's talk about sugar for a minute. Yes, we do say that it's perfectly fine to have it in your coffee or tea, on your oatmeal or yogurt, and also okay if you buy yogurt which already contains sugar. But ask yourself this: Am I having sweetened yogurt, then adding fruit to it and also having several cups of coffee or tea with sugar (when I say sugar, I mean any of the sweeteners we suggest such as honey and maple syrup). So, it's just about getting real with yourself and thinking about how much that sugar might be adding up over the day. Is there anywhere you could cut back? I'm not suggesting you eliminate sugar altogether but just be mindful of how much you are having in total.

7. Are You Switching Up Your Proteins?

Meat, especially red meat, can take the body a long time to digest. Not a reason not to eat it but have a look at how much meat you are eating and try switching up your proteins to include some fish and plant-based proteins, especially at dinner.

LET'S TALK ABOUT PRE-PACKAGED AND PROCESSED FOODS

Eating pre-packaged and processed food on occasion is nothing to worry about and can be a great convenience when needed. But just like I mentioned in regards to meat and sugar, how much is it adding up? Are you eating packaged food every day...every meal? Is there anywhere you can cut back if you feel you might be using processed foods too often?

Not all processed foods are created equal. Minimally processed foods are totally fine on plan. Things like canned beans, tuna, salad mixes in a bag, frozen vegetables etc. But when it comes to frozen prepared foods, jarred sauces, condiments etc. here are some things to keep in mind when checking the ingredients.

INGREDIENT LISTS

Reading ingredient lists can seem a bit overwhelming when you first start looking. Trust me, you will become a pro! You can go down a deep dark rabbit hole when it comes to the ingredients in processed foods, so here are some of the key things to keep in mind when shopping.

- Always avoid artificial colours, flavours or sweeteners, as well as hydrogenated oil or trans fats.

- Avoid products that contain high fructose corn syrup and watch that the ingredient list doesn't contain sugar named 3 (or more!) different ways to hide the fact that it is actually one of the top ingredients! There are over 50 different names for sugar on food labels. Some examples are: glucose, sucrose, dextrose, maltose, maltodextrin and anything ending in the word "syrup" or sugar such as "brown rice syrup" and "beet sugar".

- Always keep in mind that the first ingredient is the largest quantity ingredient and descends from there. The last ingredient being the smallest. So always look at the first 3 ingredients as they will make up the largest part of what you're eating.

- Choose the product with the least number of ingredients.

- Some of those "hard to pronounce" ingredients can be harmless and/or added in such small quantities that it's nothing to be concerned about. One example is Xanthan Gum. You might see that as an ingredient in salad dressings or sauces which is perfectly fine. It's added as a thickener and is harmless.

- When you are not sure about an ingredient, Google it on your phone while you are in the store. Or take a pic of the list and look things up when you're at home to educate yourself on what the ingredients are.

This post is another example of how to advocate for yourself. We are all adults and have to make our own choices. I am not here to hold your hand, but I am here to provide you with the information you need to make informed choices. It's your decision, and yours alone, how hard core or relaxed you want to be about this process.

To read more about the science behind how the foods we eat can benefit your body head to the Science Guide and read Hormones of Hunger and Satiety and Timing of Digestion, and Maintenance and the Microbiome.

LET'S TALK TRAVEL

How it can affect your weight loss journey and how to capitalize on it to work it to your advantage.

LET'S START WITH VACATIONS:

It's key to understand that life is stressful, too stressful for our still very primitive, working bodies. Stress can play a major role when trying to lose weight. Your body can only handle about 3 hours of stress max per day before your cortisol levels skyrocket and the next thing you know, you are exhausting your adrenals and then thyroid...leading to serious weight gain.

Members are always concerned about gaining weight when on holiday, when in fact it can do wonders for weight loss. Change in environment, less stress, abundance of good fresh foods, and some decent sleep can be exactly what the body needs to get the scale moving.

TIPS FOR TRAVEL:

- It starts at the airport...resist the urge to indulge in treats before you fly.
- Flying is super dehydrating and combined with high sugar is a recipe for carb cravings, serious bloating, and constipation once you land.
- Spend the money on healthy snacks so you are not inclined to eat the crackers and cookies or heavily salted meal they serve during the flight.
- Sometimes I buy the snacks but eat the plane food if it looks decent. I'm always happy to have the extra snacks when I land as they can come in handy.
- HYDRATE! The altitude when flying sucks the water out of you, leaving you epically dehydrated, and can have you craving carbs and sugar from the get-go...so once you land, work that water!
- Try to maintain regular eating habits as much as possible and look at any extras as just that, extra.

Generally, on vacay you are less stressed and more active in different ways, and you gotta eat right? So might as well choose foods that make you feel good.

- Don't stress if you can't follow the Plan. It's ok to have your food choices be off routine if your schedule is off from your normal weekly routine.
- Get back on track when you land by getting in the water and jump back on the basic Food Plan. As we move forward in The Program, we will be talking more about how to help the body recover from any indulgences.
- Have fun and remember you can't do anything in a week that can't be undone with a few days of being back to the basic Food Plan and on routine!

No one is expecting you to deprive yourself of any of the joys that come with being on vacation to be successful.

So, feel free to indulge. Just be mindful to balance it out. Try to get in fresh fruits, veggies and leafy greens when you can.

It's not unusual to lose weight while away on holiday, or to have your weight be up when you are back, only to have it drop right back down within days once you get back to following the Program or using Back On Track (a method which we will talk more about later). It's also not unusual for it to continue to drop to a new low afterwards.

LET'S TALK WORK FUNCTIONS AND WORK TRAVEL:

Traveling for work is not as fun but can be just as effective, as travel in general is very stimulating for the body.

- Focus on the water and keep things simple. Make the best choices you can when you can.
- Being on the road may mean making a few stops to the grocery store to pick up healthy snacks.
- Bathroom visits can be annoying, but keep in mind they are a means to an end and a key part of weight loss.
- Assess your day before it starts and plan when you can get the water in and when you need to hold off.

As we move forward, you will find it easier to plan.

TO RECAP:

Try to stay on Plan the best you can and don't stress. It's all about keeping it together when you can, balancing things out, planning ahead, and getting Back on Track when you are back.

Keep in mind that your body is not trying to or wanting to gain weight.

The key is to stay on track when you can and to be as consistent as possible. This way, you have some wiggle room for when you find yourself off or away from your daily routine.

- Consistency with supplements (if taking).
- Getting in your water when you can.
- Hitting all meals and snacks.
- Making your food choices as nutrient rich as possible.
- Being super mindful about portions, making sure you eat enough, but not too much, and allowing your body to stay focused on detox and fat loss instead of digestion.

Please take the time to head over to the Facebook Group or the Livy Method App and watch the quick video that accompanies this post.

WHAT PROGRESS IS REALLY LIKE

(An excerpt from the book Atomic Habits written by James Clear, I think will be sure to resonate)

Imagine that you have an ice cube sitting on the table in front of you. The room is cold and you can see your breath. It is currently twenty-five degrees. Ever so slowly, the room begins to heat up.

Twenty-six degrees.

Twenty-seven.

Twenty-eight.

The ice cube is still on the table in front of you.

Twenty-nine degrees.

Thirty.

Thirty-one.

Still, nothing has happened.

Then, thirty-two degrees. The ice begins to melt. A one-degree shift, seemingly no different from the temperature increases before it, has unlocked a huge change.

Breakthrough moments are often the result of many previous actions, which build up the potential required to unleash a major change. This pattern shows up everywhere.

Cancer spends 80 percent of its life undetectable, then takes over the body in months.

Bamboo can barely be seen for the first five years as it builds extensive root systems underground before exploding ninety feet into the air within six weeks.

Similarly, habits often appear to make no difference until you cross a critical threshold and unlock a new level of performance. In the early and middle stages of any quest, there is often a valley of disappointment.

You expect to make progress in a linear fashion and it's frustrating how ineffective changes can seem during the first days, weeks, and even months. It doesn't feel like you are going anywhere. It's a hallmark of any compounding process: the most powerful outcomes are delayed.

This is one of the core reasons why it is so hard to build habits that last. People make a few small changes, fail to see a tangible result and decide to stop. You think, "I've been running every day for a month, so why can't I see any change in my body?" Once this kind of thinking takes over, it's easy to let good habits fall by the wayside. But in order to make a meaningful difference, habits need to persist long enough to break through this plateau - what I call the plateau of latent potential.

If you find yourself struggling to build a good habit or break a bad one, it is not because you have lost your ability to improve. It is often because you have not yet crossed the Plateau of Latent Potential.

Complaining about not achieving success despite working hard is like complaining about an ice cube not melting when you heated it from twenty-five to thirty-one degrees. Your work was not wasted; it is just being stored. All the action happens at thirty-two degrees.

When you finally break through the Plateau of Latent Potential, people will call it an overnight success. The outside world only sees the most dramatic event rather than all that preceded it. But you know that it's work you did long ago when it seemed that you weren't making any progress, that makes the jump today possible.

You can see how this relates to what we are doing here, and as frustrating as it can be …keep going and you will get there.

LET'S TALK CELEBRATORY WEEKENDS

Because The Program covers a span of 3 months, chances are you are going to encounter those moments that are made for indulging. But with that said, they are nothing to worry about because The Program takes them into account.

We are expecting life to happen, and we are not expecting perfection, so it's more about how you want to feel after them. Meaning, how do you want to feel when it comes time to step on the scale Monday/Tuesday?

Here are some tips:

1. **Take some time to set your intention before the weekend. Are you going to stay on plan, choose to indulge, or take each day as it comes?**

   There is no right or wrong answer to this, it's all about how you want to feel when it's time to get back at it.

2. **Regardless of what you plan to do, make a point of eating normally the day of any big event or in anticipation of a big/festive meal.**

   Meaning, follow the Food Plan leading up to your event. This will help keep your digestive system stimulated so you are able to digest your meal better and feel less bloated after eating a bigger meal.

3. **Eating all meals and snacks leading up will prevent you from overeating.**

   This includes starting your day with higher protein like eggs or full fat greek yogurt, even if you usually skip it.

4. **Starting your day higher in protein and fat and minimal carbs, for example eggs over oatmeal, will get your body working harder from the get-go and give you more sustaining energy.**

   Also, if you have carbs like cereal, oatmeal or bread, you run more of a risk of setting yourself up to crave carbs and sugar all day and if there is lots of food around, you are going to be tempted by it if you are already craving it.

5. **Stay on top of your water and try to start earlier in the day.**

   If you are on the road or out and about, make a plan and get it in when you can.

And finally, keep in mind:

At the end of the day, even if you eat your face off, you can't make a pound of fat in a day, overnight, or weekend...so all you need to do is get right back on track the next day.

Please take the time to head over to the Facebook Group or the Livy Method App and watch the quick video that accompanies this post.

WEEK 4 GUIDELINES: DOWNSIZING

THIS IS NOT ABOUT CALORIES!

Week 4 has you downsizing portions in the moment so the body feels slightly unsatisfied (after weeks of eating to satisfaction) and drops fat to adjust. You are going to keep the same routine but make your portions smaller, keeping in mind hunger levels fluctuate day to day and portions are always about what they feel like, and not what they look like.

Here we are on Week 4 of The Program...the first question I must ask is, are you still with us?

If, for whatever reason you fell off or had to take time off, I want to assure you that at any given time you can pick up right where you left off. Although it is ideally followed day by day, The Program is designed in a way where you can follow at your own pace.

Any extra information you need is available in the Facebook Group and listed in descending order in the Guides section. You can also easily revisit old topics by using the Topics section.

NOW LET'S TALK DOWNSIZING

This is the point in the program that you have been working towards and waiting for.

You have spent the past 3 weeks addressing the needs of your body by giving it what it needs so it no longer feels the need to store fat.

You have worked hard to lay a strong foundation that you can now utilize to specifically get the body to focus on dropping fat!

Moving forward, this process is going to be all about the scale and your weight moving.

With that said, keep in mind we still have a long way to go and as we move forward, the formula you have been following is key and there is still very much a rhyme and a reason to each new step.

This week brings us to "DOWNSIZING"

Downsizing is my way of addressing portion sizes and decreasing the amount of insulin your body uses to break down food and ultimately, what makes you feel satisfied.

Things to keep in mind:

1.   **The routine of eating remains the same:**
   • Protein
   • Fruit
   • Lunch
   • Raw veg
   • Nuts/seed
   • Dinner

2.   **The kinds of foods you have been eating also stays the same.**

3.   **Supplements and water intake also stay the same.**

4.   **You are also still adding in and utilizing Bonus Snacks if you need them.**

5.   **The only thing that we are changing is the amount of food you are eating.**
   • You do this by simply decreasing your portion sizes by a few bites less.

The goal is to get the body's attention and because you have spent the last 3 weeks eating to the point of satisfaction, even the slightest decrease in portions will be felt by the body. The key is to SLIGHTLY decrease portions, so the body feels SLIGHTLY unsatisfied.

You may feel like your portions are already small enough, but keep in mind you have been eating to the point of satisfaction for the size of body you are now. When you lose weight, you will need less food to satisfy a smaller size frame...so think of it like you are feeding a smaller size you with less weight.

In decreasing your portions by even a few bites less, the body will not be happy. It will be looking for and asking for more. When you don't give in and give your body less than what it is used to getting to feel satisfied, it will respond by dropping the extra fat it doesn't need. It drops the extra fat in order to adjust to the amount of food you are eating so it can feel satisfied again.

HERE IS HOW IT WORKS:

1. You are going to decrease portions for each meal and snack by a few bites less than you were eating to feel satisfied.

2. The body will feel unsatisfied at the end of the day for a few days, this is normal and to be expected, so you may find yourself hungry when going to bed.

3. After a few days, when you don't give the body what it needs, it will start to drop fat to adjust the amount of food you are giving it.

4. Your body will then be looking to go into detox so it can drop the extra fat.

5. Afterwards, your weight will stabilize, and the body will spend a few days working to make the changes necessary to support the fat loss.

6. You are going to downsize for Week 4, and then for Week 5 you will be back to eating to satisfaction. Then you are going to repeat the process.

**WARNING: You do not want to decrease your portions too quickly or by too much. More is not more and will NOT get you ahead. It will only slow you down.

Again, the key is to SLIGHTLY decrease portions, so the body feels SLIGHTLY unsatisfied.

****FAQS ABOUT DOWNSIZING**

1. **Do we do this every day and for every meal and snack and for how long?**

   Yes, you are keeping to the routine and sticking to the same foods you have been eating but eat a few bites less of every meal and snack. And yes, do it every day for the week and then we will bring it back to satisfaction for Week 5. Then repeat the process for Week 6.

2. **What if my breakfast is already small?**

   - Breakfast isn't necessary to eat because when you wake up you are already full of energy and any food you eat will take hours to break down before it is of any use. So, when it comes to breakfast, if you do eat it, you are breaking the fast and turning your body on, getting it to work harder from the get-go by eating higher protein.

   - You can't feel unsatisfied from food your body doesn't need so if your breakfast is already small don't worry about downsizing. If you wake up hungry and have breakfast and have room to downsize, then you should downsize.

3. **Do we still use Bonus Snacks?**

   - Yes, if you have been using Bonus Snacks, you can still use them and downsize them as well. If you have not been using them, try not to.

   - PLEASE NOTE: Feeling unsatisfied is different than actually being hungry. You should NOT feel like you are starving or deprived, so don't hesitate to use the Bonus Snacks.

   - BUT, before you reach for that Bonus Snack, be sure to review the HUNGER Video and keep in mind even if you are hungry, adding more food to the lineup of food your body is already digesting is not always the answer.

4.   **What if I am feeling hungry at the end of the day?**

- The whole point is to feel unsatisfied, especially at the end of the day. You are decreasing the amount of insulin the body is used to getting. So, the whole point is to feel unsatisfied.

- Wrap your head around feeling unsatisfied for a few days and remind yourself this is just one phase of the program and not how it is going to be forever.

- This is just a first step in getting your body's attention, so it responds by dropping fat. You will and should be eating enough during the day, that even with the downsizing you do not need to be worried about not eating enough, even if you are hungry before bed.

5.   **Will I burn fat and ruin my metabolism by doing this?**

- NO. And for good measure, let me say that again, NO.

- This is why you spent the past few weeks giving your body what it needs so it no longer feels the need to store fat. This is also why the Formula and the routine is to stay the same. You will be eating every few hours so your body will be getting what it needs just not as much as it is used to.

6.   **What if I don't feel that I can do this?**

- Keep in mind this is a means to an end.

- You are going to have to go through different phases to get the body to work hard and drop the weight you have gained.

- Meaning, you have to understand there is a process and you need to do what you need to do to self-correct the weight you have gained. And because you have spent the last 3 weeks giving your body what it needs and strengthening the mind-body connection, your body is going to talk to you and let you know how it feels…when it's happy and when it's not. It's important to start trusting your body.

TO RECAP:

The goal for this week is to continue to be mindful and ask yourself those 4 questions before, during, and after eating and aim to eat to feel **SLIGHTLY** unsatisfied. The goal is also to be as **consistent** as possible with the Food Plan and **maximize** your efforts day to day (refer to Maximizing Post with the 20 Questions).

I have spent a great deal of my life researching the best way to lose weight in a way that adds benefit to the body. Where you not only lose your weight, but you do so in a way that is healthy, and you can easily maintain. I would never recommend anything that would be detrimental to your health or this process, so this phase is nothing to worry about.

You are working to lose weight but also to make your body healthier by increasing your metabolism, increasing your nutrient absorption, and boosting your immune system along with decreasing your insulin levels. This puts you in tune with what your body actually needs.

There is a lot to absorb here but also a super exciting time in the process so don't overthink it, have fun with it, and if you have questions make sure you let us know.

Please take the time to head over to the Facebook Group or the Livy Method App and watch the quick video that accompanies this post.

WEEK 4 GUIDELINES FAQS

1.   After asking the 4th mindfulness question, if I am feeling satisfied, should I aim to eat a little bit less so that next time I feel just a little unsatisfied?

In downsizing, the goal is to eat just a few bites less than what we need to be satisfied, so we are leaving ourselves feeling slightly unsatisfied but not still hungry. You can try making a portion similar to what you have been eating and then stop eating when you feel like you have almost had enough. Take note of how you felt or if you noticed any cues that signified you were done. If you find that you are satisfied 10 mins later, you know you can dig deeper and stop a little sooner next time. If after 10-15 min later you find you are still hungry and not just slightly unsatisfied, you can go back for a few more bites while paying attention to how you feel. Be open to your changing hunger levels at each meal and snack as the amount you eat can change day to day so assess at each meal and snack.

2.   Should I prepare a smaller portion or prepare my usual portion size and leave a few bites on my plate?

Hunger levels can change day to day and throughout the day. When packing your meals and snacks for the day, it's best to pack as you have been eating, and then be in the moment for each meal and snack asking yourself those four questions. If preparing your meal or snack from home, you can portion less after asking yourself "how is this portion for me" if you feel the portion is too much for you. Continue to ask those 4 questions and you may find that you may still leave a few bites behind. Again, be mindful of your hunger levels in the moment, as the goal is to leave yourself slightly unsatisfied.

3.   If I have never needed a bonus snack, should I continue to not eat them this week?

For those that have been using bonus snacks, you can still use them and downsize them as well. If you have not been using them, try not to add them into your routine. It is important to note that feeling unsatisfied is different than actually being hungry. You should not feel like you are starving or deprived, so don't hesitate to use the bonus snacks if you need them or if your lifestyle factors have changed or your level of activity has increased.

4.   How do I downsize my fruit snack if eating whole fruits such as an apple or a banana?

In downsizing, you are eating to be slightly unsatisfied. Some days you may only need half of a fruit to feel slightly unsatisfied, other days you may require more. Purchasing smaller sized bananas or slicing your fruit can also help when gauging your hunger level in the moment and ask those 4 questions and leave enough behind to feel slightly unsatisfied.

5.   How do I downsize my nut snack?

Continue to use the four mindfulness questions when serving your portions, even with your nut and seed snack. Keep in mind that your hunger levels can change day to day. Some days you will need more and some you will need less. If you are not hungry, be sure to still have a token amount, 4-5 bites with chewing in between.

6. My portions for snacks and meals are inconsistent. How do I figure out what a few bites less means for me?

It is normal to feel a bit unclear about what downsizing may look like for you. The fact that you are identifying that your portions for your meals and snacks are inconsistent shows that you are identifying that your hunger levels are changing. You are becoming more in tune with the portions you are eating. During downsizing, when you are eating, ask yourself, "How do I feel and how would I feel if I stopped now." If the answer is that you feel like you could eat a few more bites, then you can stop. If you find you are still hungry 10-15min later you can always have a few bites more.

7. I have not been feeling hungry, how do I downsize when I have already been taking token bites or eating very small portions?

As our portions naturally begin to adjust to the changes we are making, you may perceive your portions to be smaller than when you started. You still want to be getting in token bites and not purposefully making your portions too small. If you are not hungry and only having token amounts then you wouldn't have to downsize your 4-5 token bites. You still want to make your meals nutrient-rich so that each bite is giving your body what it needs.

8. Will downsizing impact my energy levels or exercise performance?

When following the Program, it can be normal for your energy levels to fluctuate, but for the most part our energy levels should be forward moving and downsizing will not impact your energy levels or exercise performance. Our bodies can keep us low energy when it is focused on other things, especially while in detox when the scale is moving, stress, being more active, your body fighting a cold or virus and for a variety of other reasons. Keep in mind even with downsizing we are eating 6 times a day, 8 times if adding in bonus snacks, eating nutrient rich meals and snacks and we are only eating a few bites less to feel slightly unsatisfied, so your body is still getting everything it needs throughout the day.

9. What is the difference between feeling hungry and feeling unsatisfied? Any tips for managing these feelings?

You have been eating to satisfaction for a few weeks now, so during downsizing even the slightest decrease in portions can be felt by the body. How we feel hunger varies from person to person and also depends on how loudly our body communicates its needs. Hunger can leave you feeling distracted until you give your body what it needs. Sometimes having a glass of water can calm your feeling of hunger. If so, it means your body was looking for water, but if you are really hungry that feeling won't go away until you eat. Feeling unsatisfied is a feeling that you could have eaten more, you are slightly unsatisfied with your meal or snack, you could have eaten a few more token bites, but you are not feeling distracted. Changing up your routine, having herbal tea or going for a walk are examples of how you can manage your unsatisfied feelings.

10. I struggle to differentiate between being hungry and wanting food because of the taste. Any tips?

As we move through the program, continuing to ask those 4 questions, and recognizing how our bodies feel after eating you will be able to differentiate true hunger and satisfaction from wanting more of something because you like the taste of it. You can always save some of your food to enjoy later. Reminding yourself of your end goal can help to keep you focused on not eating more than what is needed in the moment.

LET'S TALK FAT

We talk a lot about fat in The Program but always in very general terms; like helping the body get rid of fat or focusing on fat loss. But we don't really talk about the different kinds of fat and what fat is used for.

Did you know there are actually three different types of fat cells in the body: white, brown, and beige. They can be stored as essential, subcutaneous, or visceral fat.

Each type of fat serves a different role. Some promote healthy metabolism and hormone levels, while others contribute to health issues.

LET'S TALK WHITE FAT:

White fat is what makes up most of the fat in your body and is also what makes you visibly fat.

It's made up of large, white, cells that are stored under the skin or around the organs in the belly, arms, buttocks, and thighs. These fat cells are the body's way of storing energy for later use.

White fat cells contain large lipid droplets and are involved with the body's endocrine system:

- Metabolism
- Growth and development
- Emotions and mood
- Fertility and sexual function
- Sleep
- Blood pressure

White fat cells are found just beneath the skin (called subcutaneous fat). It's the type of fat that makes you look fat and tends to accumulate around the hips, butt, thighs and arms and is attributed to cellulite.

Contrary to popular belief, this is not the fat that is linked to health issues. That title belongs to visceral white fat.

WHAT IS VISCERAL WHITE FAT?

Visceral fat is the fat that accumulates around the belly, located in the abdominal cavity, and intertwined around your organs. It's this kind of fat that can increase your risk for a number of diseases.

Now, believe it or not, there is a third kind of white fat, this fat is called ectopic fat.

Ectopic fat refers to the fat that the body stores when it runs out of places to store it. Usually found in locations not normally associated with fat storage, like your liver (Fatty liver for example).

Ectopic fat can interfere with cellular function in the body, which, in turn, can affect organ function. Some of you may know it well as it's also associated with insulin resistance.

Although the body needs some white fat to function, too much white fat can have detrimental effects, and can put you at risk for health issues like type 2 diabetes, heart disease, high blood pressure, stroke, hormone imbalances, pregnancy complications, kidney disease, liver disease & cancer.

LET'S TALK BROWN FAT:

Brown fat is found in smaller quantities in the body than white fat. It gets its brown colour from iron, is denser than white fat and helps to regulate body temperature. This process is called thermogenesis. During this process, the brown fat also burns calories.

Brown fat tends to be stored around organs like your heart, liver, kidneys, and pancreas, as well as your shoulder blades and spinal cord.

Babies, for example, are born with a lot of brown fat to help regulate body temp (stored between shoulder blades).

This type of fat burns fatty acids to keep you warm. This is also why when following a program like The Livy Method, you may find ketones in your blood while losing weight.

This is not indicative of the body being in ketosis like people tend to believe, but more so of the body naturally burning fat as it's designed to do for purposes other than weight loss.

LET'S TALK BEIGE FAT:

Ok, so here's where things get a bit weird.

Beige fat is basically white fat that has been coerced by the body to act more like brown fat.

Beige fat (also known as brite fat), is relatively new in terms of research. It's believed that certain hormones and enzymes get released when the body is "stressed", for example when you are cold or even when you exercise, which can cause the body to convert white fat into acting more like brown fat.

These beige fat cells can do the job of white and brown fat cells. Similar to brown fat, beige cells can help burn fat rather than store it.

The question now of course would be how do we increase brown or beige fat cells in the body and decrease white fat cells?

The Program itself addresses the white fat cells so you already have that covered!

In terms of increasing brown fat cells, more and more research is being done on the effects of cooling your body temperature, as exposing your body to cold temperatures may help recruit more brown fat cells.

For example, taking a cold shower or having an ice bath. Turning the thermostat down or going outside in cold weather are other ways to cool your body and possibly create more brown fat.

Just keep in mind before you start purposely freezing your butt off, that the research on this is still fairly new!

Other methods suggested for increasing brown fat cells include eating more often (being sure to eat enough) and exercising to help increase metabolism, which of course we also cover on plan.

Now that we have talked about the different kinds of fat...Let's talk about the three different ways the body stores fat.

1.   **Essential Fat:**

Essential fat is necessary for a healthy, normal functioning body. This fat is found in your brain, bone marrow, nerves & membranes that protect your organs.

Essential fat plays a major role in hormone regulation, including the hormones that control fertility, vitamin & nutrient absorption, and regulating body temperature.

2.   **Subcutaneous Fat:**

Subcutaneous fat refers to the fat stored under the skin. It's a combination of white, brown & beige fat cells. Most of your body fat is subcutaneous.

It's the fat that you can grab & pinch. It's the fat that makes you "look" fat. Most notably, subcutaneous fat is the body's method of storing energy for later use.

3.   **Visceral Fat:**

Visceral fat, also known as "belly fat," is the white fat that's stored in your abdomen and around all of your major organs, such as the liver, kidneys, pancreas, intestines, and heart.

Too much visceral fat can increase your risk for health issues like diabetes, heart disease, stroke, artery and even some cancers.

LET'S TALK BENEFITS OF FAT:

Because as much as fat gets a bad rap, it does have its uses and benefits, such as:

- Regulating body temp
- Helps to balance hormones
- Key for reproductive health

- Ensures vitamin storage
- Important for brain health & neurological function
- Essential for healthy metabolism
- Helps to balance blood sugar

NOW LET'S TALK RISKS ASSOCIATED WITH FAT:

Having too much white fat, particularly white visceral fat, can be detrimental to your health & can increase your risk for the following health conditions:

- heart disease
- stroke
- coronary artery disease
- atherosclerosis
- pregnancy complications
- type 2 diabetes
- hormone imbalances
- some cancers

LASTLY, LET'S TALK WHAT HAPPENS WHEN YOU GAIN AND LOSE WEIGHT:

Contrary to popular belief, the total number of fat cells you have remains unchanged when we gain and lose weight. When you gain weight, fat cells expand and then shrink when you lose.

You cannot get rid of fat cells unless you have them surgically removed by way of liposuction for example. Key to note here, when you have liposuction and gain weight back, it will come back in the places where you still have fat cells, which can make for a very odd appearance.

Like all cells, fat cells do die off but are replaced with new ones every year. Once you become an adult (age of 20) the number of fat cells you have essentially stays the same.

Keep in mind this info doesn't really affect your weight loss journey and there is nothing that needs to be done with it. It is more of an FYI in the hopes of helping you guys have a deeper level of the complexities of fat & fat loss.

To read more in depth about Fat please read The Science of Fat and Fat loss in our Science Guide.

LET'S TALK SUPPORTING THE BODY IN DETOX

Throughout this Process, we have been, and will continue to use, a variety of similar techniques to help keep the body focused on detox.

"Detox" being the loose term I use to describe when the body is specifically focused on and in the process of dropping/releasing fat.

Moving forward, you will hear me talk about Supporting the Body in Detox. This refers to things you can do to help the body stay in detox for as long as possible to better capitalize on fat loss.

Outlined below are the different techniques. They are all quite similar. What sets them apart from each other is the **INTENTION** behind them, as sometimes the smallest tweak can make all the difference.

This can seem a bit confusing but is really nothing to be concerned about. This just helps to make the program a more individual process along the way. Think of it as a way to stay on top of what's happening day to day to keep things moving forward and the scale moving down.

Even if you just followed The Program as is, you will have success, so there is nothing to stress about. A lot of the time when implementing these techniques, your body is already doing what it needs to do. This just helps give you an idea of how you can step up and support the body even more.

Since we are working on DOWNSIZING, let's talk about how this would relate to Week 4.

The technique behind downsizing is to follow The Formula but to purposely eat a few bites less to leave yourself feeling unsatisfied.

The intention behind this is to get your body's attention and get it to take action. Do this by:

- Being consistent with supplements
- Getting extra water in
- Hitting all meals and snacks
- Purposely eating smaller portions to get the body's attention and piss it off
- Adding in bonus snacks and using heavier carbs at lunch and dinner as needed but still eating to feel unsatisfied in the moment
- Eating dinner as early as possible
- Going to bed as early as possible
- Maximizing

When in DETOX (scale moving), the focus then becomes:

- Being consistent with supplements
- Getting extra water

- Hitting all meals and snacks
- Eating even if you are not hungry, eat a token amount to stimulate the digestive system and keep things moving
- Keeping portions on the smaller side to allow the body to stay focused on detox
- Being lighter on the carbs and heavier on the leafy greens at lunch and dinner
- Choosing easier to digest protein like fish as opposed to red meat.
- Eating as early as possible
- Going to bed earlier to help improve quality of sleep
- Moving your body but keeping it light, think walks after dinner. Nothing too heavy that will cause damage and sidetrack the body into focusing on repairing and rebuilding instead of detoxing.

When the scale starts to move, the intention here is to keep the body focused on detox for as long as possible to capitalize on fat loss.

1.   When your MENSTRUAL CYCLE hits:

This is a great opportunity for you to capitalize on the body's natural detox process. Your period each month is a time where the body looks to reset, to balance hormones and to get rid of any fat it doesn't need. The goal is to:

- Be consistent with supplements (Increase the calm mag)
- Drink extra water
- Hit all meals and snacks
- Keep portions on the smaller side to allow the body to stay focused on the task at hand
- Go lighter on the carbs and heavier on the leafy greens at lunch and dinner for increased roughage to help keep moving things in and out
- Eat dinner as early as possible
- Go to bed earlier to help the body get extra rest

The intention here is to help the body stay focused on the task at hand and capitalize on the natural detox process.

2.   When you are SICK:

Most people associate being sick with weight loss, when in fact with This Process, it's normal for your weight to go up (not real gain). Sickness always brings a natural detox, so there is no need to force the Formula when the body is already focused on the elimination process.

When fighting a cold or flu or any virus, the body will retain water and keep you low energy while trying to get the virus out. It will also retain and require a lot of water, which leads to the scale being up.

Also, when sick, your body won't be interested in eating, so it's normal to not be hungry.

The intention here is to help your body recover as quickly as possible and to give it what it needs so you can capitalize on the natural detox process that comes with sickness:

- Be consistent with supplements
- Add in immune support, if needed
- Add in extra water
- Be in the moment with meals and snacks, if not hungry, skip
- Keep portions on the smaller side to allow the body to stay focused on the task at hand, which is getting the virus out
- Avoid heavier carbs and go for easy to digest foods like soup to help keep energy up but not divert resources from healing
- Go to bed earlier and take naps to help the body get the rest it needs to heal

Once your appetite comes back, you can get back on track and then resume The Program. Typically, weight will drop back down and keep dropping once you start to feel better.

As you can see, the Process is similar with each situation but the intention is different. For example, when it comes to portions:

- When **Downsizing**, you are mindful of portions and keep them on the lighter side to piss the body off and get it to take action
- When on your **Menstrual cycle**, you are mindful of portions and keep them on the lighter side to help the body stay focused on the task at hand
- With any kind of **Sickness** or event that affects your appetite, you are mindful of portions and keep them on the lighter side to help the body stay focused on healing
- **Detox** in general...Once the scale is moving, you are mindful of portions and keep them on the lighter side to help the body stay focused on detox

Keep it simple, check in on where your body is at and what it is focused on, and be sure to use each technique as needed. Don't overthink it, show up day to day and assess where you are at and what your body needs in the moment to help keep things moving.

Please take the time to head over to the Facebook Group or the Livy Method App and watch the quick video that accompanies this post.

To learn more about the science behind our body's natural detox process please head to the Detox post in the Science Guide.

LET'S TALK SKIN AND WEIGHT LOSS

It's key to understand that when it comes to loose skin and weight loss, it's all about how you lose it. I talk about this more extensively in the Detox Post.

When doing a traditional quick fix, burn the fat diet, you can lose weight fast. The downside is that the body takes fat from where it least needs it. This creates "pockets" or certain areas where you lose more fat than in other areas.

This is great because you can look like you have lost a lot of weight in certain areas...but it's not so great for the skin.

The key to minimizing loose skin is how you lose your weight. When you detox the fat out naturally by peeing, pooping, breathing, and sweating, you release the fat in layers. This overall gradual loss, which we use with the Livy Method, makes it much easier for the body to regenerate your skin around your new sized body frame.

Here are my top tips for helping the skin during and after weight loss:

1. Dry brushing

It's like a loofah except you don't get it wet. Dry brushing is beneficial because it stimulates the nervous system, helps to increase overall circulation, but more importantly, helps to remove dead skin cells, which promotes regeneration and leaves the skin feeling invigorated.

Most experts recommend dry brushing in the morning, rather than before bed, because they believe it has energizing qualities.

Start at your feet and brush upward toward the heart. Similarly, with your arms, begin at the hands and work upward. Use firm, small strokes upward or work in a circular motion. For the stomach, work in a clockwise direction.

Dry brushing or any kind of exfoliation should be gentle on the skin, so avoid being too harsh. Ideally, dry brushing is done 1-2 times a week.

2. Collagen

Collagen is what keeps our skin from sagging, giving us that plump & youthful look. Collagen starts to decrease in the body by 1% per year after the age of 21.

Adding in a collagen supplement like the "Withinus" brand (use code **GINA15**) or the "Deep Marine Collagen" (use code **GINA20**) helps to promote the production of proteins that help structure your skin, including elastin and fibrillin.

Collagen is also found in the connective tissues of animals. Thus, foods like chicken skin, pork skin, beef, and fish are natural sources of collagen. Additionally, foods that contain gelatin, such as bone broth, also provide collagen.

Here is a list of some more food sources that either contain collagen or help promote collagen production by providing key building blocks.

- Fish
- Chicken
- Egg whites
- Citrus Fruits
- Berries
- Red and yellow vegetables
- Garlic
- White tea
- Leafy greens
- Cashews
- Tomatoes
- Bell peppers
- Beans
- Avocados
- Soy
- Also herbs high in collagen include: Chinese knotweed, horsetail, gynostemma
- Herbs that help to produce collagen include: gotukola, bala, and ashwagandha

It's hard to get what the body needs naturally so adding in a supplement is your best bet when concerned about skin issues.

Keep in mind, not all collagen supplements are created equal.

Although there are no established guidelines regarding how much collagen you should take, studies show that dosages between 2.5–15 grams of collagen peptides per day are considered safe and effective.

A better-quality product like Deep Marine or Within-Us Marine sourced collagen recommends 5 grams of powder, whereas less expensive brands might have you taking more. Something to consider when purchasing your product of choice.

You may also want to read the ingredients label, as some products may contain additional ingredients to support skin health, including silica, hyaluronic acid, or vitamin C.

Finally, be sure to opt for high quality supplements purchased from a reputable retailer. As with most things, you get what you pay for.

3.   Use natural oils and creams.

Because fat stores are full of toxins from the products you use, the foods you consume and also from the environment, you want to avoid adding in more toxins by using creams on your skin that contain perfumes, dyes and synthetic ingredients.

When a cream, lotion or oil is applied to the skin, the ingredients are absorbed into the bloodstream. From there, they have a direct effect on many of the body's processes. Meaning, if the ingredients are beneficial, they'll have beneficial effects. If they are a detriment, they'll have adverse effects on the body.

Ingredients to look out for include: parabens, sulfates, petrochemicals, synthetic dyes, propylene glycol, and triclosan.

Some of my favorite natural oils to use on your body:

Olive oil

The antioxidants in olive oil help to soothe the skin and repair damaged cells due to excessive dryness. It can also help in preventing age related wrinkles and fine lines.

Grapeseed oil

Because it contains high levels of vitamin E, this oil may contribute to better skin and reducing UV damage.

Coconut oil

Coconut oil is a powerful antioxidant that works to eliminate free radicals that can damage your skin. In addition, coconut oil hydrates and moisturizes your skin, which prevents sagging. Coconut oil can clog pores so best to use on the body and not the face.

Almond oil

It's highly emollient, which means it helps to balance the absorption of moisture and water loss. Because it is also antibacterial and full of vitamin A, almond oil can be used to treat acne and some skin conditions. Its concentration of vitamin E can also help to heal sun damage, reduce the signs of aging, and fade scars.

Lastly, the things I didn't mention are all the things you are doing on Plan. Making nutrient rich food choices, adding in supplements, being hydrated, moving your body, managing your stress and getting quality sleep!

Keep in mind, right now you have your body focused on making change. A lot of the repairing of the skin happens after you have lost weight, when your body is working on stabilizing & maintaining your weight.

Just like when you cut your hand & your body repairs the skin, the same happens when you lose weight. Although it takes a while, your skin will regenerate around your new frame and anything you can do to help it along the way adds up and can make a difference.

In the coming weeks, we will be talking more extensively about skin care and skin issues with skin care experts, where you will have the opportunity to ask further questions about things like cellulite, crepey and loose skin, and skin care in general, so be sure to check into the group for that.

Please take the time to head over to the Facebook Group or the Livy Method App and watch the quick video that accompanies this post.

WEEK 5 GUIDELINES: MAXIMIZING AND EATING TO SATISFACTION PART 2

Introducing MAXIMIZING! This is all of the other things you can do to help the body focus on fat loss besides food, water, and any supplements..

- Duration - 7 Days
- Intention - to have all of your choices fall in line with your goal.
- Goal - to help the body focus on fat loss and help it follow through and get the fat out.

This is an exciting time as we embark on the middle part of The Program. I hope you are enjoying the process and still as motivated as the day you started!

Over the past month, the strong foundation has been laid and the hard work is done. Now is the time to focus on the scale and maximize everything you can do to get & keep that scale moving!

FIRST THINGS FIRST:

As always, I want to remind you that even if you have fallen off plan, are behind, or have lost your motivation, it's not too late to get back on track.

Remember, this program takes into account off days, off weeks, holidays, and also those frustrating days where you feel like throwing in the towel.

If you are not sure how to get back at it, please let us know and we'll help you get back on track!

NOW, LET'S TALK WEEK 5!

This week we are taking a break from Downsizing and instead will be Maximizing and Eating to Satisfaction.

This means digging your heels in and relentlessly doing everything you can do to get the body to focus on detox, and stay in detox mode for as long as possible.

It means stepping up your game like never before, and taking everything you have learned and not just implementing it, but also building on it so you can take things to the next level.

The goal is to take things to the NEXT LEVEL when eating to satisfaction, and maximizing to help the body focus on, and follow through on getting the body to release the fat.

This week also helps to continue to naturally decrease your insulin sensitivity levels and get even more in tune to your portions.

Think of this week as taking everything you have learned up to this point and using it to maximize your efforts and help the body focus on fat loss.

Week 5 is a key week because it's a jumping off point for the next downsizing week.

WHEN MAXIMIZING YOU ARE FOCUSING ON:

- Drinking your water and adjusting day to day.
- Consistency with supplements (if taking).
- Hitting all meals and snacks.
- Making your food choices as nutrient rich as possible.
- Being super mindful about portions, making sure you eat enough, but not too much, and allowing your body to stay focused on detox and fat loss instead of digestion.

PLEASE NOTE: Eating to Satisfaction now in Week 5 is with a slightly different intention than in the first few weeks.

For week 5, we are still asking the 4 Questions asked with mindfulness:

- Before you eat, ask yourself if you are even hungry?
- How am I feeling while eating?
- How do I feel when I'm done?
- How do I feel 10 mins later?

You asked these questions during Mindfulness & Downsizing, and now you will do the same with Satisfaction & Maximizing.

The goal is to not feel full or hungry. It's to feel like you have had JUST ENOUGH or could eat a bit more.

If you find that 10-15 minutes after eating to satisfaction you feel full, then play around with the portions. Eat what you think is enough and if you are too hungry, you can always eat more later.

We are trying to lose weight and continue to decrease insulin sensitivity levels, so portions are key.

You will have noticed that after the past few weeks your portions may have naturally decreased. They will continue to be a focus, so make sure you are tuning in to them to avoid overeating.

There is a lot to focus on during this week.

THINGS TO NOTE:

Expect the scale to move.

Remember each stage and phase is meant to get the body's attention and to get it to take action. Each week is designed to help get the body into detox and keep it there as long as possible, so your body can drop fat.

- Step 1: Get the body to focus on fat loss.
- Step 2: Create the perfect environment for the body to follow through with fat loss.
- Step 3: Support the body in detox and keep it there for as long as possible.

Obviously, there will be plateaus or stabilizing periods as they are a normal part of the process, but from this point moving forward, you should expect to see the numbers on the scale drop, even when eating to satisfaction and regardless of the stage and phase you are in.

Sometimes, there is a delayed reaction before the numbers show on the scale, so stick with it and keep working. Think of the end game. Getting caught up on the day-to-day numbers can sidetrack you and impact your final number.

In Week 5, you are moving from Downsizing to Eating to Satisfaction while maximizing everything you can do to keep the body focused on detox.

This is the week where people always ask if they will lose or even gain weight by going back to eating back to satisfaction.

Weight loss isn't always about eating less.

At this point, the body wants the fat gone as much as you do. The goal is to continue to support the body and give it what it needs, so it can focus on fat loss and get the fat out.

This Program is designed to help you lose weight. So, you don't need to spend any time worrying about gaining or not losing if you are following it.

This Program is successful because of my approach to weight loss. So, although it may look or feel different from the diets you have done before, that's because this isn't a diet. It's a method for helping address why the body is storing fat, so you can help it focus on fat loss and lose weight finally and forever.

Some side notes:

- If you have been off track, this is a great week to turn things around and get back on track by eating to satisfaction and continuing to max out everything you need to do to keep things moving.

- There is never a reason to go back and repeat steps. As long as you are attempting to make the changes you need to make each week, there is no need to repeat steps. Repeating steps can just end up confusing your body and make you feel like you're spinning your wheels.

- The Program is meant to be very forward moving where one week leads into the next. The best thing you can do is to take things day by day and maximize your efforts along the way.

MOVING FORWARD:

There is lots to talk about in the coming days and some exciting weeks ahead, so continue to keep up with the Guides and check into the Facebook Group day to day.

Moving forward, the Check In Video is going to be more on the instructional side, so be sure not to miss it as I will be reviewing key elements of The Program day to day.

It's going to be a fun few weeks as you get closer and closer to reaching your goals! Continue to show up to maximize each day!

Please take the time to head over to the Facebook Group or the Livy Method App and watch the quick video that accompanies this post.

WEEK 5 GUIDELINES FAQS

1.   What is the difference between this week and Week 3: Consistency and Mindfulness?

Week 3 the goal was to be as consistent as possible to allow the body time to calm down and adjust from the changes you had made over the first few weeks. Follow the food plan, make nutrient rich choices, continue to eat to satisfaction, add in any supplements, work the water and we were introduced to the 4 mindfulness questions. The goal this week is to take things to the next level when eating to satisfaction, and maximizing to help the body focus on, and follow through on getting fat out. You are continuing to ask those 4 questions and are back to eating to satisfaction with a slightly different intention than in the first few weeks. The goal is to not feel full or hungry. It's to feel like you have had just enough or could eat a bit more.

2.   If I am maximizing, should I take out the heavier carbs even if my body wants them?

You are looking to continue to ask yourself those 4 questions and be in tune with what your body is asking for. If you feel your body needs the heavier carbs then you can add them in. The best time to add them is to your lunch so that your body can use the energy from them throughout the day.

3.   If I did not maximize downsizing last week, should I redo it?

Recognizing that you could have done better is a great sign that you are becoming more in tune with your portion sizes. It is not recommended to go back and redo weeks unless you were on a break from the Program or fell off completely and didn't downsize any of your meals or snacks. If this is the case then yes, you want to go back and pick up where you left off, and move forward completing each day of the week.

4.   What is the difference between being full and being satisfied?

Many members before this Program didn't have a clear understanding of what it means to feel satisfied. For many, eating to satisfaction could mean eating until the plate is cleaned, or needing to loosen their belt. By following the Food Plan, asking the four questions and becoming mindful of how you are feeling after eating will all help with learning the difference between full and satisfied. Being satisfied means that 10-15 minutes after eating you are not hungry and feel like you haven't eaten. You are just left feeling satisfied. Whereas being full can leave you feeling bloated and uncomfortable with a feeling that you ate too much. This Program is designed to strengthen your mind body connection so that moving forward your body will let you know where it's at by how it feels.

5.   I have still not lost a large amount of weight, is this normal?

It can be normal for your weight to have not moved or to have only moved slightly. In the first few weeks, the focus is on giving the body what it needs so that the ideal environment can be created for the body to shift its focus onto fat loss. The fact that you have lost weight lets you know that your body is willing to drop the weight. Continue being consistent with your food, water and supplements and doing all the things to keep supporting your body. Pay attention to non-scale victories, as they are a sign that your body is busy working behind the scenes and making changes. Many members have found that they've seen bigger drops on the scale in the latter half of the program.

6.   If I went off Plan for a week, should I repeat that week or move forwards to the next one?

This Program is forward moving where each week leads into the next, so it's important that you follow the Program and put the time into completing the 91 days of the program. If you didn't follow the program at all then you will want to go back to where you left off and move forward from there. If you kind of followed the week but had an off day or added in extra bits and bites, it's best to keep moving forward with the group and work at being all in moving forward.

LET'S TALK SELF-SABOTAGE

As much as some of you want to lose weight, at this point in The Program you might start looking for a way out, a reason to give up, a reason to quit... and that's where self-sabotage can rear its ugly head. Rest assured it is perfectly normal and very common, but you will never be able to reach your weight loss goals if you don't take some time to look at this and start to pick it apart.

WHAT IS SELF-SABOTAGE?

Self-sabotage is choosing (consciously or unconsciously) to do something that undermines your success and gets in the way of you reaching your goal. The two main reasons people end up sabotaging their weight loss goals are *lack of self-esteem and fear.*

Lack of self-esteem leads to negative thoughts and self-talk. When you feel worthless, don't like yourself, don't believe you deserve success, or that you have what it takes to be successful, it creates such negativity in your mindset. Negative self-talk can be strong and take over without you even realizing it. Before you know it you are saying to yourself or feeling like "I'll never be able to do this" "it's too hard," "I'm going to fail anyway so might as well just quit," ''I'll never be able to do this," etc. ...sound familiar? This way of thinking can cause you to stop showing up every day, giving it your all, or you could end up giving up altogether.

This kind of negative chatter then feeds into your fears - the other reason you sabotage yourself.

COMMON FEARS THAT CAN LEAD TO SELF-SABOTAGING BEHAVIOURS:

Not all fears are obvious and many can be happening subconsciously. Have a look at this list and see if any of these resonate with you whether you are aware of them or not.

- **Fear of Change** - We all feel comfy and cozy in the familiar. It's hard to step outside of your comfort zone into the unknown. You may have no idea what losing weight will feel like physically or emotionally.

- **Failure and embarrassment** - Are you afraid of failing at another attempt at weight loss so might as well just give up now? Are you worried you will be embarrassed to admit you have quit yet another attempt to lose weight?

- **Changing body type** - Are you afraid of what your body might look like once you have lost the weight? A body you aren't familiar with?

- **Losing Your Comfort Foods** - "What am I going to do without my comfort foods? I can't handle stress without them. I don't want to stop enjoying food!"

- **New Clothes** - "I won't even know how to shop for clothes or know what to buy! I don't have money for new clothes anyway."

- **Relationships** - "Will people be jealous of me or uncomfortable around me if they have weight to lose? Will my friends and family look at me differently or treat me differently?"

- **Fear of your abilities** - Not believing in yourself is a big one. This plays into the negative self-talk. "I can't do this" "I'm just a failure" "I just suck at this".

- **Fear of the new YOU** - Who am I without the weight? I'm afraid of becoming someone I don't know anymore. Who am I if I'm not the "fat friend"..or sister/brother, or grandma/ grandpa, or mother/father...?"

- **Looking for people to tell you what you want to hear** - seeking out the "me too" mentality instead of listening to a good "kick in the pants".

Do any of those things resonate with you? The above examples play into both categories of Fear of Failure and Fear of Success, but it's important to break those down so you can really dig into what thoughts are really holding you back. Fear of Failure or Fear of Success are more blanket statements that don't really get to the bottom of anything, so let's dig deeper.

You're probably also confused as to why you do such things. Especially when you're so desperate to lose weight "Why would I fear success when I've wanted to lose weight for so long?!".

Some self-sabotaging behaviours, when it comes to weight loss are obvious, like eating foods you know you shouldn't, overeating, not drinking enough water, not having your snacks etc. However, there are other behaviours that can also get in the way of reaching your goals. It's important to look at those as well.

- **Focusing on the end result instead of the journey** - Are you so focused on that goal weight that you aren't paying attention to all the other positive changes that are happening?

- **Procrastinating** - Are you avoiding doing the things you know you need to do?

- **Trying to rush results** - Are you frustrated all the time because the scale isn't moving as fast as you want it to?

- **Focusing on the scale** - Is the number on the scale going down the only thing you are thinking about? Are you stressing every time it goes up or doesn't come down as fast as you want?

- **Overthinking things and becoming overwhelmed** - Overthinking things causes unnecessary stress and ultimately makes you feel overwhelmed. Then you are tired and ready to give up... [enter stage right: negative self-talk].

- **Avoiding accountability** - Are you avoiding showing up every day and being real with yourself about what you are or are not doing?

- **Not taking responsibility and blaming others** - Are you blaming your behaviours on your family? (I'm a busy single mom), work? (I'm just too busy), on the program? (It's just not right for me, I don't like the approach).

- **Comparing yourself to everyone else** - "Everyone else is losing weight and I'm not so obviously this doesn't work for me."

- **Perfectionism** - Are you focused so much on doing everything perfectly that it's stressing you out? Do you beat yourself up every time you feel like you weren't perfect? ...leading to negative self-talk? This too causes stress and makes it easier to give up.

- **Not asking for help** - Are you avoiding asking for help, whether it's from the group or family or friends? Maybe you need extra support from your family but are afraid to ask. Maybe you don't want to ask in the group because you know you won't get the answer you want to hear.

OKAY... SO NOW WHAT?

Now, you are going to get yourself a piece of paper and a pen and go through these questions below.

1.   Ask yourself "What am I afraid of?"

Make a list of your own fears. Even if you are repeating some of the examples I gave above, writing them down in your own words helps it to sink in. You may also have your own fears or self-sabotaging behaviours that aren't listed above.

2.   What are my triggers?

What makes you turn to food other than nutritional requirements? What emotions are coming up? Angry, sad, stressed, bored, happy...can all be reasons you want to eat. Write them all down. What are you feeling, or what is happening, when you want to turn to food?

3.   How does it make you feel when you turn to food?

Does it make you feel better? Maybe it does, in the moment, but does it last? How does it make you feel about yourself? Write down all the negative self-talk you use when you engage in self-sabotaging behaviours. Get that negative voice out on paper so you can really take a look at it.

4.   Make a list of things you can do instead of turning to food.

Maybe it's taking a walk, cuddling with your pet, taking a bath, having a nice soothing tea, listening to a FB Live with Gina! Maybe it's deep breathing, meditation, yoga, listening to your favourite music and dancing it out. Whatever you can think of, that is an alternative to food. Give yourself a few options. Make a separate copy of it for easy access when you feel like you might be heading for the cookie jar.

5.   How will choosing something that's in line with your goals make you feel?

Maybe you don't know yet because you haven't tried, but that's okay. Write down how you think it will make you feel. After you've tried something, you can go back and add to it. Add to that how you will feel about yourself for making a different choice. How will the dialogue in your head change? No more "shit-talk" right? Huh...funny how that works!

6.   Make a list of positive self-talk/affirmations.

"You got this!" "You can face your fears head on" "It's okay to have a bad day but I can turn this around." "I don't need to be perfect" "I can and will crush this!" Pay attention to how you feel as you write these down as compared to how you felt when writing down the negative thoughts. Post this list somewhere you can see it and read it often. Say these things to yourself every morning and every night before you go to bed.

7.   What is your WHY?

Write down all the reasons why you want to lose weight. How will your life be better once you've achieved your goal? Look back on that list anytime you are starting to feel you need some motivation.

Increasing awareness of your triggers and changing your negative self-talk is a solid first step in changing your patterns. These types of behaviours can't be changed overnight and for some are so deeply rooted that it might take more than a few lists to undo. Some of you might find that seeking out a therapist is something you need to do, and that's okay. You need to do what you need to do to stop the habit loop of self-sabotage if you want to reach your goals.

Take the time for yourself. You deserve it!

For more information on Self-sabotage head to the Science Guide and read The Psychology of Effort.

TROUBLESHOOTING: USING THE 20 QUESTIONS FROM THE MAXIMIZING POST

Troubleshooting Worksheet: Using the 20 Questions from the Maximizing Post

INSTRUCTIONS:

- Read the questions.

- Make note of the things you are doing.

- Make note of the things you can still do to help with the process.

- I suggest you give yourself an HONEST score from 1- 10 on the things you are DOING, not TRYING.

- Using your score, highlight areas of opportunity that you can focus on that will amount to getting you to that perfect 10.

- Once you achieve your 10, then you can rest assured that what your body needs is time.

- Check into the Facebook Group for a printable PDF of the 20 Questions as well as our Maximizing and 20 Questions Checklist.

20 QUESTIONS TO ASK YOURSELF:

1. **Are you doing everything you can to create the ideal environment for your body to focus on fat loss? SCORE   /10**

   - Are you following the program 100% day in and day out? Like actually, because there is a difference between trying and doing.

   - Are you being as consistent as possible, day in and day out?

   - Have you watched these videos that break down the rhyme & reason behind the order of the meals and snacks?

        1. The Livy Method
        2. The Food Plan
        3. Let's Talk Detox
        4. Let's Talk about the Scale
        5. Let's Talk Weight Loss
        6. Let's Talk Hunger

KEY TAKEAWAY AND TIPS:

- Check into the Facebook Group every day and asking all the questions you need.

- Review the information over and over again until you are super clear on it.

- Make all the tweaks you need to make day to day.

- Drink enough water for you, hit all your meals and snacks, take your supplements, get enough sleep, manage your stress, and maximize your efforts.

- What more can you do to create the ideal environment for your body to focus on fat loss?

2.   Has your body had time to consistently focus on fat loss?   SCORE /10

- Meaning has your body had days and weeks of working the plan where nothing trumps the body from focusing on fat loss? Day in and day out? Or have you had some off days and/or off weekends?

- Be real about the time your body has had to focus on fat loss. Have you been hit or miss with following The Food Plan, sick or stressed out, or are there things you are dealing with physically or mentally that need to be taken into account?

KEY TAKEAWAY AND TIPS:

- Keep a checklist.

- Set reminders for food/water/supplements.

- Set intentions in the morning, check in mid-day, and reflect on your situation at night.

- What more can you do to be more consistent?

3.   Have you had the flu or a cold or any other sickness that your body is dealing with, or had to deal with and focus on?   SCORE /10

- Is your body more focused on healing right now?

- Are you taking antibiotics or meds that might mess with digestion or make you dehydrated that you need to address?

- Are you following the Sickness Protocol?

KEY TAKEAWAY AND TIPS:

- Follow the Sickness Protocol if and when needed.

- Be patient with your body and recognize where it's at and what it needs.

- What more can you do to help your body deal with your sickness?

4. **Are you managing your stress levels?** **SCORE /10**

- Are you meditating, deep breathing, stretching, moving your body, going for walks, taking Epsom salt baths and so on. And if so, for how long and how often?

- Have you read the post on managing stress?

KEY TAKEAWAY AND TIPS:

- Are you really doing all you can do to help the body manage your stress? Stress can play a major role in preventing the body from focusing on fat loss. Managing your stress can go a long way in getting the scale to move.

- What more can you do to help manage your stress?

5. **Are you getting lots of deep & REM sleep?** **SCORE /10**

- Are you helping your body prepare for sleep by eating earlier in the evening, going to bed earlier, keeping lights low and avoiding stimulants like TV and phone, taking a relaxing bath, keeping a journal by your bed?

- Have you read the post on sleep?

KEY TAKEAWAY AND TIPS:

- Your body makes change and detoxes when you sleep. Every little bit you can do to help improve your sleep will add up and make a difference.

- Are you actually making changes? Or still staying up late? What more can you do to help improve your overall sleep?

6. **Are you drinking enough water?** **SCORE /10**

- Not just a set amount, but adjusting it according to the body's demands? (Not just "more than before" or "lots") Are you drinking enough?

- Are you spreading it out and sipping on it for maximum absorption & utilization?

- Are you adding in salt or trace minerals?

- Have you read all of the posts on water?

KEY TAKEAWAY AND TIPS:

- Because we utilize the body's natural detox response to get the fat out, you need to be sure you are drinking enough water for the body to be able to focus on fat loss.

- Are you maximizing your efforts to get your water in? Setting reminders, having a good water bottle, keeping track of your water intake through apps, elastics, or other methods.

- Are you adding different elements to your meals? Veg, protein, greens, healthy fats? (Not just grabbing what's convenient or easy or what you like or love. Think most bang for your buck and maximum value).

- Have you read the Making Your Meals Nutrient Rich Post?

- Get real honest here…you don't get points for drinking more than you used to, you get points for drinking as much as you actually need.

- How much daily water are you actually drinking and what else can you do to improve in this area?

7.	Are you making your food as nutrient rich as possible?	SCORE /10

- • Are you adding different elements to your meals? Veg, protein, greens, healthy fats? (Not just grabbing what's convenient or easy or what you like or love. think most bang for your buck and maximum value).

- • Have you read the Making Your Meals Nutrient Rich Post?

KEY TAKEAWAY AND TIPS:

- Make sure your foods are nutrient rich to ensure your body is getting the nutrients it needs so it doesn't feel the need to store fat.

- What else can you do to make your foods as nutrient rich as possible?

8.	Are you exercising? Are you moving your body?	SCORE /10

- • If so, what are you doing and how often? Are you getting your heart rate up?

- • Are you making an effort to be more active?

- • Are you taking the stairs, parking further away, participating and not just sitting on the sidelines?

- • Are you factoring in time for the body to repair and rebuild any damage from your workouts?

- • Have you read the post on exercise?

KEY TAKEAWAY AND TIPS:

- Are you being mindful to move? Is there anything else you can do to move more or make your efforts more effective

- For example, if you only have time to walk your dog 3 times/week, you can maximize that by choosing a route that's uphill, walk with your arms above your heart to increase heart rate, perhaps carry light weights, pick up the pace, stop and do some squats along the way, etc.

9.	Are you helping the body while in detox?	SCORE /10

- Watching portions, keeping food light, drinking lots of water, eating early at night and getting lots of sleep and maximizing everything else you can and need to do?
- Have you watched the Detox Video and read the Supporting the Body in Detox Post?

KEY TAKEAWAY AND TIPS:

- Have you made an effort to really understand and help the body Maximize when it's in detox? What else can you do to help support the body while in detox?

10. Are you taking medications or have health issues that need to be factored in?
SCORE /10

- You can lose weight regardless of your health issues, but they will impact your journey. So, if there are things you can do to help the body adjust to medications and help to address or heal the issue, it will help when it comes to the scale.
- Are you keeping up with appointments like your Chiropractor or Therapist?

KEY TAKEAWAY AND TIPS:

- Be sure to work hand in hand with your doctor, pharmacist, or health practitioner when it comes to your medications.
- Get your blood work done.
- Addressing your health issues above and beyond what we are doing on The Program. For example, seeking out a hormone expert, thyroid expert, cross referencing foods that can help decrease inflammation in the body, etc.
- Have you looked into other ways you can help your body heal or deal with your health issues?

11. Are you missing any organs?   SCORE /10

- Are you missing any organs? Kidneys, gallbladders, thyroids, liver, have you had a hysterectomy, etc.?
- Are you helping the body compensate for missing organs by adding in the bile salts or digestive bitters if missing your gallbladder?
- Are you going the extra mile to help your body manage any deficiencies?

KEY TAKEAWAY AND TIPS

- You know your body best and what you are dealing with so you can better help support your body in all its needs, not just weight loss.
- Anything you can do to help the body better address any health issues you have will help with weight loss. What else can you do to better support any missing organs?

12. Do you have hormone issues you need to address? Or that needs to be factored in? SCORE /10

- Are you seeing a specialist or adding in supplements that can help?

- Have you looked into addressing hormonal issues you may be dealing with?

KEY TAKEAWAY AND TIPS:

- Your hormones can have an impact on your weight loss journey. However, there is a lot you can do to help manage your hormones outside of what we focus on in the groups. Is there anything else you can do to help balance your hormones?

13. Have you had your blood work done? SCORE /10

- Do you have any deficiencies that could be affecting your body's ability to function properly?

- Have you seen or checked in with your doctor recently?

- Have you had a physical done recently?

KEY TAKEAWAY AND TIPS:

- Check into the Facebook Group for a link to a Healthline article about blood tests.

- Knowing what is going on in all areas of health in regards to your body can give you great insight into the things you can do to maximize your efforts when it comes to weight loss.

14. Are you taking all the supplements and taking them consistently? SCORE /10

- They all work together and are all key in weight loss. Are you maximizing your efforts by adding them in?

- Are you consistent with taking them?

- Have you read all the posts on supplements?

KEY TAKEAWAYS AND TIPS:

- The supplements are suggested for a rhyme and a reason. They help with this program and this process.

- Have you booked a consultation with your pharmacist to discuss your supplements?

- Do you have a gameplan for when you are going to take them?

- Have you truly considered all the supplements, asked all the questions, and are you sure you have added in everything you need? Is there anything else you can do?

15. **Is your body changing? Has your body been focusing on repair and rebuild and making change?** **SCORE /10**

- What changes have you seen that can't be seen on the scale and is your body changing shape and size?

KEY TAKEAWAY AND TIPS:

- Pay attention to what your body is focused on and when. The non-scale victories can be just as key because your body is always working and it can't all be about weight loss.

- List some of your favourite non-scale victories here.

16. **Are you eating a lot of red meat and meat in general or are you switching between veg proteins, seafood, fish, and meat?** **SCORE /10**

- Be mindful about those quality protein choices.

- Are you making an effort to maximize your food choices?

- Are you choosing the best options or are you stuck on eating what you like and love?

KEY TAKEAWAY AND TIPS:

- Although there are nutrients in meat that we benefit from, meat in general can be hard to digest. It's a great idea to be adding in a variety of protein including plant based.

- What else can you do to maximize your efforts to include a variety of different protein sources in your diet?

17. **Do you have any digestive issues?** **SCORE /10**

- Have you added in the supplements to help?

- Are you maximizing your food choices to help your body better digest and process your food?

- Are you eating things you are sensitive to like dairy or gluten?

- Are you keeping a journal and taking notes on how your body is responding to your food choices?

KEY TAKEAWAY AND TIPS:

- Anything you do to help with digestion will help with weight loss. Is there anything else you can do to maximize your efforts?

18. **Do you have issues with bowel movements and if so, what are you doing to address them?**
SCORE   /10

- Have you added in the supplements to help and are you maximizing your food choices?

- Are you making the best choices possible?

- Are you adding leafy greens to your meals and mindful to add in fibre rich foods?

KEY TAKEAWAY AND TIPS:

- Review the Bowel Movement Post and let us know if you have any questions. Although bowel movements may be all over the place – from being loose to feeling constipated – anything you can do to help with the food moving in and out of the body will help with this process.

- What else can you do to help support the body when it comes to bowel movements?

19. **Are you sabotaging yourself?**   **SCORE /10**

- Do you continue to get in your own way of reaching your goals?

- Are you making choices that take you further away, not closer to, your goals?

- Are you indulging in your frustration?

- Are you having real conversations with yourself?

KEY TAKEAWAY AND TIPS:

- Sabotage is real. Be sure to review the Sabotage Post for more things you can do to help with self-sabotage.

- Get real with yourself. If you recognize you are sabotaging yourself, what else can you do to help prevent it and work through it?

20. **Do you genuinely believe you have what it takes to follow through and finish?**
SCORE: /10

- Do you have faith that you can lose the weight?

- What is your WHY? What is motivating you to keep showing up and to follow through till the end?

- Do you truly see yourself still here at the end?

KEY TAKEAWAY AND TIPS:

- Having a strong "why" and a strong visual of the end game can make all the difference when it comes to following through and finishing your weight loss journey.

- What else can you do to make sure you will be a success story at the end of our 12 weeks? Do you need to reexamine your WHY?

LET'S TALK SETTING INTENTIONS

This week started the conversation with a post on self-sabotage. Sabotage can mean different things for different people. Some people sabotage out of fear of failure, some out of fear of success. And some for a variety of other reasons.

Regardless, Setting Your Intentions can do a lot for helping to keep you on track each day regardless of any subconscious attempt to self-sabotage.

Setting Your Intentions in the morning is like making a declaration that you are still working towards your goal.

A reminder to yourself that the plan is to make choices that fall in line with reaching your goal, which in turn can help to keep the goal you are working towards in the forefront of your mind.

Especially in today's world with all the extra stress everyone is dealing with in their day to day, your goal of trying to also lose weight can get lost in translation some days.

Setting Your Intention first thing in the morning, checking in on yourself mid-day, and reviewing your choices at the end of the day, can help to keep you accountable to yourself.

So even if you are continually getting in your own way, this will help you to counteract that. Visualization is also key; it works like a blueprint or a guide for your body to follow.

Visualization can be done on a small-scale, day to day by visualizing and harmonizing your daily tasks, and it can also be done on a larger scale in terms of visualizing the end game and reaching your ultimate goal.

Studies show that you don't have to actually experience something for it to feel real to your body. So, if you want to take it a step further, try to also imagine what reaching your goal will "feel" like.

Making your goal feel tangible can help reinforce the belief that you are going to reach your goal.

Please take the time to head over to the Facebook Group or the Livy Method App and watch the quick video that accompanies this post.

WEEK 6 GUIDELINES: DOWNSIZE AGAIN

This week, you are repeating the Downsizing process while being even more in tune to your body's needs. I hope you are enjoying the process and are excited about the weeks to come as we move forward towards the second half of The Program! It is even more important to stay focused as there is a lot more to cover and a lot more weight to lose!

THIS WEEK WE ARE GOING TO DOWNSIZE AGAIN.

Now, I know some of you may be wondering how you are going to downsize if your portions are already getting pretty small. Remember, when it comes to downsizing, you are only eating a few bites less from what you were eating to feel satisfied. It's about what the portions feel like when you eat, not what they look like.

It is important to keep in mind, the downsizing phase is just one of many techniques designed to get the body's attention to take action and focus on dropping fat.

The real secret to The Program and to your success is consistency with the food, the supplements, and the water, while maximizing everything you can to keep things progressing and take things to the next level.

With downsizing, the idea is to give the body slightly less food so that it feels more inclined to get rid of any extra fat it doesn't need by downsizing and adjusting to the amount of food that is coming in. This only works because of the strong foundation you created in the first few weeks by giving the body what it needs and eating to the point of satisfaction.

With downsizing, it is essential that you continue to eat all the meals and snacks that the body has come to rely on.

With the first round of downsizing in week 4, you were decreasing portions by a few bites for a week. This was more of a practice round for you to get a sense of how it works and test the waters when it comes to eating smaller portions.

In Week 6, you are going to take things to the next level by being mindful with the portions, maximizing everything you can to keep the scale moving, and cracking down on and testing the body a little harder now that you understand the process.

The idea is to get your body's attention and get it to focus on detox and dropping fat when normally detox and fat loss is low on the list of the body's priorities day to day.

In getting the body's attention, you may feel unsatisfied to the point where you will notice and may need to step outside your comfort zone.

Keep in mind the idea is to feel "slightly" unsatisfied. The goal is NOT to feel hungry like you are starving and depriving your body...it's just enough of a decrease to leave it wanting more.

Also keep in mind that you will be dealing with fluctuating hunger levels and a variety of variables that need to be factored in at any given time.

There will be some days where the body will be naturally hungrier than other days. Where one day you might be hungry every 30 minutes, and then the next day 4 hours can go by and you won't be hungry at all. Be sure to watch the Hunger Video posted in the Facebook Group or in the Livy Method App.

This is normal and to be expected. On the days you are not hungry, you still want to eat a token amount. You may find after a few bites, you will start to feel hungry, in which case, you still want to leave yourself feeling unsatisfied.

It should also be noted that, although the whole point of downsizing is to see the scale move, the drop in weight may not go hand in hand with downsizing day to day. Just because you eat less doesn't mean the scale will move right away. Depending on where your body is at, and what it is currently focused on, there can be a delayed reaction in the reflection on the scale. Therefore, it is very important that you stay as consistent as possible and relentlessly MAXIMIZE and stay on top of everything you need to keep the scale moving.

ON A FINAL NOTE: Keep in mind that how you are eating now is only a means to an end. How and what you eat will change and evolve as we move forward in the weeks to come.

A LOOK AHEAD: Other stages in the program will include eating more and more often and then eating more in tune with your body's needs based on day-to-day requirements. Eventually you will be going off this structured way of eating and working on Personalizing The Plan for your own individual needs. But for now, be as consistent as you can with The Process.

If you are unsure or need a refresher on Downsizing, be sure to review your notes from Week 4 and ask any questions you need.

This is the last week you will be purposely reducing portions as we will not be Downsizing again, so do your best to be all in!

Please take the time to head over to the Facebook Group or the Livy Method App and watch the quick video that accompanies this post.

WEEK 6 GUIDELINES FAQS

1.   I am struggling with downsizing. Any tips on how to fine tune the process?

It's important to keep in mind, the downsizing phase is just one of the tweaks designed to get the body's attention to take action and focus on dropping fat and this is the last week we are downsizing. This week of downsizing we are taking things to the next level by being mindful with our portions, Maximizing everything we can to keep the scale moving, and cracking down on and testing the body a little harder. Keep in mind that you are eating 6 times a day, nutrient rich foods. You can reduce your portions a little more than the first week and if you find after 10-15 minutes you are still hungry you can always go back for more. Try and have fun this week and see how your body responds. Continue to ask those 4 questions, and keep your end goal in mind.

2.   I am eating to slightly less than satisfaction but am really hungry shortly after. Any tips?

If you are finding yourself hungry shortly after eating, make sure that the foods you are eating are nutrient rich, that you are adding protein and good fats to your meals and veg snack and incorporate eating breakfast if that is something you tend to skip. Keep asking yourself those 4 mindfulness questions. If you are feeling like you are still hungry after your meals or snacks, this may be a signal that you need to eat more. Remember that, in downsizing, the goal is to feel slightly unsatisfied and not distractedly hungry.

3.   Do we downsize both our snacks and our meals this week?

When downsizing, you want to try and downsize all of your meals and snacks if possible. Hunger levels will be different every day, so the amount you need each day will change. If you are not hungry and have only token bites then you don't need to downsize those.

4.   When downsizing, if I start getting full before my last few bites should I stop eating?

You want to be in tune with your hunger level and ask those 4 questions with each meal and snack. If you are noticing that you are starting to feel full, stop eating and pay attention to how you feel 10-15min after you have eaten. If you find that you feel full, then you know you have room to reduce a little more.

5.   I get symptoms such as headaches during downsizing. Is this normal or a result of hunger?

Headaches can be a side effect of detox. However, side effects from the Program should never be severe, so if you're concerned, be sure to check in with your healthcare provider. In terms of hunger, feeling unsatisfied is normal for downsizing week as a result of eating slightly less than satisfaction. However because we are eating 6 times a day, nutrient rich food, we are not depriving ourselves of nutrients.

6. **I am going on vacation and will not be able to downsize, should I eat to satisfaction instead this week?**

Vacations can do wonders for weight loss. Change of environment, less stress, abundance of good fresh foods and some decent sleep can be exactly what the body needs to get the scale moving. If you find you are unable to follow the week while away, then try to maintain regular eating habits as much as possible and look at any extras as just that, extra. Once you are back you can pick up from where you left off and follow through with the week downsizing.

LET'S TALK SECONDARY SUPPLEMENTS

The following are suggested supplements that can help speed up the fat loss process. With that said, they are not a mandatory part of the process or make or break when it comes to reaching your goals.

Always remember that if you have any concerns adding in any supplements, be sure to have a conversation with your healthcare provider.

If you are struggling with your weight and have yet to use or add in the basic supplements, those are what you should start with first.

This list is for those of you who may be interested in taking things to the next level when it comes to your health and wellness.

You may be wondering why I haven't mentioned these supplements in length before now. That is because the first part of this process is to give the body what it needs so it no longer feels the need to store fat. As we move forward, it's about helping the body focus on detox and getting the fat out.

In making that the focus, your body has been working hard to re-wire and re-work how it has come to function over the years. In order to make real foundational change, it was important to give the body the time it needed to make its own connections and figure out how to re-wire and re-work things on its own.

Now that you have spent the past 5 weeks laying a strong foundation, there are supplements you can add that can help take things to the next level and in a sense, speed up the process.

By no means are these suggested supplements necessary to reach your goal. Nor do you need to rush out and buy them right away to be successful.

The health food stores are full of products that promise increased fat loss, but at the end of the day, none of them will work unless your body functions properly to begin with. If you are still here, chances are your body is now working on making you as healthy as possible so it can benefit from the added support.

Read over the information and decide if you think any of the listed supplements could be a benefit to you.

MCT OIL

MCT oil is a medium-chain triglyceride (MCT) which I started using about 15 years ago to help natural bodybuilders and professional athletes shed excess fat fast.

Coconut oil is a great source of healthy fat containing 65% MCT's, but it is important to note that when I am referring to adding in MCT oil as a supplement, I am talking about the derivative of MCT's from coconut oil...so not coconut oil itself.

The reason why MCT oil is so great for fat loss is because it works like the old thermogenic supplements people used to take to burn fat, but without the harmful effects.

Unlike every other fat source that needs to be broken down, digested, and stored before it is of any use to the body, MCT oil is easily digested and sent directly to your liver where it has a thermogenic effect and the ability to support your metabolism (the rate at which your body functions and burns calories).

MCT's are instantly utilized for fuel instead of being stored as fat, so it helps to calm the mind (since your brain is floating in cholesterol, it needs good fat for energy to function) but keeps the body revved up and working extra hard.

Normally, MCT is a great add-in during the cooler/winter months where the body is in hibernation mode and you are looking to get it revved up.

Look for MCT oil derived from 100% coconut oil, NOT coconut oil itself.

You can take it straight up, in oil form, add to coffee and shakes, or use as a dressing on salads.

DOSE

Use as directed, although I suggest starting with 1 teaspoon and working your way up to a tablespoon per serving...to a max of 3 servings per day.

WHEN TO TAKE

Ideally, you can use it in the morning, around 3:00/4:00 pm, and then after dinner.

Side effects can include digestive upset if you use too much too soon, so I cannot express how important it is to use less instead of more, and work your way up.

Please also make sure to continue taking your omega 3 supplements, as MCT oil is not an essential fatty acid.

ADAPTOGENS

Adaptogens are supplements derived from plants that can help our bodies manage and recover from stress. They support the body's ability to cope with stress and help it to return to a balanced state when we experience stressful situations.

Your adrenals produce and control cortisol, the stress hormone. When you are stressed, your adrenals can produce too much cortisol or not enough. Cortisol is known as the stress hormone because of the body's stress response, although it is about more than just stress. Most of the cells in your body have cortisol receptors that use it for a variety of functions including: regulating blood sugar, reducing inflammation, regulating metabolism, and memory function.

We care about cortisol because too much or not enough, signals the need to store fat in the body.

COMMON EXAMPLES OF ADAPTOGENS:

- Ashwaganda
- Ginseng
- Reishi
- Rhodiola
- Schisandra
- Holy Basil

THESE ARE SIGNS YOU CAN BENEFIT FROM ADAPTOGENS:

- Feeling tired; struggling to wake up in the morning
- Trouble falling asleep
- Anxiety, or feeling on edge
- Mood swings
- Depression
- Weight gain
- Autoimmune issues
- Brain fog
- Body aches
- Hair loss
- Lightheaded

These symptoms are pretty general, which is one of the challenges because there are many variables that affect how your body functions.

DOSE

Follow the directions on your product's label for dosage.

WHEN TO TAKE

Take as directed and be sure to check with your healthcare provider.

*Be sure to check in with your healthcare provider if you are taking any antidepressant medications.

TURMERIC

The primary antioxidant in Turmeric the spice is curcumin, which is an anti-inflammatory. While increasing your intake of turmeric isn't a lone strategy for weight loss, it may help you address the inflammation associated with extra fat and help with metabolism.

Carrying extra fat creates low grade inflammation in the body that puts you at a higher risk of developing chronic diseases, like heart disease and type 2 diabetes.

Curcumin, which is an antioxidant in turmeric, suppresses the inflammatory messaging in many cells, including pancreatic, fat and muscle cells. This can help curb insulin resistance, high blood sugar, high cholesterol levels, and other metabolic conditions resulting from excess fat.

We care because when your body isn't fighting so much inflammation, it's easier to focus on weight loss.

Turmeric is a readily available spice, and adding it to your diet has no side effects unless you have an allergy, so it can easily be added to foods.

However, in order to get the amount of curcumin necessary to aid in weight loss you would have to use a lot of it. Therefore, if you want to experience the full effects, you need to take a supplement that contains significant amounts of curcumin.

WHAT TO LOOK FOR

Curcumin is poorly absorbed into the bloodstream, so it is better absorbed with black pepper. Black pepper contains piperine, which is a natural substance that enhances the absorption of curcumin by as much as 2,000%.

The best curcumin supplements contain piperine, which substantially increases the absorption and therefore effectiveness.

DOSE

Follow the directions on your product's label for dosage.

WHEN TO TAKE

Follow the directions on your product's label.

**NOTE: Turmeric, especially taken as a supplement, can interact with certain medications, so always consult your healthcare provider when considering adding it to your diet. Turmeric can increase your risk of bleeding if you're on blood thinners, interfere with the action of drugs that reduce stomach acid and increase the risk of low blood sugar when taken with certain diabetes drugs. Turmeric is also contraindicated if you have gallstones or obstruction of the bile passages. **

TRACE MINERALS

Most of us are familiar with the vitamins we need and know how essential they are to our health and wellness. But even with taking a supplement, or choosing nutrient rich food, many people are not getting in enough trace minerals. Even though trace minerals are only required in small amounts, they are indeed essential. Not only for good health, but also weight loss.

There are two classes of minerals:

1. Major
2. Trace

Major minerals include: calcium, potassium, chloride, phosphorus, magnesium, sodium, and selenium. Trace minerals include chromium, germanium, manganese, rubidium, vanadium, cobalt, iron, molybdenum, zinc, copper, lithium, nickel, and silica.

Minerals are needed for important metabolic functions in the body and mineral deficiencies are involved in metabolic disorders that cause diseases including hypertension, headaches, depression, heart disease, insulin resistance, and obesity.

An important part of a successful correction of the metabolism to achieve weight loss is addressing the mineral deficiency and replacing them in the correct way. Most of the over-the-counter multivitamins do not have the required amounts of minerals, especially the trace minerals.

Because on the program you are drinking lots of water, adding in trace minerals can also help prevent low sodium levels and balance minerals caused from drinking too fast, drinking too much in a short period of time, and sweating.

DOSE

Follow recommendations on your product's label.

WHEN TO TAKE

Add to your water following directions on your product's label.

COQ10

The primary role of CoQ10 is as an antioxidant. Your diet consists of antioxidants from a wide variety of sources, including fruits and vegetables.

The main source of dietary CoQ10 is from fatty fish such as mackerel, along with whole-grain foods. Your body also requires CoQ10 to produce energy from the carbohydrates and fat you eat in your diet.

CoQ10 assists in the production of energy by the cells. A deficiency can contribute to lower energy levels and a slower metabolism. Many people believe that CoQ10 production decreases with age, which can help explain one of the reasons why it can be harder to lose weight as you get older.

The CoQ10 can enhance healthy weight loss because it helps to support increased metabolic function. In addition, it can work to decrease body fat while boosting energy levels by maximizing your body's ability to convert food to fuel.

It's also great for the skin. Lack of CoQ10 results in decreased production of collagen and elastin. Collagen is important because it makes your skin firm, while elastin gives your skin flexibility. The loss of collagen and elastin causes your skin to wrinkle and sag.

DOSE

90–200 mg of CoQ10 per day is recommended, though some conditions may require higher doses of 300–600 mg. It is a relatively well tolerated and safe supplement.

WHEN TO TAKE

CoQ10 is fat soluble, so it should be taken with a meal containing fat so your body can absorb it. Also, taking CoQ10 at night may help with the body's ability to use and absorb it.

Take as directed and for more information, check in with your pharmacist/doctor.

**NOTE: Check with your doctor if you are on blood thinning or blood pressure medications. **

B COMPLEX

Vitamin B Complex is a group of water-soluble vitamins, which play a very important role in maintaining the growth and the metabolism of cells in the body.

When it comes to weight loss, B12 is among the MOST IMPORTANT because it helps the body convert fats and proteins into energy. B12 is mainly found in red meat, chicken, fish, dairy and eggs.

A B Complex can help the body maintain sufficient levels of a variety of B vitamins so that it can efficiently burn carbohydrates, fats, and proteins and help the body maintain energy, stamina, and control appetite.

B-vitamins are water-soluble, meaning they are not stored in the body. Though they don't stick around long, B-vitamins are vital for supporting a variety of bodily functions. Most people get the right amount of B-vitamins through diet, but others may need to supplement these important vitamins through pills or shots.

Each B-vitamin supports different bodily functions, so your doctor will be able to pinpoint the supplements you need and help you decide between B12 vs. B complex.

Typically, it is B1, B6 & B12 that is the issue.

- B1 (thiamine): Helps convert nutrients into energy, making it essential to your metabolic system. It strengthens the immune system and supports nerve function. Naturally found in pork, sunflower seeds and wheat germ.

- B2 (riboflavin): Riboflavin works with thiamine to convert food to energy, while also serving as an antioxidant. Naturally found in organ meats, beef, and mushrooms.

- B3 (niacin): Niacin helps your cells communicate and plays a role in metabolism and DNA production. Naturally found in chicken, tuna, and lentils.

- B5 (pantothenic acid): Converts food to energy, supports hormone and cholesterol production. Naturally found in liver, fish, yogurt, and avocado.

- B6 (pyridoxine): Facilitates energy production, regulates hormone activity, blood glucose levels, hemoglobin production and aids in the creation of neurotransmitters. Found naturally in chickpeas, salmon, and potatoes.

- B7 (biotin): Biotin specifically helps metabolize carbohydrates and fats. Can be found naturally in yeast, eggs, salmon, cheese, and liver.

- B9 (folate): Folate metabolizes amino acids, assists in the formation of blood cells, and helps your cells develop and divide properly. Found naturally in leafy greens, liver, and beans.

- B12 (cobalamin): Involved in neurological function, DNA production, and red blood cell development. Found naturally in animal sources like meat, eggs, seafood, and dairy.

DOSE

Range varies depending on the B vitamin. Follow directions on your product's label.

WHEN TO TAKE

B vitamins can boost energy, so it is best to take them earlier in your day and with a meal.

L-THEANINE

L-theanine is an amino acid found in both green and black tea leaves. It is also found in mushrooms, available in pill or tablet form.

It is thought to work by decreasing brain chemicals that contribute to stress and anxiety while increasing brain chemicals that encourage a sense of calm. L-theanine elevates levels of GABA, as well as serotonin and dopamine. These chemicals are known as neurotransmitters, and they work in the brain to regulate emotions, mood, concentration, alertness, and sleep as well as appetite, energy, and other cognitive skills. Increasing levels of these calming brain chemicals promotes relaxation and can help with sleep. Some research also suggests that L-theanine may improve the function of the body's immune system and help to improve inflammation in the intestinal system.

There are no known side effects of taking L-theanine. It's safe to take the supplement and/or drink teas that contain L-theanine.

Due to its calming effects, L-theanine may help lower blood pressure so you may want to keep that in mind and consult with your doctor if you have low blood pressure.

Women who are pregnant or breastfeeding should consult their health care practitioner before adding L-theanine or supplementing with green or black tea.

If you are using the Natural Calm "Calmful Sleep," it contains L-theanine. You can use magnesium and L-theanine together.

DOSE

Dose ranges from 100-400mg. Start with a smaller dose and work up.

WHEN TO TAKE

Follow the directions on your product's label.

As with all the suggestions I make, please be sure to check with your doctor if you have any concerns.

Please take the time to head over to the Facebook Group or the Livy Method App and watch the quick video that accompanies this post.

LET'S TALK NON-SCALE VICTORIES

One of our Program Specialists, Krystyna Recoskie, put together this post to talk about the importance of non-scale victories. She has lost 35 lbs., is now in Maintenance, and continues to see her body change with new non-scale victories!

Non-scale victories (NSVs) refer to any changes that have improved your health and well-being but are not related to the scale. To take it one step further, it is any change that you are proud of that is positive and brings you joy in your weight loss journey. It doesn't matter how big or how small they may be, if YOU feel that something has changed for the better, that is something to be celebrated!

Throughout this program, we can become discouraged at times, especially if the scale is not moving. This is why we need to bring self-awareness and lean into the NSV's that are happening. If you only focus on the number the scale shows, you won't notice them! The outcome of your success is not only determined by the piece of metal, or glass lying on the floor. There are so many different things that improve during our journey to finally and forever, and we need to pay attention to those as well.

So why are the NSVs important? As Gina has mentioned before, "Your energy is your vibe." The energy you put into this program is going to affect your success. Your self-talk, and how you think and feel has a HUGE impact on this process and can impact your overall goal. Think of yourself as your own personal coach. If you are constantly giving yourself negative feedback, where will the motivation come from? Keeping a positive vibe and keeping your NSVs in the forefront of your mind throughout this process will help you realize all of your successes that have to be celebrated, motivate you, and is what will get you through the messy middle of weight loss. Remember, as long as you keep showing up for yourself, you WILL be successful in this program.

Here are some NSV examples, but remember, they can be different for everyone. Anything that you find that has improved when it comes to your health and wellness is a NSV that is worth celebrating!

- Body changing - the scale may not be moving, but your clothes feel looser. Sometimes the scale can be a bit behind when it comes to losing fat in layers.

- Improved and more regular bowel movements

- Better sleep

- More positive attitude

- Learning new information - so much info and guest speakers available to help improve your knowledge.

- Increased energy

- Being able and motivated to do things that you could not previously do. For example, exercising, taking the stairs instead of the elevator or cooking more meals.

- Mindful eating - This one is huge! Think about your improved relationship with food. Taking the time to enjoy it. Mindfully paying attention to your portions. Being IN TUNE with your body and understanding when to eat, when not to eat, and what to eat.

- Developing positive eating habits and associations

- Wedding rings fitting again

- Increased libido

- Improved complexion (hydrated skin!)

- Decreased inflammation

- Decreased or discontinued medications

- Improvement in blood pressure, sugar levels, etc.

- Positive changes in menstruation

When you are feeling discouraged, review your NSVs. Try writing them down and keep adding to the list as the program moves on. Keep them in a place where you can visually see them, so you are reminded daily and so they motivate you to keep pushing towards your goals.

Feed the positive vibes of your body and mind! Look at all of your NSVs and celebrate! The weight loss will come. This journey is about so much more than just losing weight - it is about overall health and wellness, and increasing your positive energy and vibe in life. You have given yourself a beautiful gift here - finally and forever weight loss. Keep showing up. Keep being kind to yourself, and keep celebrating those non-scale victories!

SCALE NOT MOVING? LET'S TALK 4 MAIN REASONS WHY YOUR WEIGHT MIGHT BE SLOWER TO MOVE

The human body is not meant to store excess fat. Every extra pound of fat is hard on the body, so contrary to popular belief…your body is not looking to make you fat.

Weight gain is much more complicated than just the foods you are eating. If you are following the food plan, you are not going to gain weight. Just be mindful that for many reasons, the scale is going to fluctuate throughout this process.

With that said, this program and process will work for anyone who is human and has a body. I've never met anyone I couldn't help lose weight, as long as they were willing to put the time in and do the work necessary to make changes.

The reality is for some, weight loss will come easier and for others, they will have to work a little harder and dig a little deeper because they have some underlying issues their body is dealing with.

If your weight is dropping and or your body is changing and you are noticing non scale victories like better energy, sleeping better, and even pooping better, then chances are you are doing great and your body is responding well to the process.

There are always things you can do to level up your efforts so continue to be engaged in the conversation as we continue to focus on maximizing as we move forward with this process.

If your weight isn't dropping and your body isn't changing and you are not noticing any non-scale victories, then chances are you have some issues you need to address.

4 MAIN REASONS WHY YOUR WEIGHT MIGHT NOT BE MOVING:

1: INFLAMMATION

Inflammation is an issue because weight gain is associated with increased inflammation in the body, which can lead to insulin resistance.

Insulin resistance is an issue when it comes to weight loss because it leads to higher blood sugar levels, as well as fatty liver, which can further contribute to insulin resistance.

It's key to note, there are different types of inflammation which can be caused by a variety of conditions, so it's best to check in with your health care provider as this is just a general overview.

Causes of inflammation:

- Hormonal issues like insulin resistance, Hashimotos and high cortisol
- Digestive issues including food sensitivities or allergies

- Autoimmune diseases like arthritis, lupus, psoriasis
- Medications
- Stress
- Lifestyle & environment/exposure to chemicals and irritants

It is worth pointing out there are also foods that can cause or contribute to inflammation.

These include:

- Sugar
- Refined carbohydrates
- Alcohol
- Processed meats
- Trans fats

These are foods we try to minimize and things we address while following the program. But if your body isn't responding in the way it should, then a visit to your health care provider to further investigate can be just what you need to get the scale moving.

2: FOOD SENSITIVITIES

When it comes to food allergies, you generally know when you have them as they tend to be pretty noticeable and, in some cases, extreme. Symptoms often involve swelling, itching and wheezing and can require immediate attention and medication.

Food sensitivity, on the other hand, is usually GI-related. They can happen when the body has a hard time digesting certain foods and can affect the weight loss process simply because they make people feel unwell.

They can also cause bloating and discomfort that may mimic weight gain, which doesn't help when it comes to staying motivated.

Food intolerance symptoms usually begin about half an hour after eating or drinking, but in some cases, you might not notice them for a few days after consuming.

Symptoms include:

- Nausea
- Stomach pain
- Gas, cramps or bloating
- Vomiting

- Heartburn
- Diarrhea
- Headaches
- Irritability or nervousness

As you progress through the program, you will become very in tune to your body's needs. Keeping a journal or using the Livy Method App to track how your body is dealing with the foods you eat can help give you insight into any food sensitivities you might have.

3: GUT DYSBIOSIS

I'm hesitant to use this word because it seems to be the new buzzword of the year, so it's key to keep in mind this is a general term used to describe when the bacteria in your digestive system becomes unbalanced.

There can be many causes and a variety of symptoms, so if you feel there is something off with your digestion, be sure to consult with your health care provider.

Causes of Dysbiosis:

- Consuming processed foods, including sugar & artificial sweeteners like sucralose, food additives, preservatives & artificial ingredients
- Chemicals like pesticides on unwashed fruit and veg
- Environmental toxins, skin care products
- Alcohol
- Any new medications added in
- Use of antibiotics that affect your microbiome
- Parasites
- Poor oral hygiene
- High levels of stress or anxiety

Some symptoms can include:

- Nausea, upset stomach
- Constipation
- Diarrhea
- Bad breath
- Trouble urinating

- Vaginal or rectal itching

- Bloating

- Extreme fatigue

- Chest pain

- Rashes

- Trouble concentrating

- Anxiety

There are tests your health care provider can perform to diagnose. And there are medications and different types of treatment including changes in lifestyle (like following the plan) that can help.

4: HORMONAL HEALTH

When people think of hormones, they tend to think of sex hormones, when in reality there are 50 different types of hormones that factors into your weight loss journey. These hormones control a number of functions in the body including; heart rate, appetite, sleep cycles, metabolism, mood, and of course sexual health to name a few.

Hormones are key to the weight loss conversation because your body storing fat and releasing it are regulated by certain hormones in the body. Hormones also influence your energy expenditure (or the number of calories your body burns on a daily basis, not that we care or talk about calories).

Hormones work like chemical messengers that can make or break your weight-loss efforts. While following the program, we leverage the benefits of certain hormones while minimizing the downside of others. For example, following a balanced diet that feeds into your satiety hormone (Leptin) and minimizing the need for as much insulin as your body is used to using, which are things you are already doing by following the Food Plan.

Please note: I am NOT highlighting these 4 things to say that you can't lose weight if you are dealing with them. It's more so to highlight that if the scale isn't moving, there can be underlying issues the body needs to focus on more than others in order to help it start focusing on weight loss.

If you suspect you are dealing with any of these issues, have faith the program will help to address them and continue to maximize your efforts. But it is also worthwhile to work with your health care provider to level up in these areas, which can be a game changer when it comes to the scale.

Hope that helps, be sure to check into the Support Group for more info or if you have any questions. Head to the Science Guide and check out The Set Point Theory for more information on factors that can affect how quickly we lose weight.

WEEK 7 GUIDELINES: MAXIMIZING & FEEDING THE METABOLISM

Consistently working the Food Plan and Maximizing your efforts to help the body focus on fat loss. This week also has us introducing Feeding the Metabolism mid-week.

As we move into Week 7, we are going to move on from Downsizing, bring it back to Eating to Satisfaction and Maximizing for 3 days and then completely shift gears for the last 4 days.

DAYS 1-3 YOU ARE MAXIMIZING

Keep in mind that with Maximizing and Eating to Satisfaction, you are relentlessly doing everything you can to get the body to focus on detox and stay there as long as possible.

WHEN MAXIMIZING, YOU ARE FOCUSING ON:

- Drinking enough water.
- Being consistent with any supplements you are taking.
- Hitting all of your meals and snacks.
- Making your food choices as nutrient rich as possible.
- Being super mindful about portions. Make sure you eat enough, but not too much, allowing your body to stay focused on detox and fat loss instead of digestion.
- Avoiding eating too late in the evening. It will mess with sleep and the detox process.
- Managing stress levels, getting lots of rest, going to bed earlier, going for walks, deep breathing, moving the body and meditation.

- Being more active, adjusting workouts and adding in more movement by taking the stairs or parking further away.

DAYS 4 - 7 YOU ARE GOING TO INTRODUCE FEEDING THE METABOLISM.

Please note: There will be a post and video posted on Wednesday to further explain this tweak.

LET"S TALK FEEDING THE METABOLISM

Feeding the metabolism is meant to be used as another way to utilize your digestive system to help feed into your increasing metabolism by eating more often.

A higher metabolism means you are using more energy and burning more calories on a daily basis.

A body with a nice high metabolism looks to be as efficient as possible and looks at any extra stored fat as a hindrance and something it needs to get rid of.

In Feeding the Metabolism, you are going to continue to be super consistent with the supplements, the water, and the food. You will also continue to follow the Food Plan.

The tweak is to split your meals into 2 portions, eating the second portion 30 minutes later. This will have you eating more often and keeps the digestive system working hard all day and have you more in tune with your portion sizes.

You can do this with one meal or all of your meals. You can also do this with your snacks.

FOR EXAMPLE: Prepare a lunch portion that looks right for you and divide it in two. Eat one portion, continuing to be mindful of how you feel. A half an hour later, give or take, you will have the second portion. If you aren't hungry for the second portion, make sure you still have a token amount.

Keep in mind there is no hard and fast rule for this. You can split up all of your meals and snacks, some of your meals and snacks, or even just one.

The goal is to eat more often than what your body is used to. So, it can be once more a day to 6 more times a day, and that can change from day to day.

TO TAKE IT ONE STEP FURTHER: It is ideal when dividing meals to separate your protein from your carbs.

Protein is better digested on its own because it does not require as much insulin to process versus heavier carbs. As an example, for lunch eat your protein first and then eat your veggies later.

Do the same with vegetable protein. For example, with chickpeas, which are a protein and carb, there is still a benefit from separating them from the extra vegetables.

Healthy fats and leafy greens can be eaten with either portion, or both.

PLEASE NOTE: When it comes to soups, stews, chili etc., where it's harder to separate the protein, just separate the portion into 2 servings and don't worry about separating the protein.

There is no right or wrong or specific time frame with this. You can eat as often as you can manage or just a few times more, and the number of times can be different each day.

- Keep in mind you are still working to maximize everything that you are doing.

- Continue to get the water in.

- Be consistent with all supplements as well as fine tuning and adjusting when needed.

- Getting as much sleep as you can since it is vital for the body to be able to detox and make changes.

- Adding in exercise or moving your body and being more active.

- Managing stress levels, meditating, deep breathing, adding in yoga and going for walks.

When it comes to PORTIONS, you want to be mindful of giving the body what it needs but also mindful not to match hunger levels. You are still looking to lose weight, so you will want to keep your portions in check. This is where you need to step up your mindfulness (i.e., Keep asking yourself those 4 mindfulness questions when eating).

You don't want to purposely decrease portions to the point you stress your body like we did with downsizing. BUT, if you overeat the first portion, or even eat to feel satisfied, you will feel like you are overeating with the second portion. There is some tweaking to do here so it's important that you are paying attention.

You may find with eating more often; you are either not as hungry or hungrier. Both are beneficial responses from the body. At this point, your body wants your fat gone just as much as you do so it will be looking to get rid of it. All you need to do is stay on top of doing everything you can do to maximize your results.

TO RECAP:

Days 1-3 you are Eating to Satisfaction and Maximizing. Days 4-7 you will implement Feeding the Metabolism.

It is not okay to switch up the order of Eating to Satisfaction with Feeding the Metabolism. Everything is for a rhyme and a reason, so if you start rearranging the order of things, you aren't following The Program as designed, and may not get the desired results.

Remember you can split up all or some of your meals and snacks. Do the best you can. This is only for a few days. We will be posting a separate post and video explaining this tweak more before we start the Feeding the Metabolism portion.

We are only on Week 7, we have 6 weeks left to cover a lot of ground and lose a lot more weight, so stay strong and stay in the game!

Please take the time to head over to the Facebook Group or the Livy Method App and watch the quick video that accompanies this post. Head over to the Science Guide and read The Migrating Motor Complex (MMC) and Hunger for more information.

WEEK 7 GUIDELINES FAQS

1.   I work full time and struggle to split my meals and snacks throughout the day. Any tips?

Some members find that setting timers/alarms as reminders to eat really helps with this process. For Feeding the Metabolism, you don't need to split all your meals and snacks for the tweak to be effective. Do the best you can while at work and maximize splitting the other meals when at home.

2.   Do I eat 30 minutes after starting or finishing my last portion?

It's 30 minutes after your last bite of your last meal or snack. Setting timers/alarms as reminders to eat can really help.

3.   Do I have to wait until mid-week to start the splitting process? Or can I start at the beginning of the week?

To maximize your efforts, it's best to follow the Program as designed. Feeding the Metabolism works best off the heels of maximizing and eating to satisfaction. To recap, days 1-3 you are eating to satisfaction and Maximizing. Days 4-7 you will implement Feeding The Metabolism. It is not recommended to switch up the order. Everything is for a rhyme and a reason, and if you do switch up the order of this tweak, you may not get the desired results.

4.   Do I have to split the same meals each day?

The great thing about this tweak is that there is no hard and fast rule. You can split all of your meals and snacks, or even just one of them in a day for this tweak to be effective. This can change day to day.

5.   What if I am not hungry for the second half of my meal/snack?

If after 30 minutes you find you are not hungry for the second portion, you still want to eat a token amount of 4-5 bites with lots of chewing to stimulate digestion. It also puts you in tune with your portion, recognizing that your first portion was enough to satisfy you. You may find with eating more often, you are either not as hungry or hungrier. Both are normal and beneficial responses from the body.

6.   If I am already eating token bites for most of my snacks, how do I split them?

If you are not hungry for a meal/snack, and are having only token bites, 4-5 bites with chewing in between, then you wouldn't need to split those meals or snacks. Be open to your changing hunger levels as you can find that you may be hungry for your next meal or snack. The goal is just to eat more often than what your body is used to, so split the portions or the meals and/or snacks that you are hungry for.

7.   **Which would maximize our efforts the most, dividing a couple portions daily or dividing ALL portions daily?**

It would be ideal to divide all of your portions for each meal/snack to make your body work as hard as possible. However, you can ultimately choose which meals and snacks you would like to split each day depending on convenience and your changing hunger levels.

8.   **If I normally skip breakfast do I start with splitting my morning fruit?**

As always, breakfast is optional when following the Plan, but can be a great benefit to have. If you are not having breakfast, you can start by splitting your morning fruit snack if you are able to. Keep in mind that even splitting one meal or snack is still working the tweak, but eating more often keeps the digestive system working hard all day.

9.   **I am confused about how I should be splitting my meals and snacks. Any tips or advice?**

There is no hard and fast rule for this. You can split up all of your meals or just one of your meals, and the same rules apply with the snacks. To take it one step further, it is ideal when dividing meals to separate your protein from your carbs. Healthy fats and greens can be eaten with either portion, or both. If it is too difficult to separate your meal components, just separate the portion into 2 servings.

LET'S REVISIT THE TOPIC OF WATER

Water and how much you need to drink continues to be a hot topic around here.

So, let's revisit how much you need and why relevant to where you are now in this process.

Key takeaways when it comes to water:

- Everyone is different & every day is different…consider your body's needs and adjust day to day to find the right amount.

- When the scale is bouncing up and down the same few pounds this is usually a sign the body is trying to detox but needs more water …try increasing by a few cups.

- When you crave carbs and sugar specifically, this is usually a sign you are dehydrated and the body is trying to get you to eat high water content foods like fruit. So, when craving sugar, bump up your water intake.

- It's normal to be extra hungry and extra thirsty heading into the evening right before your weight is about to drop. Drink more water to help support detox.

- When you are drinking lots of water but your lips are dry and or you are thirsty, this is a sign your body is asking for even more water…you can trust your body so drink more.

- If the scale is moving and you find the water hard to drink or particularly unappealing this can be a sign you are in active detox, so support the body and the scale dropping by drinking more.

- If you drop weight and the next day the scale is the same or even up, this can be a sign the body is retaining water to continue to drop, so support the body's needs and drink more water to keep the scale moving.

- If the more water you drink, the more you have to pee…that can be a sign you are still dehydrated. Once properly hydrated you will be able to go longer periods of time without having to go to the bathroom as often. Try drinking earlier in the day and spreading it out.

Why water is key:

- Unlike traditional diets that force your body to burn fat by way of eating less or exercising more, the Livy Method uses the body's natural detox process to help release the fat, so water is key in helping that happen.

How much do you need?

- The average person needs at least 2.7 - 3.5 liters of water for basic body functions like digestion, pumping blood through your veins, sweating, bowel movements etc. (see original post for the source).

- To help the body get into detox mode (focus on fat loss), you need to drink above and beyond what it needs for basic body functions.
- Since your goal here is weight loss, aim for 3.5 liters. You can adjust from there depending on your height, weight and other factors listed below.

When to drink more than 3.5 liters:

- Your body is in detox
- You are fighting an illness
- You have your period
- You take medication that causes weight gain or dehydration
- You work or live in a dry environment
- You exercise or are active enough to sweat
- You drink alcohol
- You eat salty food
- You are taller than average (over 5'5" for women, 5'9" for men)
- You have more weight to lose

How do you know you are drinking enough?

- You no longer feel thirsty
- You no longer have dry mouth or lips
- Your trips to the bathroom have decreased (they will increase until you are properly hydrated)

How much is too much?

- Too much water is not really a concern for most people. Over-hydration and water intoxication happen when you drink more water than your kidneys can get rid of through urine. As long as you are not drinking more than a liter an hour you will be fine.

What about low sodium?

- Unless you are older and take medication that can deplete or are at risk for low sodium levels, this isn't really an issue.
- It's not drinking the extra water that can cause low sodium, it's the lack of sodium. Your muscles need salt to work properly, so you want to make sure you are getting enough salt in your diet.
- To prevent low sodium levels, add a pinch of pink Himalayan, Celtic or Sea salt to your

warm water and lemon or ACV in the morning. This will add in minerals and electrolytes as well as support hormone and adrenal function. Or you can purchase trace minerals to add to your water

Tips for increasing water intake:

- Increase slowly.
- Start early and spread your water drinking throughout the day.
- Sip and don't chug a large amount at once.
- Make it fun! Make it a challenge!
- Start drinking early in your day. Most people find it easier to get the majority in the first half of the day.
- Sip, don't guzzle or it will go right through you.
- Get a good water bottle.
- Track your water (and other fluids such as coffee, tea, bone broth) intake by using an app.
- Set reminders to drink.
- Add fresh or frozen fruit, cucumber slices, and/or fresh herbs or ginger.
- Stop drinking after dinner, so it doesn't mess with your sleep.

When it comes to water, it's not about drinking more and more. It's about drinking enough. Do what's right for you and always consult with your doctor if you have any concerns.

Once you have lost the weight and are in maintenance you can adjust and scale back on the amount you are drinking to maintain hydration without having to push more for the sake of weight loss.

To read more about how water can support the weight loss process please read Detox and The Science of Fat and Fat Loss in the Science Guide.

LET'S TALK FEEDING THE METABOLISM

Here we are on Week 7

- Day 1-3 has you Eating to Satisfaction and Maximizing.
- Day 4-7 you are going to introduce Feeding the Metabolism.

Feeding the Metabolism is meant to be used as another way to utilize your digestive system to help maximize your metabolism by eating more often.

A higher metabolism means you are using more energy and burning more calories on a daily basis.

A body with a nice high metabolism looks to be as efficient as possible and looks at any extra stored fat as a hindrance and something it needs to get rid of.

LET'S TALK TWEAKS:

In Feeding the Metabolism, you are going to continue to be super consistent with the supplements, the water and the food.

You are also going to continue to follow the Food Plan.

The only thing that changes is you are going to split your meals up into smaller portions and eat as often as possible to keep the digestive system working hard all day.

- For example, you can split your breakfast into 2 portions, your lunch into 2 portions, and dinner into 2 portions.
- You can also split snacks into 2 portions each.

As you can see, this will have you eating a lot more often.

Keep in mind there is no hard and fast rule for this. You can split up all of your meals or some of your meals or just one of your meals, and the same rules apply with the Snacks.

- The goal is to eat more often than what you are used to eating. This can be 1 more time a day or 5 more times a day, and that can change day to day.
- To take it one step further, it is ideal when dividing meals to separate your protein from your carbs.
- Protein is better digested on its own without the need for insulin, which is required to break down carbs.

As an example, for lunch, eat your protein first and then eat your veggies a half hour later.

With veg protein you can still do the same. With chickpeas for example, which are a protein and carb, there is still a benefit from separating them from the extra veg.

Healthy fats and greens can be eaten with either portion, or both.

For something like soup, where it's harder to separate the protein, just separate the portion into 2 servings.

THINGS TO KEEP IN MIND:

- There is no right or wrong way to do this.
- You do however want to wait 30 minutes between portions.
- You can eat as often as you can manage or just a few times more.
- Keep in mind you are still working to Maximize everything that you are doing.
- Continue to get the water in.
- Be consistent with all supplements as well as fine tuning and adjusting when needed.
- Getting as much sleep as you can since it is vital for the body to be able to detox and make changes.
- Adding in exercise or moving your body and being more active.
- Managing stress levels, meditating, deep breathing, adding in yoga and going for walks.

When it comes to PORTIONS, you want to be mindful of giving the body what it needs, but also mindful of not matching hunger levels or overeating.

You are still looking to lose weight, so you will want to keep your portions in check.

This is where you need to step up your mindfulness. Remember to ask yourself those 4 Mindfulness Questions at every meal and snack. You want to eat, but be mindful of portions. The goal is to eat just enough so when you walk away, you are feeling satisfied and not full or stuffed.

With breaking up your portions into smaller portions, keep in mind chances are your body will be getting more than enough food because you will be eating more often. With that said, you may find with eating more often, you are either not as hungry or hungrier. Both are normal and beneficial responses from the body.

TO RECAP:

- Be super mindful of portions, eat the first half and then take note of how you feel 15 mins later and be super mindful when eating the second half.
- If you find yourself not hungry for the second half, then just eat a token amount. This can be

an indication that you may still be eating too much of your first portion. So there's room to play around with that.

- Ideally, you want to wait 30 minutes before consuming the second portion.

At this point, your body wants your fat gone just as much as you do so it will be looking to get rid of it. All you need to do is stay on top of doing everything you can do to maximize your results.

Please take the time to head over to the Facebook Group or the Livy Method App and watch the quick video that accompanies this post. Head over to the Science Guide and read The Migrating Motor Complex (MMC) and Hunger for more information.

LET'S REVISIT EXERCISE

Exercise is a great compliment to the program, it's great for heart health, bone density, stress release, as well as toning and shaping your changing body.

Earlier in the program we talked about how to incorporate it and tweak it so it is more conducive to fat loss. Because as great as exercise can be for your health and wellness, it's not the best weight loss tool. Which is one reason why it's not a mandatory component of the program. But given where we are at in the program with your body working hard to maximize your metabolism. It's not unusual for you to start thinking about moving more as your body gives you access to more energy.

Your metabolism is the rate at which your body functions day to day or to simplify, how much energy you use and calories you naturally burn on a daily basis. When the body feels a need to store fat, it keeps you in "reserve mode" and limits the amount of energy you can use.

Now that you're feeling more energetic let's talk about the best way to implement exercises that will fall in line with your weight loss goals:

- If you are new to exercise, I suggest you start by simply being more active.
- I know it sounds cliché, but things like taking the stairs and parking further away when getting groceries, going for walks or doing some push-ups or squats in your kitchen, can add up and have a big impact.
- If you are looking for something more intense, there are a lot of great home workout options. It's best to start slow to minimize the stress on the body and build up to it.
- Whatever you choose to do, it should be something you enjoy so you make a positive association to exercise moving forward and it becomes something you look forward to doing.
- You also want to walk away from any exercise feeling good and energized, not tired, taxed or drained.

You have to remember you are working towards getting the body to focus on detox and fat loss. If you work out too hard and you create too much damage in the body, it will have no choice but to focus on repairing and rebuilding instead of detox and fat loss.

When you lift weights, the goal is to rip and tear your muscle and create damage so the body works hard to fix the damage and repair the muscle making it stronger, which leaves you more toned. And that's great. However, that can very easily keep your body in a state of repair and rebuild instead of focusing on fat loss.

THIS BRINGS US TO THE TOPIC OF REST:

- If you are going to work out to the point of being sore, you need to make sure you are giving your body adequate time to repair and rebuild, or you will run the risk of over-training.

- Overtraining happens when the body can't catch up to the damage that's been done, leaving your body feeling weak and in a deficit, which in turn can cause the body to feel the need to hold on to fat or store more fat for easy energy.

LET'S TALK CARDIO OR GETTING YOUR HEART RATE UP:

- When it comes to exercise and weight loss, it's all about the message you are sending to the body.

- Your physical brain that runs your body doesn't see what you are doing for exercise, it only interprets what you are doing based on your movements and heart rate.

- This is where you can use the body's natural FIGHT or FLIGHT response to maximize your results.

- Getting your heart rate up as high as you can for as long as you can, even if just for a few minutes, evokes the FIGHT or FLIGHT response in the body and immediately sends a message for the body to work to make you stronger.

The body's sole responsibility is to keep you alive so if you repeatedly evoke the fight or flight response, your body will look to make you as strong and efficient as possible.

In wanting to be as efficient as possible, your body will look to get rid of any extra fat that could be slowing you down.

This makes Cardio (exercise that gets your heart rate up) very effective for fat loss.

Cardio doesn't have to be running, it can be walking fast, skipping, swimming, dancing, lifting lighter weights with higher reps, sports activities, and anything else that helps get your heart rate up.

With cardio you are basically taking the muscle you already have in your body and using it to move your body, which will get your heart rate up without creating damage, making it a complement to the weight loss program.

WHEN IT COMES TO LIFTING WEIGHTS, THINGS CAN GET TRICKY:

- When it comes to lifting weights, you are purposely creating damage in the body so the body repairs the damage and makes the muscle stronger.

- That is great for bone density, building muscle and shaping your body, but not great for fat loss.

- That doesn't mean you can't continue to lift weights, especially if that is something you enjoy. I would, however, suggest you lift a little lighter using higher repetitions, to use the muscle you do have to help to get your heart rate up with minimal damage.

During sleep is when the body detoxes and/or makes change, it doesn't do both at the same time. So if your body is always sore, then your body is always focusing on repairing the damage that is making you sore. Leaving very little to no time left to focus on detox.

With that said, you may think I'm not a fan of exercise or I'm suggesting you don't exercise....so let me be clear in saying, exercise is absolutely a benefit with this program.

The message I'm trying to get across is that you need to be smart about it and understand the message that is being sent to the body when you exercise and be mindful to support your body's needs and be sure to get enough rest between workouts.

HERE ARE MY EXERCISE FAVES FOR FAT LOSS:

- Walking because it's also conducive to healing and the least stressful type of exercise you can do.
- Anything outside, because it stimulates the brain and works the body while communing with nature and relieving stress.
- Dance or Boxing/Martial arts type classes that move the body in different ways other than side to side and up and down, while evoking the fight response.
- Biking or spinning is great for getting your heart rate up and evoking the flight response.
- Resistance training using your own body weight.

Let us know if you have any questions and be sure to check with your Health Care Provider before starting any new routine.

Please take time to head over to the Facebook Group or the Livy Method App and check out Gina's Easy Toning Exercises that will be posted throughout the week. For more information on exercise and weight loss check out The Science of Fat and Fat Loss in the Science Guide.

FOOD FACTS - ANTI-INFLAMMATORY FOODS

WHAT IS INFLAMMATION?

Inflammation is the body's normal reaction to injuries and infection. Short term bouts of inflammation called "acute inflammation" is just your body's way of protecting yourself and is doing its job just fine.

However, too much inflammation, and for too long, isn't a good thing. When this happens, the body thinks it's under constant attack so the immune system continues fighting back, indefinitely. Research has shown that chronic inflammation is linked to many diseases like arthritis, diabetes, heart disease, cancer and bowel diseases like Crohn's disease.

CAN CERTAIN FOODS HELP REDUCE INFLAMMATION?

A diet rich in anti-inflammatory foods isn't a magic cure when dealing with chronic inflammation. Medication and other treatments are important so be sure to be working with your healthcare practitioner. However, the combination of treatment and changes in diet can have a noticeable impact on low-grade inflammation.

FOODS THAT CAN HELP LOWER INFLAMMATION

The good news is, anti-inflammatory foods tend to be the same foods that help keep you healthy in other ways as well! So even if you don't suffer from inflammation, it's a great idea to add more of these nutrient rich foods into your diet!

- **Vegetables** - especially broccoli, Brussels sprouts, cauliflower, and bok choy
- **Leafy greens** - kale, spinach, and romaine lettuce. The darker the better!
- **Fresh fruit** - Intense colours are a sign that fruits are high in antioxidants. Look for dark blues & purples, like blackberries, plums and grapes. Bright reds, oranges and yellows like pomegranate, apples, raspberries, strawberries, papaya, mango and pineapple
- **Plant-based proteins** - bump up those beans and lentils!
- **Fatty fish** - salmon, sardines, albacore tuna, herring, lake trout, and mackerel
- **Whole grains** - oatmeal, dark rices, barley, wheat kernels etc.
- **Foods with healthy fats** - olive oil, avocados, nuts, and seeds (especially walnuts, almonds, hemp, flax, and chia seeds)
- **Other foods/beverages high in antioxidants** - Ginger, turmeric, green tea, coffee and red wine (in moderation)

WHAT FOODS MAKE INFLAMMATION WORSE?

- Refined carbohydrates, such as white bread, pastries, and sweets
- Foods and drinks that are high in sugar, including excessive alcohol, soda and other sugary beverages
- Red meat
- Dairy
- Processed meat, such as hot dogs and sausages
- Fried foods
- Artificial food additives often found in highly processed foods and fast food
- Any foods that you may have a sensitivity to

BOTTOM LINE IS...

- Eat more plants
- Focus on antioxidants
- Consume Omega 3s
- Eat less red meat
- Cut out highly processed and sugary foods

If you are following the program, you have likely added in lots of great anti-inflammatory foods already. This is just another way to get you thinking about how you could level up your efforts. Whether you suffer from inflammation or not, adding in anti-inflammatory foods increases your health in general and can help prevent any inflammation from getting out of control.

LET'S REVISIT ALCOHOL

It is important to note that your tolerance to alcohol can change while following the plan.

Meaning that, if it used to take you 2 glasses of wine before you felt the effects, you should not be surprised if, after following the plan and losing weight, that you are unable to consume as much as you did before.

When your metabolism increases, your body works more efficiently. When you combine that with significant weight loss, you may notice that your tolerance can change.

If you like to enjoy an alcoholic beverage every now and then, let's revisit these tips to help minimize the impact on your body and the scale:

WINE

- Choose red wine over white. Although both are fine, red has more antioxidants and is slightly better for you. That isn't a reason to give up your white if that's what you prefer.

ROSE & CHAMPAGNES

- A little higher in sugar so don't be surprised if you wake up with a headache but also totally fine to have.

BEER/CIDERS

- Avoid "light" or "low-cal" beer. Light beer may have less calories but turns to sugar faster. That is an issue because we are not worried about calories, we are more concerned about how it breaks down in the body and affects your insulin levels and digestive system. Darker beers like Guinness are higher in nutrient value but any of your regular, all-natural ales, lagers, pilsners etc. are totally fine.

- When it comes to Ciders the same rules apply. Be mindful of added sugars and artificial ingredients.

- Non-alcoholic beer/ciders is counted as an extra, just as juice would be. Be mindful of the ingredients and if there is a small alcohol percentage, you may want to add in some extra water.

HARD LIQUOR

- When it comes to the hard stuff, be mindful about what you are using as a mix. Try to avoid pop/soda, including diet and flavoured juice.

- Stick with carbonated water, mixed with a splash of natural juices, tomato juice or Clamato etc. If you enjoy something like rye and coke or gin and tonic once every now and then, it's no big deal.

The issue with alcohol is more the food you eat with it. If you are following the plan this is a non-issue but sometimes you might be at a party and be mindfully indulging. Here's a couple of things to keep in mind if you are:

- Drinking alcohol slows down the metabolism & your digestive system, so you want to avoid any heavy carbs like bread and pasta and stick to more protein, fats (like cheese and nuts) and veggies.

- Keep in mind alcohol can affect weight loss in other ways. For example, interrupting your sleep, messing with estrogen levels, causing dehydration, and causing you to crave both sugar and salt the next day.

- Alcohol increases the production of galanin, a neuropeptide in the brain, which causes you to crave greasy food. Pair that with the effects of dehydration that causes you to crave sugar and you are ready to eat your face off the next day!

- Bumping up good fats like oils, nuts, seeds, and avocados, increasing your water along with having a banana, which is high in potassium, first thing the next day will help the body metabolize the alcohol and reduce the galanin.

- Drinking can also affect the good bacteria in your digestive system, so if your stomach always feels off the next day, try adding in or doubling up on your probiotic.

MY FINAL AND MOST IMPORTANT TIP:

The best thing you can do to offset negative effects of alcohol consumption is to add in that extra water of one cup per drink. Besides that, enjoy your beverages!

WEEK 8 GUIDELINES: FEEDING THE METABOLISM

Continuing to maximize your efforts and making the body work hard for food again. This also supports the body's need to be efficient and maximize your metabolism.

First, let me say congrats for making it this far in the Process. It is no small feat to continue to stay so focused on reaching your goals and to keep showing up for yourself each & every day!

It's an exciting place to be on this journey. After spending so much time addressing the body's needs and helping it stay focused on fat loss, your body is now in a place where it wants the fat gone just as much as you do.

Essentially, moving forward weight loss should get easier as your body is looking to function at more optimal levels & make you as healthy as possible and you are more in tune than ever to your body's needs and know what it needs to stay focused on fat loss.

LET'S TALK WEEK 8

Week 8 is the same as week 7. We will be doing Maximizing and Eating to Satisfaction for the first **THREE** days followed by Feeding the Metabolism for **FOUR** days.

If you feel like you didn't have the chance to work Week 7 to the best of your ability, then this is your second chance. For a refresher, please review the Week 7 Guidelines and check out the video on Feeding the Metabolism, found in the Facebook Group or the Livy Method App.

OVERVIEW:

DAYS 1-3

- Back to satisfaction but with an emphasis on portions, eating just enough and being mindful not to match hunger levels.

DAYS 4-7

Feeding the Metabolism:

- Hitting all meals and snacks.

- Making foods nutrient rich.

- Breaking up meals and snacks into 2 portions.

- If you are taking it one step further, separating protein from carbs (fats & greens can be included with protein or carbs).

- Super mindful of portions and adjusting to hunger levels day to day.

This will be the last week we will be following the basic food formula. Moving forward, we will be changing things up to adapt to the changes your body is making.

A LOOK AHEAD:

Week 9 - HIGHER PROTEIN AND FAT REVAMP

Week 10 - REVAMP Part 2

Week 11 - PERSONALIZING THE FOOD PLAN

Week 12 - MAINTENANCE & EATING OFF ROUTINE

Remember to focus on MAXIMIZING and doing all the other things, besides the food, water & any supplements, that you can be focusing on to help speed up the fat loss process.

We have a lot of time left to lose a lot of weight. Your focus moving forward should be following through and finishing just as strong, if not stronger than when you started. Your body is on your side, so continue to be all in to maximize your results in the time frame we have left.

Please take the time to head over to the Facebook Group or the Livy Method App and watch the quick video that accompanies this post.

WEEK 8 GUIDELINES FAQS

1.   Is it normal to be hungry during the Feeding The Metabolism tweak?

It is totally normal to feel hungry during the Feeding The Metabolism tweak. You may find with eating more often, you are either not as hungry as usual or feel hungrier. Both are normal and beneficial responses from the body.

2.   How should I seperate my meals properly?

Similar to week 7, there is no hard and fast rule for this. You can split up all of your meals or just one of your meals, and the same rules apply with the snacks. To take it one step further, it is ideal when dividing meals to separate your protein from your carbs. Healthy fats and greens can be eaten with either portion, or both. If it is too difficult to separate your meal components, just separate the portion into 2 servings.

3.   Can I eat the second portion after 30 minutes have passed, or should I skip it?

With Feeding the Metabolism, you want to eat your second portion 30 minutes after you have finished your first portion. If you are not hungry for that second portion then you want to have 4-5 token bites with chewing in between. Keep in mind that you can split up all of your meals and snacks, some of your meals and snacks, or even just one.

4.   What does it mean to be "mindful not to match hunger levels"?

Not matching hunger levels means you are eating just enough. You are still looking to lose weight, so you want to keep your portions in check and continue to ask those 4 mindfulness questions. You want to walk away from your meal or snack feeling like you have eaten just enough with no physical feelings of having eaten. You shouldn't feel full or stuffed 15 minutes later. You don't want to feel hungry, but you don't want to eat to satisfaction, like the first weeks of the program.

5.   What is an example of splitting protein from carbs?

By separating your protein from your carbs you are taking it one step further during Feeding the Metabolism. For example, eat your protein first, whether that is an animal or plant based protein, and eat your carbs for 30 min later for your second portion. Carbs are fruit, vegetables, heavier root veg, rice and grains, to name a few. For carbs like beans, lentils and chickpeas, which are both protein and carbs, it's still beneficial to separate them when you can. Good fats and leafy greens can be eaten with either or both portions. When it comes to soups, stews, chili's, etc., foods that are harder to separate out the protein, just divide your meal into 2 servings.

6.   I am experiencing a plateau this week, any tips?

There can be many reasons that your body is experiencing a plateau or stabilizing period. These stabilizing periods are really important for the body to solidify the weight you have lost and allow time for your body to adjust to the weight it has lost. Keep being all in and maximize your efforts and expect to see that scale move. We are either actively losing weight or our bodies are stabilizing and making change, our body won't do both at the same time. Focus on your non scale victories, as plateaus are often when we see the most change.

7.   I am not hungry for the second portion, any tips?

If after 30 minutes you find you are not hungry for the second portion of your meal or snack, you still want to eat a token amount of 4-5 bites with lots of chewing to stimulate digestion. Take note of how you feel and you may find that you can adjust your first portion accordingly. Remember to continue to engage in the four mindfulness questions at every meal and snack.

LET'S REVISIT THE SCALE

We have talked a lot about the scale over these past few months, the ups, the downs and the plateaus.

When it comes to the scale, the key thing to note is….it is going to fluctuate. Your weight loss journey will **NOT** be a straight line down.

When using the scale, it is more about the downward trend and understanding all the ups, downs and plateaus along the way.

THINGS TO KEEP IN MIND:

- When it comes to the scale using My Method, a drop is always a drop. When the scale moves down you can count on it being because of actual fat loss and that is your true weight.

- When the scale goes up it's not real weight gain. When following the plan weight gain is always superficial based on what you did or didn't eat or drink the day before. (Check out the Why is My Weight Up Post, and the 4 Reasons Why Your Weight is Up Post for more reasons your weight can be up)

- It is normal when you drop fat to have your weight go down & then have it go back up again on the scale as your body retains water before the cells have time to shrink. It retains water because it is in detox mode and looking to drop even more, so be sure to stay on top of drinking your water.

- It is normal to wake up feeling like you have lost weight, only to have the scale showing the same number as the day before or in some cases it might even be up. This is usually a sign you are about to drop.

- It's normal to feel bloated and gross and have your weight be up the day before you see a drop on the scale. This is just the body retaining water preparing for a drop.

- If your weight is bouncing up and down the same few pounds, that usually means your body needs more water to get into detox.

- You are going to have plateaus. Plateaus are part of the process and happen when the body is adjusting to weight you have lost or is focused on making change.

- You need and want plateaus; they are necessary to help the body solidify the weight you have lost which will factor in to making your weight loss easier to maintain.

    **** If you are looking to break a plateau refer to the troubleshooting post. ***

WHEN TO WEIGH IN:

- Weigh yourself in the morning after you go to the bathroom.

- Avoid weighing in at night as weight can fluctuate up to 10 pounds after a day of eating, which of course is not real weight gain.

- If you are weighing yourself, make sure you are doing it consistently. If you weigh in once a week, for example, you are only getting a snapshot and you may miss the fluctuations that you can use to understand your body's reaction as you move along in your journey. Either weigh in every day to use the scale as a tool, or skip the scale altogether.

WHAT KIND OF SCALE DO YOU NEED:

- Nothing fancy, any scale will work.

- A digital scale is ideal as you can see the small fluctuations, which can be helpful.

- I'm not a fan of scales that track water, weight, or fat % as I don't not believe they are accurate; however, you can use them if you like.

OTHER THINGS TO KEEP IN MIND:

- It's key to understand that the body doesn't care about how much you want the scale to move. It has no concept of time or your desire to lose weight as fast as possible.

- Your body also has no concept of any number you want to reach on the scale.

- Continue showing up and remember that your body is on your side and that it wants to get rid of the fat just as much as you do.

LET'S TALK ABOUT GOALS:

What is a good weight for you?

- Without sounding cliché, I really do think it's when you feel comfortable in your skin. A good base line I use for clients is your lowest weight after the age of 21, that you were able to easily maintain.

- That doesn't mean if you have always carried extra weight that you can't weigh less than you ever have, because you totally can. I always say weight loss is a side effect of being healthy. A properly functioning body has no need for excess fat, so given the opportunity and the time, it will be more than happy to get rid of it.

- It is good to set a target weight as a goal, but I find most people underestimate their goals out of fear of failing. Group members are always setting new goals along the way and that's ok because it's a process.

- Because the body is not meant to store excess fat, there is no reason why you wouldn't be able to lose all of your weight.

- You also don't need to worry about losing too much weight as we are focused on helping the body get rid of fat that no longer serves a purpose in the healthiest of ways.

TO RECAP:

- As frustrating as it can be sometimes, the scale is a very helpful tool for weight loss and nothing to be feared.

- Best time to weigh yourself is first thing in the morning, ideally after going to the bathroom. Later in the day the scale will always read higher.

- Weight up does not mean you gained weight. It is normal for your weight to fluctuate whether you are losing weight or not.

- A new low on the scale is always real weight loss and is your actual weight.

- It's normal for the scale to be up and is usually a sign you are about to drop.

- It's normal to "feel like" you have lost weight but have the scale up or the same. This also can be a sign you are about to drop.

- It's also normal to feel bloated and gross and have your weight up the day before it shows a drop on scale.

- Weight loss is never a straight line down. The scale is going to go up and down whether you like it or not. It's a normal part of the process and it is natural for weight to fluctuate even after you have finished losing weight.

Now that you have had some time to experience using the scale with this process, I hope this helps to not only explain, but also to normalize the ups, the downs and the plateaus when it comes to the scale while trying to reach your finally and forever weight loss goals.

SELF-SABOTAGE PART 2

Self-sabotage refers to behaviors or thought patterns that hold you back and prevent you from doing what you want to do and/or achieving your goals.

At this point in The Program, self-sabotage can start to rear its ugly head, once again, and the reasons can be a bit different than earlier on in the process. Let's take a look at some of these and see if we can pinpoint some areas where you might be struggling. These are just a few examples with some suggestions on how you can start to address them. Awareness is the first step to change so let's get to it!

1. **I'm Rewarding Myself For Reaching A Milestone - Many of us have been taught to use food as a reward so this one can be a tough one to break. But it is possible!**

    Make a list of things other than food that you can reward yourself with. Here are some ideas to get you started:

    - A new book or magazine.

    - A new skin care product or something for the bath.

    - Treat yourself to a special coffee or tea at your favourite café with a book or a friend.

    - Schedule yourself some "ME" time, whatever that looks like for you.

2. **I've Lost A Good Chunk Of Weight So I Deserve A Break** - This is similar to #1 but a different excuse. Many people who are successful on Plan but haven't yet reached their goals think it's okay to start adding in bits and bites and start half-assing the process. This can be a slippery slope. Try to stay all in until you reach your goals and go through the maintenance period to solidify the weight you have lost. Don't put yourself into the situation where you lose a bunch of weight and then spend the next several years trying to lose that last 10 lbs! If you need a break, take a mindful break. Allow yourself a "vacation". Make a plan, give it a timeline, and get right back in the game. Get it done and move on to your *finally and forever*!

3. **I'm Bored** - Bored with the food plan, the foods, the routine, the focus? Boredom is no joke and a very common reason why some people might give up.

    How about changing up some of the foods you are eating? Try a new fruit or vegetable you've always wondered about. Maybe find a new recipe to try. There are lots of great ideas and recipes to try over in the Recipe Share Pages in the Facebook Group. Or just try something new in general. A new hobby, a new exercise routine, take a class, learn something new!

4. **I Have 'Program Fatigue'** - You're starting to lose your enthusiasm or ambition to lose weight and maybe just plain tired of having to think about it! Take a moment to think back to when you started and how pumped and excited you were! Why were you so excited? What is your "WHY"? Revisit that and make a list. Watch some of the Facebook Lives for motivation and inspiration. Even if you don't have time to watch all of them, checking in to watch part of one each day can really help. If you are just plain tired of having to think about it, try simplifying

your meals and snacks as much as possible so there isn't much thinking involved. Prep some food on the weekends so you are prepared, set timers and reminders on your phone for your food, water and supplements. Make things as much of a "no-brainer" as you can.

5. **I'm Just Going To Enjoy The Break And Get Back In The Game In The Next Group** - There's still time to lose weight between now and the next Group! Think about how you will feel come the start date and you look back at all the time you could have been continuing with the process. Remember that even if the scale slows down because you indulge a bit more over the break, you will still have kept up the momentum, which is what weight loss is built on. This will put you in a much better position when starting the next Group or continuing your journey however you chose.

6. **The Scale Hasn't Moved, Or Is Moving Too Slowly So This Program Just Doesn't Work For Me** - If you give up now, what will you do next? Try another burn the fat diet, lose some weight, and then gain it all back plus more? Remember, even if you haven't lost any weight yet you are only making your body healthier and working towards it, eventually feeling comfortable letting go of the fat. There is no way around it, only through. Dig deeper to find what is causing your body to hold onto fat. Most often, it is an underlying health issue that can be addressed under the guidance of a healthcare professional.

7. **Future-tripping!** - You are worried about what lies ahead. How will I keep the weight off?" "What does life after weight loss look like?" "I don't trust that I can follow through and reach my goals." "I don't trust myself to not go back to my old eating habits".

Peering into an imagined future and predicting the outcome is a major form of self-sabotage. Focusing on what you don't know isn't going to get you anywhere. Work on staying in the moment. Focus on what you need to do day to day. Practice gratitude for all you have accomplished and trust yourself to be able to handle whatever the future holds. Consider joining the next Group even if you have reached your goal to help you stay on track through maintenance. The extra support can be very helpful to not feel like you are on your own.

8. **Are You Too Focused On Numbers And The Scale Not Reaching The Number You Had Planned For The Timeframe?** - Your brain cares about numbers, not your body. As long as you are doing the things you need to do your body will work at its own pace. Trust that your body is doing everything it needs to be doing to make you healthier. Make a list of all your non-scale victories for a reminder of all the other things you have accomplished. Do this every day to continually remind yourself. Try to take the focus off of the numbers and put it on how you feel.

SELF-SABOTAGE is no joke and often goes unnoticed if you don't take the time to stop and think. Sometimes all it takes is a little reminder of what tricks the brain can play on us to wake us to our senses! Take a step back and reflect on the things listed above. Make some lists, do some journaling, and get your head back in the game!

If you would like to dig deeper, be sure to go back and check out the first post on Self-Sabotage for even more insight and inspiration. Also be sure to head to the Science Guide and read The Psychology of Effort.

LET'S REVISIT WHY MY WEIGHT IS UP?

While following the Plan, remember that your weight might go up for various reasons, none of which will have anything to do with actual weight gain.

Let me first say…when following the Plan, and eating all meals and snacks, making foods nutrient rich and eating to satisfaction (or even overeating) you are NOT going to gain weight.

The body is not inclined to want to store fat, in fact it's quite the opposite. The body wants your fat gone as much as you do!

It's important to understand that throughout this Program, your weight is going to naturally fluctuate, no matter what you do.

REASONS YOUR WEIGHT CAN BE UP:

- Stress
- Lack of sleep
- Salty food
- Hard to digest food (like red meat, although not a reason to not eat it)
- Dehydration
- Body fighting an illness
- Body sore from a workout
- Body reacting to change in routine
- Body reacting to change in food
- Body reacting to new medication or change in medications
- Body reacting to any new supplements or change in supplements
- Deficiencies like being low in iron
- Hormones balancing
- PMS
- Your scale needing new batteries
- And the most important reason is that your body is detoxing and your weight is about to drop.

**If you haven't seen it yet, take time to review the scale post and watch the video as it's important to understand what real weight loss looks like on the scale. **

If you are doing all of the things and you are not seeing any movement on the scale, your body just may need time. If you feel as though something else may be going on, remember the 4 Reasons Why Your Weight Might Be Slower To Move:

- Inflammation
- Food sensitivities
- Gut Dysbiosis
- Hormonal health

In this case, best to follow up with your healthcare provider or a naturopath for more insight. Review the post in the Week 6 guides for more information.

If you stick around and keep showing up, you are going to be successful and lose your weight regardless of the little ups along the way. The ups are normal and to be expected.

Although we do like to have fun around here, weight loss can have its frustrating moments so we don't want anyone stressing about the scale any more than they need to...or even at all!

Hope this helps. Embrace the little ups because they always lead to the big drops!

LET'S REVISIT PROTEINS, CARBS, AND FATS

As we embark on Week 9 the Higher Protein and Fat Revamp, I thought it would be timely to revisit the protein, carbs and fats list.

Remember, it's not an exhaustive list and keep in mind you don't need to worry about serving sizes or percentages. This is just to give you examples of what foods fall under each category.

SOURCES OF CARBS

(Foods that break down into energy)

- Fruit
- Vegetables
- Heavier Root Veg like potatoes, squash, cassava, plantain
- Naturally occurring sugar found in things like beans and lentils and chickpeas...
- Oatmeal and whole grain cereal like hemp hearts and buckwheat
- Rice and grains like black rice & quinoa, barley
- Ryvita crackers and Ezekiel bread

SOURCES OF PROTEIN

(Feeds the muscles helping to repair and rebuild along with maintain and build muscle mass)

- Fish
- Meat (Any Meat)
- Eggs
- Seafood
- Beans, lentils, legumes
- Nuts and Seeds
- Incomplete protein like oatmeal, quinoa and dark rice (not to be used as main source)
- Dairy - cheese, yogurt, milk products (not to be used as main source of protein)
- Tofu
- Protein Powder (look for all natural without any artificial colour, flavor and sweeteners)

SOURCES OF PLANT BASED PROTEIN

(As you can see below, there is protein found in lots of things besides animal sources)

- Broccoli - 2.6g per 1 cup
- Asparagus - 2.4g per 1 cup
- Peas - 9g per 1 cup
- Cauliflower - 2g per 1 cup
- Brussels - 3g per 1 cup
- Bok choy - 1g per 1 cup
- Spinach, collard greens - 1g per 1 cup
- Mung bean sprouts - 2.5g per 1 cup
- Beans (kidney, pinto, black beans, chick peas etc.) - 7.5g per 1/2 cup
- Lentils - 9g per 1/2 cup
- Quinoa - 4g per 1/2 cup
- Tempeh - 11g per 1/2 cup
- Tofu - 7g per 1/2 cup
- Buckwheat - 6g per 1 cup
- Soy beans/Edamame - 10g per 1/2 cup
- Hemp seeds/hearts - 10g per 3 tbsp
- Pumpkin seeds - 5g per oz
- Chia - 4g per 2 tbsp
- Nut butter -15g per 2 tbsp
- Hummus - 7g per 2 tbsp
- Spirulina - 4g per 1 tbsp

Keep in mind you DO NOT need to worry about these measurements. They are for reference only and to point out the fact that some proteins have carbs in them, some vegetables have protein in them, and that protein adds up.

As long as you are following the Plan as outlined, you are getting enough and the right mix of everything you need.

SOURCES OF FATS

(Essential for cellular function, providing alternative energy and brain fuel)

- Fish/Fish oil
- Omega 3 and or 369
- Alternative oils like olive oil, coconut oil, avocado oil, grape seed oil, flax and hemp oil
- Salad dressings with good quality oils
- Olives
- Avocado
- Nuts/Nut butters
- Seeds/Seed butters
- Hemp hearts
- Dairy...like yogurt, cheese, butter

This is not a complete list, it is just to give you an idea of the kind of foods I'm suggesting when talking about incorporating proteins, carbs and fats to your meals.

FOOD FACTS - CRUCIFEROUS VEGETABLES!

Did you know that the word "cruciferous" originates from the Latin word for "cross bearing"? That's because the flower petals resemble a cross.

Cruciferous - [KROO] + [SIF] - [UH] - [RHUS]

Not sure what cruciferous vegetables are?

Here's a list of the most common ones:

- Arugula
- Bok choy
- Broccoli
- Brussels sprouts
- Cabbage
- Cauliflower
- Collard greens
- Kale
- Radish
- Turnips

These tasty veggies are packed with folate, vitamins C, E, and K and also loaded with fiber. Fiber helps to make these vegetables filling. So a little goes a long way!

Did you know that cruciferous vegetables support many areas of our health, like detoxification, anti-oxidant protection, and control of inflammation? They help neutralize and eliminate toxins, providing more energy, improved health, and the power to aid in the reduction of some serious illnesses like cancers, autoimmunity, and neurodegenerative disorders.

Without getting too "sciencey" about it, they contain a sulfur rich substance called sulforaphane which is a powerful antioxidant. Sulforaphane is only activated when these vegetables are chopped or chewed. The action of "damaging" by chopping or chewing mixes the enzymes together with other components that produce the sulforaphane.

Sulforaphane can't be formed after cooking, so if you want to get the most out of your cruciferous veggies you can chop and "rest" your veggies for 40 minutes before cooking. This allows time for the enzymes to mix and the sulforaphane to be formed. Once it's there it won't be destroyed by cooking.

Cruciferous vegetables are super versatile! They can all be enjoyed raw or cooked, added to salads, soups, stir frys, stews, roasted, steamed, sauteed, pureed...you name it!

Here are some ideas of how to easily incorporate more of these amazing veggies into your diet!

ARUGULA

It's zesty and peppery and can be enjoyed cooked or raw!

Perfect as a leafy green side dish simply drizzled with olive oil or your favourite dressing. Or toss it in your favourite soup or stir fry to add some extra zesty leafy greens.

Did you know that arugula is one of the easiest leafy greens to grow yourself? Just toss some seeds in a planter or your garden and watch them grow! They will continue to reproduce as you cut them so they can last all season long!

BROCCOLI AND CAULIFLOWER

These versatile veggies are delicious prepared in so many different ways! You can steam, roast, and grate into a "rice". Or why not try pureeing a combination of both together for a beautiful and tasty mashed potato substitute! Pick up some broccoli sprouts to add to salads for an even bigger boost of the powerful sulforaphane!

BRUSSELS SPROUTS

Brussels Sprouts are versatile. You can roast them which helps to bring out the sweetness. Add some parmesan cheese on top to make them even more delicious! You can also steam, or pan fry them. Brussels sprouts are equally delicious raw and make a great coleslaw or addition to any salad. Just slice them thinly or run them through a food processor and add your favourite coleslaw dressing!

CABBAGE, COLLARD GREENS AND KALE

All of the above are equally good cooked or raw. Cabbage is perfect for coleslaw of course but did you know it's also great cut into "steaks" brushed with olive oil and roasted in the oven? Collard greens make a great wrap instead of using bread, but they are also delicious chopped and fried with some oil and garlic for an amazing and easy leafy green side dish. Kale will not wilt for days so is perfect for make-ahead salads. Remove the tough stems, slice into ribbons and toss with your favourite dressing! Bok choy is a perfect addition to stir frys, soups and stews!

TURNIP & RADISH

Thinly sliced radish is a welcome peppery addition to any salad but did you know they are also delicious roasted? Roasting them releases the sweetness and mellows out the peppery bite. Turnips are totally underrated! They are very versatile and can be enjoyed raw or cooked. Boil or steam and mash as a potato substitute. Grate them raw into salads and soups or roast them on their own or with a mixture of your favourite roasted veggies to bring out their sweetness.

LET'S REVISIT TRAVEL

Although travelling can make it tricky to stay on plan it does have its advantages when it comes to weight loss.

LET'S START WITH VACATIONS:

It's key to understand that life is stressful, too stressful for our still very primitive, working bodies. Stress can play a major role when trying to lose weight.

Members are always concerned about gaining weight when on holiday, when in fact it can do wonders for weight loss. Change in environment, less stress, abundance of good fresh foods, and some decent sleep can be exactly what the body needs to get the scale moving.

TIPS FOR TRAVEL:

- It starts at the airport...resist the urge to indulge in treats before you fly.
- Flying is super dehydrating and combined with high sugar is a recipe for carb cravings, serious bloating, and constipation once you land.
- Spend the money on healthy snacks so you are not inclined to eat the crackers and cookies or heavily salted meal they serve during the flight.
- Sometimes I buy the snacks but eat the plane food if it looks decent. I'm always happy to have the extra snacks when I land as they can come in handy.
- **HYDRATE!** The altitude when flying sucks the water out of you, leaving you epically dehydrated, and can have you craving carbs and sugar from the get-go...so once you land, work that water!
- Try to maintain regular eating habits as much as possible and look at any extras as just that, extra.
- If you plan on taking supplements with you, best to bring them in their original packaging.

Generally, on vacay you are less stressed and more active in different ways, and you gotta eat right? So might as well choose foods that make you feel good.

- Don't stress if you can't follow the Food Plan. It's ok to have your food choices be off routine if your schedule is off from your normal weekly routine.
- Get back on track when you land. Start with the water and jump back on the Food Plan. As we move forward in the Program, we will be talking more about how to help the body recover from any indulgences.
- Have fun and remember you can't do anything in a week that can't be undone with a few days back on track and on routine!

No one is expecting you to deprive yourself of any of the joys that come with being on vacation to be successful. So, feel free to indulge. Just be mindful to balance it out. Try to get in fresh fruits, veggies and leafy greens when you can.

It's not unusual to lose weight while away on holiday, or to have your weight be up when you are back, only to have it drop right back down within days using Back on Track (which we will discuss in the Week 10 Guidelines). It's also not unusual for it to continue to drop to a new low afterwards.

Travel is a challenge for the body, which is great when it comes to losing and maintaining your weight.

LET'S TALK WORK FUNCTIONS AND WORK TRAVEL:

Travelling for work is not as fun but can be just as effective, as travel in general is very stimulating for the body.

- Focus on the water and keep things simple. Make the best choices you can when you can.
- Being on the road may mean making a few stops to the grocery store to pick up healthy snacks.
- Bathroom visits can be annoying, but keep in mind they are a means to an end and a key part of weight loss.
- Assess your day before it starts and plan when you can get the water in and when you need to hold off.

As we move forward, you will find it easier to plan.

TO RECAP:

Try to stay on Plan the best you can and don't stress. It's all about keeping it together when you can, balancing things out, planning ahead, and getting Back on Track when you are back.

Keep in mind that your body is not trying to or wanting to gain weight.

The key is to stay on track when you can and to be as consistent as possible. This way, you have some wiggle room for when you find yourself off or away from your daily routine.

- Be consistent with supplements (if taking).
- Get in your water when you can.
- Hit all meals and snacks.
- Make your food choices as nutrient rich as possible.
- Be super mindful about portions, making sure you eat enough, but not too much, and allowing your body to stay focused on detox and fat loss instead of digestion.

You are working to lose weight but also to make your body healthier by increasing your metabolism, increasing your nutrient absorption, and boosting your immune system along with decreasing your insulin levels. This puts you in tune with what your body actually needs.

WEEK 9 GUIDELINES: HIGHER PROTEIN & FAT REVAMP

This week is about feeding into your increasing metabolism and supporting the body working at a more optimal level.

WELCOME TO WEEK 9!

Off the heels of Feeding the Metabolism and making the body work extra hard for its food, we are going to scale back on the number of times you eat each day.

You will also be bumping up the protein and fat slightly, so your body gets more sustaining energy. I call this the **HIGHER PROTEIN AND FAT REVAMP.**

Now you may think higher fat and protein will force the body to burn fat and therefore reinforce the need to store fat. But that's not the case here.

So let me be clear, **THIS IS NOT KETO.**

We will still be incorporating nutrient rich carbs such as vegetables and fruits.

The higher protein and fat will help give you more sustained energy while we scale back on the amount of times you eat throughout the day. This will give the body easy energy which will feed into its need to easily work at a more optimal level.

You will still be following the Food Plan Formula but we will be making a few tweaks.

With where we are in the Program, your body is working hard to support your metabolism. Decreasing the number of times you are eating each day along with increasing protein and fat will feed into your increasing metabolism, which will cause the body to decrease insulin levels even further.

Portion wise, the goal is still to eat **JUST ENOUGH**, so 10 - 15 mins later you don't feel full or stuffed.

THIS WEEK'S TWEAK:

- **Breakfast** - still higher protein, ideally taking out any harder to digest carbs like bread, crackers, oatmeals and go more for fish, eggs, yogurts, protein shakes, etc.

- **Morning Snack** - can still be fruit but with added protein and fat. OR you can skip the fruit and just have protein and fat (examples below).

- **Lunch – protein is now the star of the show** with veg, leafy greens and added healthy fats. Eliminate any heavier carbs like potatoes, white rice, grains... except quinoa & black rice in small portions if needed.

- **Afternoon Snack (only one)**- There will only be one afternoon snack. You can combine the veg and nuts/seeds snack or see other ideas/options below.

- **Dinner** - **Veg is now the star of the show** with protein, leafy greens and added healthy fats. Please note the added carbs by way of the vegetables, which are now the star of the show at dinner. This will help balance out the day of eating higher protein.

Let's revisit PROTEIN & FAT sources:

PROTEIN SOURCES:

- Fish
- Meat (Any Meat)
- Eggs
- Seafood
- Beans, lentils, legumes
- Nuts and Seeds
- Dairy - cheese, yogurt, milk products
- Tofu, Tempeh
- Nut butter
- Hummus
- All-natural protein powder
- ...and don't forget about the protein in the vegetable carbs you are eating!

FAT SOURCES:

- Olives

- Avocado
- Nuts
- Seeds
- Hemp hearts
- Dairy...like yogurt, cheese, butter, sour cream etc.
- Olive oil, coconut oil, avocado oil, grape seed oil, flax and hemp oil
- Salad dressings made with good quality oils
- Omega 3 and 369
- Plus, any others you might think of

MEAL AND SNACK EXAMPLES/IDEAS:

Keep in mind these are only ideas. Feel free to come up with your own.

BREAKFAST:

- Eggs and egg whites (can add sautéed veg and/or greens)
- Yogurt with hemp hearts nuts/seeds. Can also add protein powder.
- Beans or lentils
- Veg or meat protein (can add sautéed veg)
- Higher protein cereals such as Holy Crap or Qi'a with added hemp hearts.
- Protein shakes (make sure to use natural protein powders). If adding fruit, keep it to a minimum and add in good fat by way of oils, avocados, nut butter, nuts, seeds, unsweetened coconut, coconut milk etc.

MORNING SNACK IDEAS:

- Fruit with nuts, seeds, nut butter, cheese or avocado
- Nuts and/or seeds on their own
- Yogurt
- Boiled egg
- Protein shake (If you didn't have it for breakfast) make sure to use natural protein powders. If adding fruit, keep it to a minimum and add in good fat by way of oils, avocados, coconut etc.

LUNCH:

- Take out any heavier carbs like potatoes, white rice, grains... except quinoa & black rice in small portions if needed, or other whole grains such as spelt, kamut, teff, amaranth, sorghum etc.

- Protein (any kind) with veg/leafy greens and healthy fat, in any combination of soup, salad, stew, stir fry or just straight up.

AFTERNOON SNACK IDEAS:

- Raw veg with nuts and/or seeds

- Nuts, seeds, or cheese

- Yogurt, cottage cheese (if you didn't have it in the AM)

- Raw veg with natural dips, guacamole, hummus, or nut butter

- Fruit and protein (like nuts, cheese, boiled eggs)

DINNER:

- Veg, protein, leafy greens and healthy fats (Protein should be a smaller portion and veg is now the star of the show.)

It's a few simple tweaks, so try not to overthink it. Although you want to be super mindful of portions, try to avoid purposely trying to eat less. Taking out the heavier carbs will do the work for you, so make sure to eat to satisfaction (JUST ENOUGH) and still be mindful of portions.

You may find portions may be smaller or larger this week. Both are normal responses from the body and as always, hunger levels change day to day and portions are always what they feel like and not what they look like.

Please take the time to head over to the Facebook Group or the Livy Method App and watch the quick video that accompanies this post.

WEEK 9 GUIDELINES FAQS

1.   What vegan/vegetarian protein sources are on Plan?

There are lots of high protein plant-based options available that you can have. For example, you can have tofu, beans, lentils, dairy-free yogurts, protein shakes with dairy-free "milk" etc. Be sure to check out the Grocery Checklist for more plant-based options.

2.   What protein powders/shakes are on Plan?

To maximize your efforts, it's best to have your protein shake either at breakfast or at morning snack (if you didn't have it at breakfast). Hemp and pea protein are good options. You'll want to look for protein powders that are all natural with no artificial colours, flavours, and sweeteners. Make sure to add in good fat which will balance out any carbs (fruits or veg) you add in. Be mindful about the amount of fruit you are using. Like all meals and snacks, be in tune with the portion size of your shake. With liquid nutrients it can be harder to gauge satisfaction levels. Finally, keep in mind you do not need to add in protein shakes. You can get everything you need to be successful with this week's tweak without adding them in.

3.   Can we still only have fruit for our first snack?

It's best to follow the program as designed and during this week's tweak it's best to add some protein and fat to your morning fruit snack. You can also skip the fruit and just have protein and fat.

4.   I am confused about the afternoon snack, can you clarify what this should look like?

Since we are removing one of the afternoon snacks, the easiest would be to combine your veg snack with your nuts and seeds snack. You can also have fruit with added protein, or yogurt or cottage cheese if you didn't have it in the morning. The added protein and fat with your afternoon snack will help with your sustaining energy.

5.   Should I be increasing my protein amount this week?

For this week we are only looking to bump up the protein and fat slightly, so your body gets more sustaining energy. We are not looking to add large amounts of protein, and we are still incorporating nutrient rich carbs such as vegetables and fruits. The higher protein and fat will help give you more sustained energy while we scale back on the amount of times you eat throughout the day.

6.   Are carbs completely eliminated from this tweak?

We will still be incorporating nutrient rich carbs such as vegetables and fruits for Higher Protein & Fat Revamp. Ideally take out any harder to digest carbs like bread, crackers, oatmeals; and any heavier carbs like potatoes, white rice and grains from your meals. Quinoa and black rice can still be added in small portions if needed.

7.   Do I continue to add healthy fats to my lunches and dinners?

Yes. Healthy fats are an important component of the Program. Our bodies need good fats. You will want to continue to add them in with your meals and also you can add them to your veg snack.

8.   Are we still keeping our nuts to the same amount per day?

The amount of nuts you eat for your snack can change day to day depending on your hunger level. Ask yourself those 4 mindfulness questions and determine in the moment how many you will need to feel satisfied.

9.   Do the people who were incorporating bonus snacks continue to do so?

If you have been utilizing the bonus snacks, and you need them, you can continue to do so. Be sure to make your meals nutrient rich, and add a high protein breakfast if you aren't already. Add in bonus snacks only if you have a real need for them.

10.   I've been skipping breakfast most days. Is it a good idea to eat breakfast this week to get extra protein?

As always, breakfast is optional when following the Plan, but it can be greatly beneficial to have a high protein breakfast, especially if looking to maximize. If you choose to have breakfast, ensure it is still higher protein, ideally taking out any of the carbs you may have been having like bread, crackers, and oatmeal and going for higher protein choices like fish, eggs, and yogurts.

LET'S TALK PROTEIN SHAKES

I think I have made my stance on shakes pretty clear. It's not that I'm opposed to having them, it's just when it comes to weight loss...there is a time and a place for them.

With where we are at in the process, and with the focus more on supporting the body where it is at and feeding into its increasing metabolism...protein shakes can be an easy and convenient way for the body to get what it needs so it can better focus on fat loss.

If you are thinking of adding in a shake here are some things to keep in mind:

1.   There are a variety of protein powder options out there, find one that works best for you.

SIDE NOTE: Although shakes can be the perfect place to add in your collagen powder, collagen powder is a non-essential protein (not a food source) so it doesn't replace the need for protein powder in a shake.

2.   Check the ingredients, make sure you are buying natural protein powder (not synthetic) and avoid any artificial flavour or colour or sweeteners.

3.   Make sure to add in good fat which will balance out any carbs (fruits or veg) you add in. Examples of some good fats would be:

- Liquid Omega 3 or 369 combo

- Flax oil

- Hemp oil

- Avocado

- Coconut oil/chunks, or unsweetened milk

- MCT oil

- Nut butters

- Yogurt

4.   Be mindful about the amount of fruit ratio you are using and bonus if you make them more veg based.

5.   Be in tune to the portion size of your shake, with liquid nutrients you need less than what you would eat because the breakdown process is already done for you.

Keep in mind you do NOT need to add in protein shakes. You can get everything you need to be successful with this week's tweak without adding them in.

Please take the time to head over to the Facebook Group or the Livy Method App and watch the quick video that accompanies this post.

LET'S REVISIT NUTRIENT RICH MEALS

With where we are in the program, it's easy to fall into old habits and start choosing foods that you like and love or are easy and convenient instead of choosing foods that will maximize your efforts.

Not that this program is all about salads but if you are going to eat them, make sure you load them up with tons of nutrients, think quality over quantity.

Let's use a salad as an example, but the same idea can be applied to absolutely ANY meal and even your snacks.

LET'S BREAK IT DOWN:

- Spring Mix/Greens = leafy greens + roughage + vitamins + minerals + protein
- Variety of Vegetables = fiber + vitamins
- Avocado = healthy fat + potassium + fiber
- Feta cheese = healthy fat + protein
- Nuts and Seeds = healthy fat + protein
- An all-natural vinaigrette or dressing = healthy fat when made with quality oil.

THINGS TO HAVE ON HAND THAT CAN QUICKLY BUMP UP YOUR MEALS:

- A variety of nuts and seeds - good fat and protein and an excellent addition to yogurt or oats
- Olives - good fat
- Pickled and marinated veg like artichoke heart, pickled beets, roasted red peppers, etc. - bump up your veggies.
- Good quality oils like extra virgin olive oil, nut oils, avocado and coconut oil. - good fats
- Quality salad dressings (store bought or homemade)
- Coconut milk - a great healthy fat addition to things like your morning oatmeal or cereal.
- Salsa - extra veg
- Guacamole - good fat
- Hummus - good fat plus protein
- Tuna, sardines, smoked oysters - a quick way to add protein to any meal.

Nutrient rich meals provide the most bang for your buck and give you longer lasting energy.

Even if you can just sneak in one or two extra things like a drizzle of olive oil, an extra veg, or a few nuts… it can make all the difference.

LET'S REVISIT STRESS & SLEEP

Stress factors into the weight loss process because when you are stressed your body releases a hormone called cortisol and too much cortisol can signal weight gain.

Sleep is key to the process because when you sleep is when the body makes all the changes you want to see.

Managing your stress and getting enough sleep can make all the difference when it comes to getting and keeping the scale moving.

Just by following the food plan, you are helping the body manage stress because this process helps to provide an environment where the body can focus on making change and addressing issues.

Although the basics of The Program; the food, the water and the supplements suggested all help with both stress & sleep...there are quite a few things above and beyond that you can focus on to help with this process.

TIPS FOR MANAGING STRESS:

1.   Be consistent with the basics of the program; the food, water & supplements.

2.   Practice deep breathing exercises.

3.   Get outside and commune with nature.

4.   Move your body more. Go for walks, dance, stretch, find activities you enjoy doing like sports and other leisure activities.

5.   Have a warm epsom salt bath before bed.

6.   Keep up with health issues. Seeing a Naturopathic doctor, Chiropractor, Acupuncturist, Massage Therapist and other health care providers can be helpful.

7.   Add in helpful supplements like omega 3, and add good fats to your meals along with being consistent with magnesium and any stress tonics or immune boosters you have added in.

8.   Check your attitude and be self-aware of where you are at and what you are struggling with. Help you help yourself and prioritize your body's needs.

9.   Look for things that bring you joy. Look to have fun with this process. Don't underestimate the power of having a good conversation with a friend or spending time with a loved one. Some good laughs over a glass of wine can do wonders for relieving stress.

10.   Get better sleep: The body needs deep and REM sleep to repair, rebuild and detox. You will find that following The Program will help with your overall sleep, but there are things you can do now to help make a difference when it comes to the scale.

   • Change your sleep to fall in line with the change in seasons, for example, going to sleep earlier in the fall when the sun sets earlier.

- Take naps when you feel the need. Naps are not advised in general when trying to improve sleep patterns, but when it comes to this Process, the body is working so hard on making change, it needs all the sleep it can get.

- Turn lights down low in the evening.

- Use blue light glasses.

- Stay off of screens or get off them earlier.

- Add in the calm magnesium before bed and adjust the dose as needed. It will work well with your natural melatonin production.

- Eat as early in the evening as possible.

- Keep a journal and glass of water beside the bed.

Getting enough sleep, getting a handle on your stress and helping the body manage it, can help you to use your stress as an advantage in this process.

Stress will challenge your body and with your body working for you, it will rise to the occasion; which can lead to your body wanting to be stronger and healthier, which helps put a greater focus on fat loss.

Keep in mind the goal isn't to make stress go away, it's more to recognize it, and help the body manage it, so you can capitalize on it. And when it comes to sleep you may not be able to get more sleep but you can work to improve the quality of sleep you do get.

LET'S REVISIT KEEPING A JOURNAL

It's not too late to start tracking your progress.

We have talked in the past about the benefits of keeping a journal or using our app to track things like your weight to see patterns of behavior and how your body responds to this process. Also, the importance of tracking things like how you feel physically and mentally as well as the basics like your water to help make sure you are drinking enough.

But it can be even more important with where we are at in this process now to help you capitalize on the time we have left…which btw, is still a lot of time left to lose a lot of weight!

BENEFITS OF JOURNALING:

- A journal can be a great tool to help give you insight into how your body is responding to the process.

- It can help you pick up on patterns of behavior and responses, and give you a better idea of what weight loss looks like specifically to you.

- It can help you pick up on any food sensitivities, especially if you have digestive issues. It can help you track bowel movements if you struggle in that department.

- It can help you track your body's response to the supplements you have been taking and/or anything new you are adding in or taking out.

- It can also help to track your mood and can be beneficial in helping you show up for yourself every day, by taking time to think about how you are managing your emotions and how you are feeling day to day.

THINGS TO TRACK:

- Weight in the morning
- How you are feeling physically and mentally
- Food
- Water
- Extras (added food and drink on or not on plan)
- Bowel movements if they are an issue
- Notable responses from food
- Digestive upset
- Sleep
- Medications

- Supplements
- Notable wins not food related (NSV)
- Energy day to day
- Changes taking place that aren't scale related

You can use good old pen and paper, your computer, or an app. Whatever works best for you!

We are at the point in this process where keeping a journal can be a very helpful tool to problem solve and make the most of your effort in conjunction with the info being posted in the group.

The more tools the better!

FOOD FACTS - BEANS & LENTILS

How many of you are familiar with this rhyme?

"Beans, beans the musical fruit, the more you eat, the less you toot!"

Or is it,

"Beans, beans the musical fruit, the more you eat, the more you toot?"

You may have heard it both ways! But did you notice how the 2 variations say opposite things about gassiness?

SO, WHICH ONE IS IT?

Well...sort of both. Beans and lentils *can* cause an increase in gassiness after eating. This is because of a complex sugar called raffinose, which the body can have trouble digesting. Raffinose passes through the small intestine, undigested, and into the large intestines where your gut bacteria breaks it down. This produces gas that eventually you pass.

BUT...slowly incorporating more beans and lentils into your diet allows your system to get used to them, making them more easily digested, and decreasing gassiness. Beans and lentils have also shown to enhance overall gut health by improving intestinal barrier function and increasing beneficial digestive bacteria. If you are new to adding beans and lentils to your diet, start slowly to allow your digestive system to get used to them.

WHAT ARE BEANS AND LENTILS?

We're talking about things like chickpeas, beans (kidney, pinto, navy, black, etc.), dried peas (split peas) and lentils. These are all the edible seeds of the plants in the legume family and are called "pulses".

Technically, a "legume" is the name of the whole plant including the leaves, stems, and pods. For example, a pea pod (think snap peas) is a legume but the pea inside the pod is a pulse.

Legumes and pulses are a nutritious staple of many diets around the world and have been cultivated by humans for approximately 6000 years!

SUPERFOOD?

I'm not a fan of the word *"superfood"* but when it comes to beans and lentils, I think it's appropriate. Check out all the nutrients these pulses are jam-packed with:

- Protein
- Fiber

- Folate

- Calcium

- Iron

- B vitamins

- Vitamin C

- Complex carbohydrates

- Potassium

- Antioxidants

Beans and lentils are digested slowly which gives a feeling of satiety. They also promote a slow burning, steady energy while the iron content helps transport oxygen through the body. This helps to increase your energy and support your metabolism. The high amount of fiber is excellent for managing cholesterol, digestive health, regulating energy levels, as well as helping to stabilize blood glucose levels.

ENVIRONMENTAL HEROS!

Not only are they powerhouses in the nutritional department but did you know they are also good for the environment? Legume crops have a lower carbon footprint than almost any other food group. They are considered one of the most sustainable proteins in the world as they have the ability to enrich the soil, reducing the need for chemical fertilizers, and compared to other proteins, they need only one-tenth the amount of water to grow. They are also frost and drought resistant which makes them almost indestructible!

CANNED OR DRIED?

CANNED beans and lentils are definitely more convenient but also have a higher price tag. They are already soaked and cooked so are ready to be used in fresh or cooked dishes. Just rinse and go! Canned beans can be high in sodium so something to watch out for when purchasing. Be sure to rinse them well to remove as much sodium as possible but keep in mind they will have absorbed a lot of it. Look for low or no-sodium canned beans and lentils as a better alternative.

DRIED beans are much less expensive but involve some labour. They also take up less space in your pantry. Preparing them can be a bit time consuming as they require soaking and then simmering for up to a few hours, depending on the bean. It can be helpful to prepare a whole bag at once and freezing whatever you aren't using. They freeze perfectly and are ready to use for whatever you are making! Lentils, on the other hand, don't require soaking therefore take less time to prepare.

LET'S BREAK DOWN THE COST DIFFERENCE

Here, red kidney beans are being used as an example.

(These prices are an average and in Canadian dollars)

COST

DRIED = $1.75 - 450g/1 lb.

CANNED = $1.40 - 540 ml/18 oz

YIELD

DRIED - 12 x ½ cup servings of cooked beans per bag

CANNED - 4 x ½ cup servings per can

$ PER SERVING

Dried = $0.15 per serving

Canned = $0.35 per serving

So, if you are on a budget then dried beans are the way to go!

EASY WAYS TO ADD THEM IN

Another amazing thing about beans and lentils is how versatile they are! Because they have a sort of benign flavour they get along well with virtually any ingredients, herbs, and spices. You can add them to almost anything!

- **Enjoy them as a quick salad topper** - Try roasting them with a bit of olive oil and your favorite spices to enhance their flavour!
- **Add them to soups** - Use them whole or pureed. Pureeing acts as a thickener.
- **Add to chili, curry, stew, and stir-fries** - You can use all beans for a meatless meal, or a combination of meat and pulses to cut down on your meat consumption and make it more nutrient rich.
- **Mash up** chickpeas and mix with your favourite tuna salad ingredients for a vegetarian version!
- **Use them to make tasty and nutritious dips and spreads** - Hummus is the classic but you can puree any cooked beans or lentils, add some seasonings to make a dip or spread for a leafy green wrap!
- **Have them for breakfast with or without eggs** - Fry up some black beans with a bit of chili powder and top with cheese, salsa and avocado!

LET'S REVISIT CRAVINGS

At this point, if you are following The Program, you should find any cravings you had or have are minimal. And if you do have them, they are nothing to be feared and can actually be your body giving you a heads up on its needs.

Cravings are just messages from the body. They are the body's way of communicating its needs by associating the foods that can help get it what it needs.

It's important to remember your body is on your side and it's not trying to screw you over by craving.

If you are following the Food Plan and drinking the water, any cravings should be few and far between. And if they do pop up, it's usually just a matter of making a few tweaks.

LET'S TALK SUGAR:

The key to beating sugar cravings is to understand that it's not actually sugar people are addicted to; it's the high insulin levels needed to break it down that has you reaching for sweets.

Why?

- Insulin is the hormone that allows your body to use glucose for energy. Glucose is a type of sugar found in carbs like fruits, vegetables, and naturally occurring sugar that your body uses for energy. After you eat food and your digestive system breaks it down, your pancreas releases insulin to help regulate your blood sugar.

- When you reach for the sweets or foods with high sugar content, your body can flood with too much insulin, which causes your blood glucose levels to drop. This creates a dip in energy and a desire for even more sugar.

- This can create a vicious cycle that makes taking sugar and carbs out of your diet a challenge.

WHY AM I CRAVING SO MUCH SUGAR IN THE FIRST PLACE?

Let's break it down:

1. **More is more:**

- When you have sugar, your body will immediately want more sugar. These cravings can be so intense that if you create a habit of having sugar at the same time every day, your body will begin to crave and expect it at that same time daily. This is also the reason you end up eating that whole box of cookies in one sitting!

THE FIX:

- Add some protein and fat.

- Making sure to add in healthy fats to your meals along with protein, will help to prevent any cravings along the way.

- But if you do find yourself indulging, you can neutralize sugar cravings by having some protein and fat with your sweet treat. For example, if you indulge in a cookie, you can cut the desire to eat another cookie by having a slice of cheese or a handful of nuts.

- The protein and fat will help neutralize the amount of insulin your body uses to break down the sugar and decrease your cravings, giving your will power a fighting chance to kick in and help.

2. **Dehydration is a factor:**

- When you are dehydrated and not picking up on the cues from your body to drink more, your body's next best bet is to crave foods with a high water content, like fruit. Fruits are also sweet, so you may mistake your body's cue to consume more water and instead find yourself reaching for processed carbs and sugar.

- This is why you may hear the advice to drink a glass of water before you eat to satisfy your appetite. It doesn't satisfy your appetite, but if it's water that you actually need, you may realize you are not really hungry after all.

THE FIX:

- Drink more water.

- Sip water throughout the day, aiming for a minimum of 3.5 litres a day and even more on days you exercise or are more active.

3. **You are tired:**

- When you are tired, your body goes looking for a pick-me-up, and you may find yourself reaching for something sweet.

- The same thing happens around 3 or 4 p.m. each afternoon when the body is wired to take a drop in energy and slows your circadian rhythm. What your body is really looking for is a nap. (There are places in the world that do just that, and call it the siesta.)

- In our fast-paced, high-stress world, it's not always possible to take a nice afternoon nap, so the body goes looking for easy energy by way of higher sugar to pick it up and keep it going.

THE FIX:

- Make sure to keep up with your water because when you are dehydrated it can add to your tiredness.

- Be sure to eat all your meals and especially your snacks. This will help to avoid energy levels that dip when you go for long periods of time without eating.

- When it comes to meals and snacks, be sure to choose foods that have a high nutrient value to give the body the energy it needs. And be extra mindful of portions so you don't make the body work harder than it needs to.

- With a few adjustments, you can easily beat the need for sweets and stay on track to reach your goals and not be held captive by sugar cravings anymore!

LET'S TALK SALT:

When you crave sugar, it generally means that you need more water. When you crave salt, it generally means that the body is asking for more good fat.

When you are stressed, your body is revving high, you burn energy, your brain works really hard and your body quickly gets depleted of its nutrients.

Periods of high stress can rapidly deplete your vitamin and mineral reserves. So, when you are stressed, your body is looking for more sustaining energy by way of good fat.

You don't have to be stressed for the body to need more good fat. Fat is essential for cellular function as well as brain and heart health. It also works like a transport system for your body to process and digest carbs and protein.

Your body would rather get that fat from the foods you eat than to utilize its emergency reserve. Without enough good fat coming in, your body will be reluctant to let go of the fat that makes you fat. So, one way you can speed up that fat loss process is to make sure you are getting lots of good fats in your meals and adding in an omega 3 supplement, which we will be talking more about in Week 2.

Now with that said there are times when the body craves salt because it is in need of actual salt, so be mindful to add salt to your foods or add in trace minerals. This is usually more of an issue in warmer months when electrolytes are a concern.

LET'S TALK TUMMY RUMBLINGS & HUNGER PAINS:

We are taught to believe if your tummy rumbles you must be hungry, when in fact that's not what the noise and rumblings are about. It's actually your body's natural MMC or Migrating Motor Complex. Your digestive system works like a self-cleaning oven where, in between processing and digesting food, it works to clear bacteria and food particles out of the small intestine.

Because we are eating so often during the day, the body is doing most of this work at night. As we move through the program, we will be phasing you into more natural patterns of eating which will be more in tune to your body's needs, which include the downtime it needs in between meals to self-regulate.

TO RECAP:

Cravings are nothing to stress about, though they can give you great insight into your body's needs. Usually, the smallest tweak or adjustments can make all the difference.

It's important to note it's not about controlling your cravings; it's about being in tune to them. As you progress through the program, you will become more in tune and able to differentiate between the body's needs and your wants.

You may also find yourself craving other kinds of foods and even specific foods. At the end of this process, your body will clearly let you know when it's hungry, what it's hungry for, and how much you need to eat. It's actually super cool how in tune you can become to your body and its needs.

Paying attention to those cravings can help you better meet your body's needs so that your body can focus on what you need to do to get and keep the scale moving.

To dig deeper into the science of cravings and your Migrating Motor Complex head to the Science Guide and read Hormones of Hunger and Satiety and Timing of Digestion, and The Migrating Motor Complex (MMC) and Hunger.

WEEK 10 GUIDELINES: HIGHER PROTEIN & FAT REVAMP PART 2 AND INTRODUCING BACK ON TRACK

Continuing the Higher Protein and Fat tweak while Maximizing your efforts. This is also the week we introduce the concept of Back on Track (BOT).

For this week, we are continuing the Higher Protein and Fat Revamp tweak along with Maximizing your efforts day to day. This is also where we introduce the concept of Back on Track (BOT). Back on Track refers to following the original Food Plan as a method to help the body recover from/or get Back on Track after indulging in a way that causes the scale to be up or for you to feel "off". First, let's review the basics for the Higher Protein and Fat Revamp tweak.

RECAP OF THIS WEEK'S TWEAK

- **Breakfast** - Still higher protein, ideally taking out any harder to digest carbs like bread, crackers, oatmeals and go more for fish, eggs, yogurts, protein shakes, etc. If you haven't been having breakfast, now is a good time to add it in. Since we want dinner to be the smallest meal of the day, adding in breakfast can help make sure you aren't hungry in the evening.

- **Morning Snack** - Can still be fruit but with added protein and fat. OR you can skip the fruit and just have protein and fat.

- **Lunch** - Protein is the star with veg and leafy greens. Eliminate any heavier carbs like potatoes, white rice, grains... except quinoa & black rice in small portions if needed.

- **Afternoon Snack (only one)** - There will only be one afternoon snack. You can combine the veg and nuts/seeds snack or see Week 9 Guidelines for other ideas/options.

- **Dinner** - Veg is the star with protein and leafy greens. Please note the added carbs by way of the vegetables, which are now the star of the show at dinner. You can add in any heavier carb veggies here if you feel the need for them. This will help balance out the day of eating higher protein.

- Refer to the Week 9 Guidelines for a review of the information.

LET'S TALK BACK ON TRACK

Weekends, holidays and vacays can be tricky when it comes to staying on plan because we tend to be more off routine, making it a bit more difficult to follow the routine. Add in a long/holiday or celebratory day and it can make it even harder.

You may have heard me reference getting "Back on Track". BOT refers to getting back to the basics.

Back on Track is a technique you will use after indulging in or having an "off day", "off weekend", or even an "off week" of eating as you continue to work through the rest of the program to lose, and once you are in maintenance, to help maintain your weight.

Back on Track refers to the original Food Plan Formula, the same one you have been following these first few months of the Program.

The original Food Plan has now become a familiar routine for the body that will help it reset and catch up after any "off days."

THE METHOD OF GETTING "BACK ON TRACK":

- Protein for breakfast
- Fruit for snack
- Veg, protein and leafy greens for lunch
- Raw veg snack
- Nut and seed snack
- Protein, veg and leafy greens for dinner

When eating "Back on Track," you want to eat all meals and snacks, but keep the portions on the smaller side.

This is NOT for the sake of eating less calories, but to help the body stay focused on getting rid of any backlog of food which is attributing to your weight being up.

You want to keep lunch and dinner light with more leafy greens and avoid any heavier carbs. You want to get in extra water.

You want to eat as early in the evening as possible. You want to help the body get a nice, deep sleep.

You want to move your body, go for a walk after dinner, have an epsom salt bath, and head to bed earlier. You also want to be as consistent as possible with the supplements.

If you get on the scale after indulging and your weight is up, it's important to understand that it is not real weight gain. Weight up is just from a backlog from hard to digest foods, salty food, and your body retaining water.

You will find after being "Back on Track" for a few days, your weight will drop right back down to where it was before you had your off day/s. And then you can carry on and pick up where you left off in the Program.

With that said, Back on Track is not always about the scale coming back down because sometimes your weight can be up for other reasons. In that case, you implement BOT until you "feel" BOT, which usually takes 1-3 days.

You may feel inclined to eat less or to skip meals and snacks after indulging thinking this will help you get ahead and Back on Track faster...it will not. Under-eating after over-indulging will only reinforce the need for the body to hold onto and store fat. It will also under stimulate your digestive system making it longer to get back on track.

- Keep in mind, Back on Track is NOT to be used unless you over indulged for a day or more.
- It is NOT meant to be used to manage day to day fluctuations on the scale or one "off" meal.
- It is best reserved for when you really go off the rails for a couple or more days. Not just one-off meal or indulgence.

How long you implement back on track depends on how off the rails you went, normally a day or two is plenty to help the body get back on track. Also, best to keep any indulgences to a minimum while looking to lose weight. Avoid the mentality of making this a lifestyle thing where you try to have your indulgences and lose weight too... Reserve Back on Track for the times you really need it.

Please take the time to head over to the Facebook Group or the Livy Method App and watch the quick video that accompanies this post.

WEEK 10 GUIDELINES FAQS

1.   For this tweak are we basically switching our lunch with our dinner?

In addition to continuing to bump up your proteins and fats, lunch now has protein as the main component and dinner now has veg as the main component. You can add in heavier carb veggies at dinner if you feel the need for them. Veg as the star at dinner will help balance out the day of eating higher protein.

2.   Can I add additional vegetables to leafy greens for dinner?

For this week dinner now has veg as the main component of your meal, so yes load up the veggies. You still want to add in protein, good fats and leafy greens. Lunch this week has protein as the main component.

3.   Can we begin using Back on Track (BOT) now, or is it meant for the end of the Program?

Yes Back on Track is a great technique to use after indulging in or having an off day, weekend or even an off week. This is a technique you will continue to use moving forward when needed. BOT is not meant to be used to manage day to day fluctuations on the scale or for one "off" meal.

4.   Is the Back on Track protocol something I need to follow?

Back on Track (BOT) is a technique that can be used after indulging in or having an off day, off weekend, or even an off week of eating, as you continue to work through the rest of the program to lose weight. Once you are in maintenance, BOT is a very helpful tool that can help you maintain your weight. So moving forward, if you feel you need it, use it.

5.   Do I need to follow the Back on Track protocol if only having one meal off plan?

Back on Track (BOT) is not meant to be used for only an off meal. For that add in some extra water and leafy greens the next day. You want to reserve BOT for when you have an off day, weekend or week and feel you need to use BOT for a couple of days until you feel like you are Back on Track.

LET'S REVISIT BOWEL MOVEMENTS

We have talked a lot about bowel movements over the past few weeks.

When following the program, it's normal to have your bowel movements be all over the place, meaning every shape, size and consistency, as it's normal to have bouts of constipation and also normal to have loose bowel movements.

Constipation is usually the body responding to the changes you are making (change in routine of foods and change in type of foods) and also the body taking time to make improvements in digestion that can lead to improvements in regularity - which is a good thing.

Loose bowel movements on the other hand are a normal and somewhat expected byproduct of the detox process we are piggybacking to lose weight. But can also be a sign of food sensitivities, which if you are keeping a journal, you should be picking up on.

If you have always suffered from bowel movement issues, you should see significant improvement by following the program. And once you are done helping the body focus on weight loss and are in maintenance, you will find your bowel movements will normalize giving you that S-Shaped Dr. Oz/Oprah bowel movements everyone strives for.

Your digestive health is directly associated with, and affects your bowel movements. Food goes in and it needs to go out. So, as you continue to focus on fat loss here is what you can do, above and beyond following The Program, to help improve your bowel movements:

LET'S TALK CONSTIPATION:

THE BASICS:

- Drink lots of water.
- Be sure to add leafy greens to meals.
- Add in, and regularly take, the basic supplements: Omega 3, Vit D, Probiotic, and Calm magnesium.

In addition to what is listed above in regards to the basics, which all work together on Plan, we also suggest looking into adding:

PREBIOTIC:

- Prebiotic is food for your probiotic. Prebiotic does come in pill form but is best to get in a clear fiber.
- You can also increase your intake of prebiotic foods that help with digestion like: Onions, garlic, leeks, chickpeas, lentils, kidney beans, bananas, grapefruit, bran, barley, and oats.

DIGESTIVE BITTERS:

- Digestive bitters are herbs that support digestive function by stimulating bitter receptors on the tongue, stomach, gallbladder, and pancreas.

- They work to promote digestive juices such as stomach acid, bile, and enzymes, which help to break down food and assist in the absorption of nutrients.

- Look for Canadian Digestive Bitters that come in drops you add to water.

- Take bitters about 20 minutes before a meal to signal your body to produce more saliva, bile, and stomach acid.

VITAMIN C:

- When taking higher doses of vitamin C, the extra or unabsorbed vitamin C pulls water into your intestines, which can help soften your stool.

- Take 30 mins before food in the morning, dose is dependent on the individual and can range from 90-2000 mg.

B COMPLEX:

- B12, B1 & B5 deficiency can cause constipation. If your constipation is caused by low levels of B's, increasing your daily intake of this nutrient may help ease your symptoms.

- B2 or B complex is part of the secondary supplements list.

- Not essential to weight loss, but it is key in supporting metabolic function, which can significantly help with weight loss, by helping to improve your energy.

- You may prefer to eat more foods rich in this vitamin rather than take a supplement.

EXAMPLES OF FOODS RICH IN B VITAMINS INCLUDE:

- Meat (red meat, poultry, fish)
- Beef
- Liver
- Trout
- Salmon
- Tuna fish
- Whole grains (brown rice, barley, millet)
- Eggs and dairy products (milk, cheese)
- Legumes (beans, lentils)
- Seeds and nuts (sunflower seeds, almonds)
- Dark, leafy vegetables (broccoli, spinach)
- Fruits (citrus fruits, avocados, bananas)

TRIPHALA:

- Used in Ayurvedic medicine for thousands of years, it is thought to support bowel health and aid digestion. As an antioxidant, it is also thought to detoxify the body and support the immune system.

- Triphala helps to keep the stomach, small intestine and large intestine healthy by flushing out toxins from the body.

- Triphala as a supplement, is available as a pill, and in powder form. The powder is meant to be dissolved in warm water and consumed as tea. It can taste bitter but can be mixed with honey or lemon without diminishing its effects.

- Triphala supplements have varying daily dosages based upon the manufacturer. It's important to follow package directions exactly.

- Triphala may be most effective when taken right before bed with a large glass of warm water.

- Some people prefer to take this supplement on an empty stomach, while others prefer to take it with food. Discuss these options with your healthcare provider.

EXERCISE/MOVE YOUR BODY:

- Exercise helps constipation by lowering the time it takes food to move through the large intestine. This limits the amount of water your body absorbs from the stool.

- Cardio exercise speeds up your breathing and heart rate, helping to stimulate the natural squeezing of muscles in your intestines which helps to move stool out quickly.

- Something as simple as going for a walk after dinner can make all the difference when it comes to improving digestion.

TIME AND CONSISTENCY:

- It is important to note that in most cases the body just needs time to rewire how it has come to function over the years.

- The foods you are eating, and the overall structure of The Program will help from a baseline level to address constipation issues.

- Try to keep things routine and be patient with the process, but also don't suffer. Sometimes you need to take something stronger like an over-the-counter laxative to help the body work through any backlog.

LET'S TALK LOOSE BOWEL MOVEMENTS:

Loose bowel movements can be unnerving but also a normal part of the process due to all the water you are drinking, leafy greens you are eating, as well as fiber rich foods like fruit and veggies which all contribute to a natural daily detox.

In most cases, it's nothing to be concerned about. However, here are some things you can do to address:

- Continuing to focus on digestive health. It can be a great idea to add in the prebiotic and bitters to help strengthen your digestive system.

- Keep a journal and record how you are feeling after eating meals and snacks as sometimes food sensitivities can pop up that can cause loose BM and discomfort.

- Dairy and gluten are the most common sensitivities, but it can come down to specific food choices like a kind of fruit for example, or even spicy food.

- Decrease calm magnesium. Although the calm mag is rarely the sole issue for loose BM, decreasing it slightly may help.

- If you are concerned about nutrient loss, rest assured, it's not a major concern when following the plan.

- You can add trace minerals to your water or add in a pinch of pink rock salt or Celtic salt to your warm water and lemon in the morning and/or water throughout the day.

- Add in Psyllium fiber. You never want to add in fiber while constipated as it can sometimes make the situation worse. It is however an excellent time to add in if experiencing loose bowel movements.

Psyllium is non-dependent and when added in, attaches itself to toxins stored in your fat cells and helps to draw them out. This can help make your bowel movements more binding and effective for fat loss.

- The soluble fiber also helps lower blood cholesterol levels and control blood sugar levels. You can also get this type of fiber from oats, barley, oranges, dried beans and lentils.

- Comes in pill or powder form. I personally like the pills.

- Take before bed or in between meals.

TO RECAP:

The body has been working hard to address digestive and BM issues. Given enough time, your body will continue to make significant improvements.

Although usually nothing to be concerned about, when it comes to BM issues, it is always recommended to check in with your doctor.

Some conditions including Crohn's disease, celiac disease, IBS, thyroid issues and medications can be the cause of loose BM, but if your changes in BM go hand in hand with following the program, chances are there is nothing to be concerned about and given the time, the body will sort out and address it on its own.

LET'S TALK PEOPLE'S REACTIONS TO YOUR WEIGHT LOSS

Our Director of Group Operations, Anna Blachuta, who is now down over 90 lbs. in her journey, put together this post in the hopes of providing insight into how to manage comments and reactions to your ever-changing body.

First thing is first. You are doing this Program for you. Make sure you remember that each and every day. Let that be the driving force to get you to your "finally and forever". Whatever your end game is, it's yours. All of the work that you've put into yourself by doing this so far is amazing, and you deserve to be your best self! Nothing and nobody should get in the way of you achieving your goals.

Now that the world is slowly starting to open up and we are starting to see our friends and family again, we will have to also figure out how to navigate social situations. Handling people's reactions to your changing body is going to be a big part of that.

Always remember that no opinion but yours matters when it comes to your body and your choices. Whether you're bigger, smaller or anything in between, some people will always have something to say.

Positive or negative, you will feel like you are being treated in a different way than you ever have been in the past. These reactions can make you feel so many ways. There are times that people will be celebrating your successes, times where people can be uncomfortably negative or awkward, and even some times where others may try to sabotage your achievements (we all know one or two cookie-pushers!!).

I love the cheerleaders! They're a no brainer! Those are the friends and family you need to keep close. People say that it's not during the hard times when you know who your friends are, it's the great times. The positivity and light that comes from these people is gold – hang on to it for more motivation for you to keep pushing towards your goals!

There has been a lot of discussion recently with members having negative reactions about their weight loss from their loved ones. That negativity can be tough to handle. Even if you are a generally confident person, it can feel hurtful and unnerving.

There are many reasons why friends and family can have negative reactions to your weight loss.

- Jealousy
- Fear, shame
- Genuine concern
- People don't realize how impactful their words and opinions can be
- Social awkwardness, especially post pandemic
- Changing dynamic in a relationship (i.e. you're not the fat friend/sister/brother anymore)

The negative things people do may be different for everyone. Some examples of negative reactions include:

- Not saying anything or pretending not to notice your weight loss
- Asking if you're sick
- Questioning your portions, food choices, supplements, exercise routine…
- Saying things like, "enough already" and "You've lost too much weight – stop now!"
- Pushing unwanted food your way
- Judging you when you don't want dessert, a second portion, to finish your entire meal, etc.
- Offering other weight loss programs/tips/advice
- Telling you that you were more fun (or cuter, or funnier…) when you were bigger

Sometimes, the negativity can even come from the people you trust the most in the world - like your spouse or immediate family. Comments can be direct or indirect, like questioning portions or making small body-shaming jokes or remarks. This can be hurtful from anyone, but can be even more so for someone you are meant to trust or be vulnerable with. It can make you question what you're doing and everything you have done so far.

Here are some ideas to help you navigate these conversations:

1. **Be yourself!!** Such a cliché but, in my opinion, it is the best advice anyone can hear! You are on the road to your finally and forever – your life, thoughts, feelings and day to day will change. This is wonderful! No better time than now to practice being yourself and becoming your most confident you!

2. **Don't take it personally**. There are many people right now who have gone through their own dark times, including gaining a lot of weight, especially while trying to navigate through this global pandemic. They can be socially awkward because of the lack of social situations, and their own insecurities. It can be hard for them to handle your new positive outlook and healthy new look. This is them. Not you. Enjoy your new self and move on.

3. **React with kindness and stay calm.** Take a moment to carefully think about what you want to say, and breathe. Be polite, make sure you are expressing yourself in a respectful voice, and smile. Sometimes it's not worth it to stoop down to their level; it's nice to leave a negative situation feeling like the bigger person.

4. **Remember that no two situations are the same.** Think for a moment about how you want to handle this particular situation, because it may be different from others that you've encountered in the past.

5. **Diffuse the situation with humor**. It can sometimes release the tension of an awkward conversation.

6. **Talk to the person to tell them how you are feeling.** If you are not able to have a discussion in the moment, you can always take a step back, think about what happened, and pull the person aside to tell them how you feel. Be direct. Sometimes the conversation can be difficult but it can be just as difficult for you if you are constantly hearing negative comments from those you love.

7. **Don't overthink it.** If you've confronted someone about their behaviour and they do not respond well, remember that it is not your responsibility to change people. You've done the best you can to resolve the situation. Sometimes you have to accept that they have their own issues, realize that it is no fault of your own, and let them find their own solutions.

8. **If you need a cheerleader – reach out!** Our team and many of our past and current members are happy to help to give you the boost you may need!

Experiencing negative reactions is never fun, but remember that positive reactions are far more common. Be sure to make time for those positive people in your life. However, you want to navigate the negative situations is up to you, just be strong and remember that you are working towards becoming your best you!

LET'S REVISIT SUPPLEMENTS

It is a great idea to revisit the supplement conversation since it is never too late to add them in and it is always a good idea to review them relative to where you are now in the program.

The following are basic supplements that, over the years, I have found helpful to aid in deficiencies in the body that may affect your ability to drop weight and/or can help speed up the process. Although they have many benefits, keep in mind these supplements are suggested because in my experience they can help with weight loss.

For more detailed information on each supplement, be sure to visit the original Supplement Post in Week 2 and the Secondary Supplement Post in Week 6.

Always remember that if you have any concerns adding in any supplements, be sure to have a conversation with your healthcare provider.

LET'S REVIEW THE BASIC SUPPLEMENTS:

PROBIOTICS:

A probiotic is good bacteria added to your digestive system that helps promote a healthy immune system, but more importantly for our purpose, helps with weight loss by improving digestion.

Digestion is important for weight loss because if your body is unable to process food properly and get the nutrients your body needs, it will store fat to compensate or be reluctant to let it go.

VITAMIN D, D3:

Vitamin D is beneficial for weight loss because it tricks the body into thinking it is summer year-round, eliminating the need for the body to hold on to the extra fat it feels inclined to store over the winter months. It is also essential in supporting the body's metabolism.

Low levels of vitamin D are often found in people who have weight to lose because when someone is lacking Vit D, the hypothalamus (the very small part of your brain that regulates hormonal functions, amongst other things) senses low vitamin D levels and responds by increasing body weight.

OMEGA 3:

Without enough good fat in your diet your body can be reluctant to let go of your stored fat, so one way to speed up the fat loss process is to increase your intake of essential fatty acids.

30% of your diet should come from fat and ideally 10% of that should come from omega 3. The primary source of omega 3 is fish and unless you are eating a lot of it, it can be difficult for the body to get enough.

CALM MAGNESIUM (MAGNESIUM CITRATE):

Although magnesium is responsible for over hundreds of actions in the body, it is important to us because, it not only helps to convert your foods into usable energy, it also helps calm the nerves and balance out cortisol levels (caused by stress.) This helps your body to relax, which can help with getting deep & REM sleep. Deep sleep is important because that is the kind of sleep you need for the body to best repair, rebuild, and detoxify.

DIGESTIVE BITTERS:

If you have known digestive issues, or digestive issues that are as simple as getting bloated after eating raw veg or nuts and seeds, you may want to add in some digestive bitters.

Digestive bitters help build up digestive enzymes that help with processing and getting nutrients from food. Look for Canadian bitters, not Swedish. Swedish bitters can contain a mild laxative which is not recommended.

PREBIOTIC WITH ADDED CLEAR FIBER:

If you have inflammation, digestive, or bowel movement issues, you might want to pick up a prebiotic with added clear fiber.

Prebiotic is food for the probiotic and together can help improve digestion and bowel movements.

LET'S REVIEW THE SECONDARY SUPPLEMENTS:

This list is for those of you who may be interested in taking things to the next level when it comes to your health and wellness.

MCT OIL:

MCT oil is a medium-chain triglyceride (MCT) which I started using about 15 years ago to help natural bodybuilders and professional athletes shed excess fat fast.

The reason why MCT oil is so great for fat loss is because it works like the old thermogenic supplements people used to take to burn fat, but without the harmful effects.

Unlike every other fat source that needs to be broken down, digested, and stored before it is of any use to the body, MCT oil is easily digested and sent directly to your liver where it has a thermogenic effect and the ability to support your metabolism (the rate at which your body functions and burns calories).

MCT's are instantly utilized for fuel instead of being stored as fat, so it helps to calm the mind (since your brain is floating in cholesterol, it needs good fat for energy to function) but keeps the body revved up and working extra hard.

ADAPTOGENS:

Adaptogens are supplements derived from plants that can help our bodies manage and recover from stress. They support the body's ability to cope with stress and help it to return to a balanced state when we experience stressful situations.

Your adrenals produce and control cortisol, the stress hormone. When you are stressed, your adrenals can produce too much cortisol or not enough. Cortisol is known as the stress hormone because of the body's stress response, although it is about more than just stress. Most of the cells in your body have cortisol receptors that use it for a variety of functions including: regulating blood sugar, reducing inflammation, regulating metabolism, and memory function.

We care about cortisol because too much or not enough, signals the need to store fat in the body.

TURMERIC:

The primary antioxidant in Turmeric the spice is curcumin, which is an anti-inflammatory. While increasing your intake of turmeric isn't a lone strategy for weight loss, it may help you address the inflammation associated with extra fat and help with metabolism.

Carrying extra fat creates low grade inflammation in the body that puts you at a higher risk of developing chronic diseases, like heart disease and type 2 diabetes.

NOTE: Turmeric, especially taken as a supplement, can interact with certain medications, so always consult your doctor when considering adding it to your diet. Turmeric can increase your risk of bleeding if you're on blood thinners, interfere with the action of drugs that reduce stomach acid and increase the risk of low blood sugar when taken with certain diabetes drugs. Turmeric is also contraindicated if you have gallstones or obstruction of the bile passages.

TRACE MINERALS:

Most of us are familiar with the vitamins we need and know how essential they are to our health and wellness. But even with taking a supplement, or choosing nutrient rich food, many people are not getting in enough trace minerals. Even though trace minerals are only required in small amounts, they are indeed essential. Not only for good health, but also weight loss.

THERE ARE TWO CLASSES OF MINERALS:

1. Major
2. Trace

Major minerals include: calcium, potassium, chloride, phosphorus, magnesium, sodium, and selenium. Trace minerals include chromium, germanium, manganese, rubidium, vanadium, cobalt, iron, molybdenum, zinc, copper, lithium, nickel, and silica.

Minerals are needed for important metabolic functions in the body and mineral deficiencies are involved in metabolic disorders that cause diseases including hypertension, headaches, depression, heart disease, insulin resistance, and obesity.

COQ10:

The primary role of CoQ10 is as an antioxidant. Your diet consists of antioxidants from a wide variety of sources, including fruits and vegetables.

The main source of dietary CoQ10 is from fatty fish such as mackerel, along with whole-grain foods. Your body also requires CoQ10 to produce energy from the carbohydrates and fat you eat in your diet.

CoQ10 assists in the production of energy by the cells. A deficiency can contribute to lower energy levels and a slower metabolism. Many people believe that CoQ10 production decreases with age, which can help explain one of the reasons why it can be harder to lose weight as you get older.

The CoQ10 can enhance healthy weight loss because it helps to support increased metabolic function. In addition, it can work to decrease body fat while boosting energy levels by maximizing your body's ability to convert food to fuel.

NOTE: Check with your doctor before taking CoQ10 if you are on blood thinning or blood pressure medications.

B COMPLEX:

Vitamin B complex is a group of water-soluble vitamins, which play a very important role in maintaining the growth and the metabolism of cells in the body.

When it comes to weight loss, B12 is among the MOST IMPORTANT because it helps the body convert fats and proteins into energy. B12 is mainly found in red meat, chicken, fish, dairy and eggs.

A B Complex can help the body maintain sufficient levels of a variety of B vitamins so that it can efficiently use carbohydrates, fats, and proteins and helps the body maintain energy, stamina, and appetite.

L-THEANINE:

L-theanine is an amino acid found in both green and black tea leaves and also mushrooms. It is available in pill or tablet form.

It is thought to work by decreasing brain chemicals that contribute to stress and anxiety while increasing brain chemicals that encourage a sense of calm. L-theanine elevates levels of GABA, as well as serotonin and dopamine. These chemicals are known as neurotransmitters, and they work in the brain to regulate emotions, mood, concentration, alertness, and sleep, as well as appetite, energy, and other cognitive skills. Increasing levels of these calming brain chemicals promotes relaxation and can help with sleep. Some research also suggests that L-theanine may improve the function of the body's immune system and help to improve inflammation in the intestinal system.

For More information on these supplements please visit the Let's Talk Supplements post in the Week 2 Guide and the Let's Talk Secondary Supplements post in the Week 6 Guide. As with all the suggestions, be sure to check with your healthcare provider if you have any concerns.

FOOD FACTS - FOOD FOR A HEALTHY GUT

As soon as you began the Livy Method, you started improving your gut health. You did this just by implementing the food plan which naturally begins increasing the healthy bacteria in your digestive system and decreasing the unhealthy ones.

WHAT YOU ARE ALREADY DOING

- Eating lots of fresh fruits and veggies
- Regularly eating leafy greens
- Increasing healthy fats
- Eating raw nuts and seeds
- Taking apple cider vinegar
- Adding in pre & probiotic supplements
- Eliminating, or significantly decreasing, the amount of processed foods and sugar you are consuming

WHAT IS GUT MICROBIOME?

Microbiome is a word we are hearing more and more these days. It's popping up everywhere but do you know what it means?

Microorganisms or microbes are microscopic living things like bacteria, viruses, and fungi. The gut microbiome refers to the microbes found in your digestive system and can affect many aspects of your health. Did you know there are about 100 trillion bacteria, good and bad, that live in your digestive system?

"Altogether, these microbes may weigh as much as 2–5 pounds (1–2 kg), which is roughly the weight of your brain. Together, they function as an extra organ in your body and play a huge role in your health." ~ healthline.com

We all have healthy and unhealthy microbes in our gut but when things get out of whack and the unhealthy ones start to take over, it can have a negative impact on your health. An unhealthy balance can contribute to weight gain, increased blood sugar levels, chronic inflammation, decreased cognitive function, heart disease, as well as many other areas that are currently being studied. Many things, including the foods we eat, can impact the balance of bacteria found in the digestive tract.

HOW CAN I CONTINUE TO IMPROVE OR SUPPORT MY GUT HEALTH?

If you want to go further in improving your gut health, or supporting what you've already done, there are some specific foods that can help you level up your gut microbiome. These foods help to increase healthy bacteria and decrease the ones we want less of.

HERE'S A FEW THINGS YOU CAN DO, OR DO MORE OF!

EAT A VARIETY OF FOODS, ESPECIALLY PLANT FOODS - Different foods lead to a more diverse microbiome. Maybe it's time to start experimenting with different foods you have never tried before! Also decreasing meat consumption and replacing it with plant-based proteins can help increase healthy bacteria in the gut.

EAT CRUCIFEROUS VEGGIES! - So many benefits to these super veggies including healing your gut! High levels of prebiotic fibers and the powerful antioxidant, sulforaphane help to increase the healthy bacteria in your gut. Eating a variety of these veggies raw, or cooked, contributes to a diverse microbiome.

EAT FERMENTED VEGETABLES - sauerkraut, kimchi, miso, tempeh and naturally fermented pickles (found in the refrigerated section and should say "fermented". Not the same as pickled pickles found in the aisles). Fermented foods contain more lactobacilli which is a type of bacteria that can benefit the health of your gut.

EAT OTHER FERMENTED FOODS - Yogurt, kefir & kombucha. When it comes to yogurt, look for "contains live active cultures" and avoid products with high amounts of sugar.

EAT FOODS THAT ARE HIGH IN PREBIOTIC FIBERS - Apples, asparagus, bananas, barley, dandelion greens, garlic, leeks, oats, onions & seaweed to name a few.

INCORPORATE WHOLE GRAINS - Whole grains contain lots of fiber and nondigestible carbs that make their way to the large intestine promoting the growth of beneficial bacteria.

EAT PULSES - Remember our friends beans and lentils? They are also high in prebiotic fiber and help promote a healthy digestive system!

THE BOTTOM LINE IS...

You are already doing wonders for your gut microbiome just by following the plan. These are just some tips for those of you looking to level up or maybe just make some improvements. Every little bit adds up!

To read more about gut health please head to the Science Guide and check out the Issues with Digestion and the Maintenance and the Microbiome posts.

LET'S REVISIT CELEBRATORY WEEKENDS

Keep in mind, you can be hard core about your journey and still enjoy those special moments in life on the way to reaching your goal. So, at the end of the day, it's more about how you want to feel afterwards.

Here my 5 top tips for staying on track:

1. **Take some time to set your intention before the weekend. Are you going to stay on plan, choose to indulge, or take each day as it comes?**

   * There is no right or wrong answer to this, it's all about how you want to feel when it's time to get back at it.

2. **Regardless of what you plan to do, make a point of eating normally the day of any big event or in anticipation of a big/festive meal.**

   * Meaning, follow the Food Plan leading up, which will help keep your digestive system stimulated so going into the meal, you digest it better, and feel less bloated after eating a bigger meal.

3. **Eating all meals and snacks leading up will prevent you from overeating.**

   * Including starting your day with higher protein like eggs or full fat Greek yogurt, even if you usually skip it.

4. **Starting your day higher in protein and fat and minimal carbs, for example eggs over oatmeal, will get your body working harder from the get-go and give you more sustaining energy.**

   * Also, If you have carbs like cereal, oatmeal or bread, you run more of a risk of setting yourself up to crave carbs and sugar all day and if there is lots of food around, you are going to be tempted by it if you are already craving it.

5. **Stay on top of your water and try to start earlier in the day.**

   * If you are on the road or out and about, make a plan and get it in when you can.

And finally, keep in mind:

At the end of the day, even if you eat your face off, you can't make a pound of fat in a day, overnight, or weekend...so all you need to do is get right back on track the next day.

LET'S REVISIT LEAFY GREENS

Great for your brain, your bones and weight loss.

Leafy greens are an ideal addition to meals because they are not only packed with tons of nutrients that are great for your health and cellular function, but they also help the body process food through your digestive system, which is needed for weight loss.

High in fiber and water content, leafy greens help to keep you more satisfied by feeding into your satiety hormones which keeps you feeling more satisfied on smaller portions.

Increasing leafy greens can also play a role in keeping blood sugar levels stable by feeding into GLP-1 (Glucagon-Like Peptide-1) which is a hormone produced in your gut which helps to regulate your appetite.

Darker leafy greens are also rich in sulfur-containing compounds that support your body's detoxification process.

Plus, all of the changes you have been making in your diet can affect your bowel movements. Leafy greens provide the roughage your body needs to keep you regular throughout this process.

Leafy greens can be added to meals raw, like in a salad, or you might find them more appealing cooked or sautéed and/or added to soups, stews & stir-frys.

The general rule is...if it's green and leafy it works!

However...Cabbage, Brussels sprouts, and bok choy (among others which are listed in the Grocery List) which are cruciferous vegetables can also be used as leafy greens on plan.

Cruciferous vegetables are a major source of glutathione. Glutathione is an antioxidant in your body that is involved in tissue repair and boosting your immune system. (See the Food Facts post on Cruciferous Vegetables for more information.)

If you are not a fan of eating your leafy greens, it is still key to get them in. Although they are suggested at lunch and dinner, they can also be added to breakfast and even your snacks.

You don't have to be fancy about it or get in a huge variety. It's also not a big deal if you are a bit hit and miss getting them in, as long as you are mindful to be as consistent as possible. But with that said, if you are looking to maximize your efforts...load them up!

WEEK 11 GUIDELINES: PERSONALIZING THE FOOD PLAN

This week has you taking what you have learned and tweaking the Food Plan to suit your body's changing needs day to day while helping it to focus on fat loss.

This is an exciting place to be in your Weight Loss journey!

You have followed through and done a lot of work, not only to address why your body was feeling a need to store fat, but to help your body be as healthy as possible.

I have been saying all along that counting calories and weighing and measuring your food is not normal. Neither is the formula we have been using; forcing the body to eat certain foods at certain times has been the way we got the body's attention and helped it to focus on fat loss.

We used the formula in the beginning to give the body what it needed so it no longer felt the need to store fat. Then we used that formula to get the body to focus on and go into detox as much as possible for as long as possible, when fat loss wasn't yet a priority for the body.

Then, as fat loss became more of a priority, we used the formula to feed into and support the nice, high metabolism you have created throughout the process, so your body can function at a more optimal level.

At this point, your body doesn't want the fat it was storing any more than you do, and it is more than happy to get rid of it, so you are going to use that to your advantage.

We will continue to use the original Food Plan formula when you need to get "Back on Track" after having an off day/s or indulging in foods that make you feel off. But unless you are in that situation, the formula is no longer needed.

THIS BRINGS US TO WEEK 11: PERSONALIZING THE FOOD PLAN.

This stage of the Program is the most work because it's about having faith in all the hard work you have done and the foundation you have built.

It's also about RELENTLESSLY MAXIMIZING everything you can, and need to do, to keep the body focused on fat loss until you reach your goal.

WHAT DOES PERSONALIZING THE PLAN LOOK LIKE?

You are still following all of the basic guidelines like eating higher protein at breakfast, not going longer than 3.5 to 4 hrs. without eating, still making sure to drink your water, take your supplements and maximize your efforts. The difference is you will be making your food choices based on the following:

1. WHEN TO EAT – You will still be checking in at each meal and snack time: breakfast, snack, lunch, snack, snack, dinner.

- Before every meal and snack time, ask yourself if you NEED to eat, COULD eat or SHOULD eat. You still don't want to go longer than 4 hours without eating. That is where "should I eat" comes in. If not hungry, just have a token amount and check in at the next meal or snack time.

- Keep in mind that hunger levels naturally fluctuate daily, meaning one day you might feel hungry every half hour and the next day, 3 to 4 hours will go by without being hungry.

- Trust your mind-body connection and understand that the body knows best and it will let you know when it's hungry.

2. WHAT TO EAT - (while still following the Guidelines) When you are hungry ask yourself, what exactly am I hungry for and what's the best choice for me to maximize my efforts.

- You still want to choose your meal and snack options from the same kinds of foods you have been eating all along. But rather than eating specific foods at specific times, you can now make your choices based on what's most appealing in the moment when you are hungry. For example, you may choose to have fruit in the afternoon and nuts in the morning.

3. HOW MUCH TO EAT – Continue being super in tune and mindful about portion sizes, keeping in mind you are still looking to lose weight.

- You want to continue to eat "just enough".

- You DO NOT want to be matching your hunger levels. You want your body to keep momentum and focus on detox and fat loss, rather than processing and digesting food. Smaller portions are better for digestion and keep the food moving in and out.

- Smaller portions also help lower insulin levels so that you feel more satisfied on less, while keeping energy levels maintained.

GUIDELINES:

- Check in at every meal and snack time. Try not to let more than 3.5 - 4 hours max go by without eating.

- You are NOT introducing any "new foods". You are sticking with the same kinds of foods you have been eating. For example, no bars or muffins, and still no pasta.

- Breakfast is still an option, but always a benefit. If you do have it, still go with higher protein.

- Morning snack is your choice and can be optional, depending on if and when you had breakfast.

- Lunch can be your choice and more of a snack size. You can add back in the heavier carbs, but only as needed while still trying to lose.

- Leafy greens are still a benefit, especially if BMs are still an issue.

- Afternoon snacks - you can have 1 or 2, or you can skip snacks depending on lunch and dinner times and your hunger levels (ideally no longer than 3.5 - 4 hours between eating).

- Dinner should be the smallest meal of the day, and can be more of a snack or snack-sized portion, and/or you can skip if not hungry (depending on the time of your last meal or snack). Avoid heavier carbs at this meal, unless needed.

ALWAYS MAXIMIZING:

- Water intake
- Supplements
- Being in tune to hunger levels
- Being in tune with portion sizes
- Managing stress levels
- Using your energy, being more active
- Working the parameters of the program. Meaning, still eating protein for breakfast and not eating or snacking late at night.

TO RECAP:

The purpose is to transition the body into a style of eating more conducive to helping it focus on fat loss, while feeding into its need to function more efficiently and at optimal levels.

At this point, the body wants the fat gone as much as you do, which means you no longer need to manipulate it into focusing on fat loss. In a sense, it means that day in and day out, you are maximizing everything you can do to help the body continue getting rid of fat.

People can be reluctant about this phase because they feel there is less structure. But the reality is, it is just as structured, if not more so, since you will be checking in at every meal and snack time.

It's also more work because it's about bringing everything you have learned over the past few months together and not only implementing it, but maximizing it.

TO SIMPLIFY WEEK 11:

The biggest change is; you no longer need to force the body to eat token amounts when you are not hungry unless 3.5 to 4 hours have gone by since you last ate. Pretty much everything else is the same, since you are still looking to lose weight by following the Guidelines & maximizing.

Remember, the goal is for you to not only lose your weight in a healthy and maintainable way, it's to eventually wake up, look good, feel good, and just go about your day making good food choices. The goal is to get out of the weight loss game, lose your weight, and move on.

This stage of Personalizing The Plan will not only help you to continue to drop fat, it will set you up to be able to move on and have your food choices be based on your body's needs, rather than its wants. It's to have you move forward in life and never look back, and to give you the tools you need to forever be in tune so that you never need to lose weight again.

We are not done yet! The goal is to finish as strong as you started.

Please take the time to head over to the Facebook Group or the Livy Method App and watch the quick video that accompanies this post.

WEEK 11 GUIDELINES FAQS

Personalizing the Plan...is not eating off Plan.

Week 11 is just another tweak like any other week on The Program. Be sure to read over the Guidelines...a few times. We are assuming you are not done losing weight...so each week is still all about losing and Maximizing your efforts...right to the very end.

Also, be sure to review the HUNGER & MAXIMIZING Posts and Videos as suggested for each new week. Now is NOT the time to do your own thing, if you are looking to capitalize on these last few weeks... be all in and follow the Program as designed.

Here are some common questions we get asked about Week 11.

1.   Can we add bread and pasta back in?

Keep in mind, some people have been eating bread and pasta all along and losing weight just fine. It's always been a choice. But make no mistake, it is not Maximizing your efforts while looking to lose. If you still have weight to lose, it's best to keep them to a minimum.

2.   Is it better to skip lunch or dinner?

You don't want to be skipping any meals "just because". If you are not eating a meal, it would be because you are not hungry for it. And even then, you need to take into account if you should eat based on the 30 minutes to 3.5 hours between meals and snacks.

3.   If I skip meals and snacks will my body go into starvation mode?

Not if you are following the 30 minutes to 3.5 hours between meals and snack rule. If you go past 3.5 hours and you are not hungry, then this is a case of where you "should" eat at least a token amount of the next meal or snack.

4.   Can I have a protein shake for my lunch or dinner?

Protein shakes are best to use at breakfast or snacks, but if you do use them at lunch or dinner then you are still to include the protein, veg and greens. Although you can add a bit of fruit like you would at a meal, you still want to include the components of protein, veg and greens and healthy fats in your shake.

5.   Are we still making meals nutrient rich?

Absolutely, nothing changes there! Be sure to add good fats to your meals and make them as nutrient rich as possible.

6.   Is there a 'star of the show' for lunch and dinner?

A high protein breakfast is still encouraged as a benefit, but there is no star of the show for the other meals. You want to go with what is appealing to you in the moment. Ideally you will want to add in protein, veg, healthy fats, and leafy greens and make your meals nutrient rich if you still have weight to lose to help your body focus on fat loss.

7.   What snack combinations can I have?

You still want to choose your meal and snack options from the same kinds of foods you have been eating all along. But rather than eating specific foods at specific times, you can now make your choices based on what's most appealing in the moment when you are hungry. For example, you may choose to have fruit in the afternoon and nuts in the morning. Check in at every meal and snack time. Try not to let more than 3.5 - 4 hours max go by without eating. You are not introducing any "new foods" at this point, for example, no bars or muffins, but keeping with the kind of snacks you have been eating. Morning snack is your choice and can be optional, depending on if and when you had breakfast. For the afternoon snack, you can have 1 or 2, or you can skip snacks depending on when you had lunch and dinner and your hunger levels.

TO RECAP:

You are very much still following The Plan, the only real thing that changes is you no longer have to eat token amounts if you are not hungry unless it's been 3.5-4 hours since you ate last, and you have a bit more flexibility in your food choices.

MAXIMIZING YOUR PERSONAL PLAN

Now that you have had some time to work on Personalizing The Food Plan with Week 11, it's time to take things to the next level. While Personalizing the Food Plan, you are still following the basic guidelines of The Plan.

For example, still having higher protein at breakfast, still being mindful to add in leafy greens when you can, keeping food nutrient rich, and still trying not to eat too late in the evening.

Along with Maximizing all the things you can do to keep the body focused and ready for "detox", you are checking in with yourself throughout the day to be sure you are in tune with your body's needs in the moment.

CONTINUING TO:

- Be mindful when you are hungry and when you are not.
- Be mindful of making the best choice in the moment.
- Be mindful of portion sizes, continuing to ask the four questions.
- Drink your water.
- Be consistent with supplements.
- Manage stress levels.
- Move your body.

LET'S TALK: NEXT LEVEL

When it comes to weight loss, there is a difference between eating well, eating better, and eating in a way that is conducive to weight loss. Some foods are easier to digest than others which is something to keep in mind when looking to lose weight and being in tune. In understanding how your body processes and digests certain foods, you can take things to the next level with your food choices.

For example:

Juice...and other liquid nutrients hit your body fast...making this an issue because it's hard to control Insulin levels

- Juice can be great in the summer when it's super hot or when you overexert yourself so much you need to replenish your glycogen (energy) stores fast. (Note these occasions are rare.)

Fruits... are easiest to digest so perfect when you need quick and easy energy.

- Fruits are also nutrient rich and high in fiber. If you are not looking for quick energy or are mindful of insulin levels, it's a good idea to pair with protein & fat to neutralize.

Veggies... are harder to digest than fruits but are good for stimulating the digestive system and have a high nutrient value.

- They are also great for increasing digestive enzymes and serve as an energy food, giving the body the carbs it needs without increasing insulin in the way fruit can.

Nuts and Seeds...take 2-3 hours to digest.

- High in protein and fat, they can help give you more sustaining (lasting) energy.

Fish and seafood... is easy to digest protein which can take 40 minutes - 1.5 hours.

Chicken/poultry takes approximately 2 hours

Eggs - 45 minutes

Beans and legumes - 1.5 - 2 hours

Red meat and pork...take the longest and can take 5+ hours (hard to digest but also high in B vitamins, so good to have when you crave).

Dairy...can take just as long as meat. (Dairy can be hard to digest, especially if you are sensitive to it, which is why it can be beneficial to limit.)

EXAMPLES OF HOW YOU CAN USE THIS INFORMATION TO YOUR ADVANTAGE

1. **"I'm feeling low on energy and need a quick snack, so I'll grab some nuts"**

Nuts take 2 - 3 hours to break down, whereas fruit takes 20 - 30 minutes. So, if you are looking for quick and fast energy, fruit is a better choice than nuts.

Nuts are hard to digest, which is why in the beginning of The Program, we added them as a second snack in the late afternoon, to purposely make the body work hard and keep you more satisfied longer. So, when grabbing something easy and looking for more sustained, longer lasting energy, you may want to have some nuts.

2. **You are going out for a night on the town or a late event**

Instead of having something like steak, which is harder to digest, have fish or seafood, which is much faster and easier to digest. That will give you the energy you need to enjoy your night out without interrupting your sleep later.

These are things to keep in mind when wanting to take your eating to the next level, Maximize weight loss results, and have a deeper level of understanding as to why I suggested eating certain foods at certain times. Also, why eating hard to digest food in the evening makes no sense. There is a lot to be learned from many angles when it comes to making your food choices.

LET'S TALK: TOP TIPS FOR GOOD DIGESTION:

1.   Check in at scheduled meal and snack times.

Life can get busy and it's easy to get sidetracked and forget to eat. Until it becomes second nature, it's a great idea to check in on yourself.

While on Plan, it is important to be consistent with your food choices because it has a regulating effect on your digestive system. It's also important to allow your Migrating Motor Complex to kick in and do its work in between meals.

Knowing when you are hungry and when you are not is key.

2.   Be conscious of what you eat and your portion sizes.

If you are still looking to lose, it's still key to be mindful of portions.

Too much sugar or too large of a portion stimulates the pancreas to release more of the hormone insulin, which signals weight gain. Also, it does stress the body out when you indulge. For example, eating too much not only slows the weight loss process, it's also the number one cause of indigestion. Although, it's no big deal since you can always get Back on Track.

3.   Chew your food completely and don't talk while eating.

Incomplete chewing and talking while eating can cause premature swallowing. Our digestive systems are not designed to digest large pieces of food. When we put large pieces in our stomach, it can lead to incomplete digestion and digestive discomfort.

4.   Relax while eating your meal.

This may seem super simple, but many of us are always on the go and always on the clock rushing through everything we do.

Eating when you are rushed increases your stress and slows down the digestive process. Try to create a calm atmosphere when eating.

5.   Practice good posture.

This is key especially with your ever-changing body, just from a structural point of view and making sure muscles are supporting proper alignment.

When you slouch or hunch over, extra pressure is put on the digestive organs in your abdomen. This extra pressure can cause poor digestion. You should practice sitting with your shoulders back and your chin tucked in. This will allow more room for the digestive organs and will help improve digestion.

6.   Don't eat late at night.

This is pretty standard on Plan but worth repeating why. Our bodies, including our digestive system, slow down in the evening hours as it gets ready to rest and rejuvenate. When we put food into our stomach at these late hours, there are not enough digestive enzymes to properly digest it. This undigested food sits in your stomach and will often disturb your sleep and prevent the body from focusing on detox.

7.   Take a brisk walk after eating.

Increased physical activity after a meal actually helps jump start your digestive system and increases the production of digestive enzymes. This will lead to more complete digestion of your food.

8.   Try a spinal twist.

Spinal twists allow excess toxins in the digestive system to be released, which has a calming effect. While in a cross-legged sitting position, slowly turn to the right and hold while taking 5 deep breaths, then repeat this process on the left side.

9.   Avoid ice cold drinks while eating.

Although a nice cold glass of water can be refreshing in the warmer months, ice cold drinks can slow down the digestive process.

Think of it as putting ice on a muscle. The muscle stiffens and does not function as well. Warm or room temperature water or teas will encourage proper digestion even in the warmer months.

Now, this isn't to say you can't drink cold water while eating, just be in tune to how it may be affecting your digestive system in the moment.

REMEMBER:

These tips are not meant to stress you out or to complicate the process. I'm putting out this info for those interested in Maximizing their efforts and taking things to the next level.

Rest assured, you are doing enough by being mindful with the Process and following along as designed.

We hope you are enjoying this week of Personalizing the Food Plan and trying to have fun with it as you work to take things to the next level.

To read more about the purpose of your Migrating Motor Complex head over to the Science Saturday Guide and read The Migrating Motor Complex (MMC) and Hunger.

LET'S TALK AVOIDING WEIGHT GAIN

With many of you expressing concern about gaining weight back...and rightfully so, given past experiences, I thought it would be a great idea to talk about how not to gain weight back after putting all of your time and energy into losing it.

First, it's key to understand that the way you have gone about losing weight with this Process is different from any past attempts at fat burning.

When you burn your fat off by restricting energy foods or starving and depriving your body, you leave the body with no choice but to burn its stored fat for fuel.

Although it's effective for weight loss, it also immediately reinforces the need for your body to hold onto and store fat.

Simply put, if you use your body's stored fat for energy as a method for weight loss (fat burning), your body will store it all back plus more the first chance it gets, every single time ...and it will do so thinking it's doing you a favour!

Which is why you can lose weight with a fat burning diet, but you can't maintain the loss after you go back to normal eating.

With this Process, because you have addressed the body's need to store fat and have helped the body drop fat in the healthiest of ways, that's not really a concern.

However, there are 2 main reasons why someone might gain weight back after this Process that you need to be mindful of.

1. **NOT PUTTING TIME INTO MAINTENANCE**
   - Maintenance is key. You have got to give your body time to get used to functioning at your new weight. You want your new weight to become your new norm / set point.
   - Even though you may have hit your goal and are done losing, your body is not done solidifying the weight you have lost.
   - Things like metabolism, blood flow, body temp and hormones are just a few of the things the body will need to address & adjust to be able to stabilize at your new weight.
   - There are 2 phases to Maintenance. The first is going to last 2-3 months, where you are mindful to follow your Personalized Plan and not add in things that will stress the body out. If you do indulge, you will simply implement Back On Track.
   - The second phase is where you go live your life and eat according to your body's fluctuating needs day to day. When you indulge, you will use Back on Track, but otherwise, you will just be waking up and going about your day being mindful of your food choices and how you feel.

Mindfulness moving forward is all you will need to be able to live a worry-free life when it comes to your weight.

This is also where the concept of "Check Yourself Before You Wreck Yourself" comes in. You don't gain 10 or 20lbs without noticing. Continue to be mindful and when you notice, simply check yourself and implement BOT.

2.   **NOT ADJUSTING TO SITUATIONAL CHANGE**

- For example, losing your weight at home where your routine, environment and stress levels are different than if you went back to work. The situation being you were at home all day and now you are at your place of work.

- Another example of this would be to have a change in job, where your stress levels are different. Helping the body manage new stress by bumping up omega 3, adding in MCT oil or being mindful to get to bed earlier to adjust to your new schedule, are a few examples of what you can do to help minimize the impact of situational change.

- It's key to help the body adjust and adapt to change. Change in environment for example; needing more water in a dryer environment than you are used to. Adjusting to stress as noted above, or even a change in the times you are able to eat. For example, having more business meetings or a job that restricts when you can eat.

- The goal is to minimize the impact on the body by helping it adjust to physical or emotional stress/change.

I'm going to add a 3rd element to be mindful of, which is seasonal change.

3.   **SEASONAL CHANGE**

- This one is all about not forcing yourself to eat salads when you are craving heavier carbs. In the cooler months, for example, be sure to be in tune to your body's needs. Heavier carbs, fatty meats, along with hot and spicy foods are more appealing for a reason. They help to create heat in the body which helps to eliminate the need for the body to store extra fat to keep you warm.

- Alternatively, be sure to decrease the heavier carbs & bump up fruits and cooling foods like salads and veg in the warmer months.

- Try to eat a seasonally sourced diet or incorporate seasonal foods WHEN possible.

THINGS TO AVOID TO PREVENT WEIGHT GAIN:

- Making a habit of going all day without eating. If this happens every now and then, it's no big deal. But if you make it a habit (like for weeks & months)... the body will pick up on this and start storing fat.

- Trying not to eat all day in anticipation of a bigger meal later in the day. This only reinforces the need for fat when you starve the body followed by overeating, which leads to increased insulin levels & signals weight gain.

- Not eating the next day after indulging. Although you may not feel like eating much after a day of indulging, it's key to help stimulate the digestive system to help get rid of any backlog.

- Falling back into old habits like thinking less is more and trying to control your body instead of being in tune to it.

- Over exercising and not giving the body enough rest in between workouts can lead to the body feeling a need to store fat to compensate.

- Not prioritizing your body's needs like managing stress and getting enough sleep.

- Not replenishing the body or helping it heal after illness. For example, not taking probiotics after antibiotics or pushing it to recover too soon.

- Not drinking enough water. Although you don't need to be drinking as much water, once you lose you do want to be mindful of being hydrated so your body can function properly.

- Not being mindful of your body's ongoing and ever-changing needs.

As you can see, easily maintaining your weight truly is about being mindful and continuing to be in tune to your body's needs while you navigate and enjoy life.

It's not as hard as you think and a little effort goes a long way in terms of living a worry-free life when it comes to your weight.

Please take the time to head over to the Facebook Group or the Livy Method App and watch the quick video that accompanies this post.

WEEK 12 GUIDELINES: MAINTENANCE AND MINDFULNESS

This week we will be having discussions on moving forward after you are done losing and how to proceed if you have more weight to lose after the Group is done.

As we enter the final week of the Fall session, it's time to talk about Maintenance for those of you who have reached your goal, or are getting close.

To be clear, Maintenance is for those of you who are done losing & are no longer working towards getting the body to drop more fat.

For those of you still looking to lose, continue with your Personalized Food Plan and later this week we will be discussing next steps for continuing your weight loss journey.

There are two stages of Maintenance:

STAGE 1 - MAINTENANCE: LASTS FOR 2 TO 3 MONTHS

This is when you have reached your goal and are now looking to solidify the weight you have lost so you can easily maintain it moving forward.

During this phase, you might look forward to adding back in all the foods you have gone without over the past few months.

HOWEVER, you still want to be mindful of choosing foods that will challenge the digestive system and cause stress internally.

This is even more important with all the added stress you may be under these days. The goal for the first stage of Maintenance is to give your body time to adjust and get used to functioning at your new weight. In other words, the goal is for your new weight to become the new normal for your body.

- During this FIRST Maintenance stage you will continue with your Personalized Food Plan but in a more relaxed manner because you are not looking to lose weight.

- Every now and then you can add in some of your old favorites but be sure to get "Back on Track" and help your body balance it out.

- It's best to keep any indulgences few and far between for the next few months.

- Just because the body is done dropping fat, doesn't mean it is done doing the work to support it.

SIDE NOTE:

For anyone concerned about loose skin, this is a great time to help that along.

Try dry brushing, adding in collagen & using natural oils and creams, as the skin takes twice the amount of time to regenerate around your new frame. Your skin cells will be regenerating as your body continues to work on addressing any issues above and beyond weight loss.

With your body now minimizing its focus on fat loss, it can allocate resources to other areas of the body when it comes to repairing, rebuilding, regenerating, and rejuvenating.

You have done a lot of work up until now. Your body is now working harder and will continue to do so, so the goal is to keep it working at these optimum levels.

STAGE 2 - MINDFULNESS: THIS WILL BE ONGOING

This is when you are not giving much thought to what you are eating or not eating, and you start to move on and live your life by being in tune to your body's needs.

- You should now have faith in all your hard work by being able to wake up and go about your day, making good food choices in the moment.

- You should be in a place where your internal dialogue, and that space in your brain reserved for obsessing about what you eat and don't eat, is non-existent or getting close to it.

- This is where you move on and enjoy your life without worrying about what you are going to eat or not eat, or having to lose weight.

But, with that said, this is also where you implement the concept of "Check Yourself Before You Wreck Yourself".

CHECK YOURSELF BEFORE YOU WRECK YOURSELF

Although you have lost weight in a healthy way that has you in tune to your body's needs, it's not a magic pill.

Moving forward, you will always need to be mindful of the choices you make, understanding how your choices will affect your body, and then self-correcting, balancing out, and getting Back On Track to minimize the effect.

I've been able to easily maintain my weight for over 25 years. My weight has fluctuated up and down naturally and sometimes more than others, but for the most part, it's just a matter of going by how I feel.

If I make crappy food choices, I feel crappy, then I just get Back On Track. I never indulge without understanding how I will feel after. This may seem like work but after a while, it just becomes second nature.

Maintenance really is as simple as that.

You want to allow your body the time it needs to adjust to its new weight and continue to be in tune to your body's needs, being mindful of the messages you are sending and receiving.

LET'S TALK WATER AND SUPPLEMENTS

Once you reach Maintenance, you can re-evaluate the supplements you are taking. You may choose to leave some in or switch some of them up. Please note, taking out the supplements WILL NOT cause you to gain weight. At this point, you will just be keeping them in for their health and wellness benefits.

In regards to water, because you are no longer looking to lose weight, you only need enough water to keep you hydrated.

STILL LOOKING TO LOSE??

For those of you still working towards your goal, later this week we will be talking about a game plan moving forward.

For now, continue with Personalizing the Plan and Maximizing your efforts and be sure to let us know if you have any questions.

Please note:

If you are done losing but want to join the next Group, I will be discussing the benefits of redoing the process to help solidify the weight you have lost and help the body level up in terms of health and wellness...when we discuss next steps later this week.

Please take the time to head over to the Facebook Group or the Livy Method App and watch the quick video that accompanies this post.

WEEK 12 GUIDELINES FAQS

1. **I need a longer break before starting another Program, any suggestions?**

It's totally fine to feel that you need more time. You can always sign up for the next group, but start when you are ready. You can continue to use Option 2 of Personalizing The Plan until you are ready. Bridging the Gap by following the original Food Plan is also something you can choose, especially if you find you are at capacity and you are still looking to lose weight. Go with whatever works best for you.

2. **I struggled to fully commit the time and effort needed to work on myself during this Program, any advice for moving forwards?**

It's progress over perfection, and life can sometimes hold us back from being able to fully commit to something. Following the program, even without being all in is still beneficial, as it's a step forward to you reaching your goal of finally and forever. Keep showing up for yourself, have patience with yourself, and do the best that you can each day. Life is always happening and there is always something that can keep us from being able to fully commit. Deciding that you are worth the time and effort to focus on your goal of weight loss and living your best life, can really help.

3. **Do you recommend that I strictly follow the original Food Plan, or can I implement more of a Personalized Plan?**

It's best to choose how you are going to proceed and stick with it. You may find that some days Personalizing The Plan can very closely resemble the original Food Plan. Personalizing The Plan (PTP) is an effective method for reaching your goal, and you can think of it as following a food plan specifically designed for you. It would be preferable to continue PTP in preparation for doing a complete reset in the next group while continuing to ask yourself the four mindfulness questions. However if you feel like you don't have the capacity to be checking in at each meal and snack you can totally use Bridging the Gap by following the original Food Plan until the next group.

4. **When I am done with my weight loss and the maintenance period, should I continue to eat multiple snacks a day?**

After consolidating your weight loss for 2-3 months, you are ready to move on to the second stage of mindfulness and live your life! You will have the confidence in your body to tell you what it needs, whilst being mindful of the food choices you make. So if you need to continue to have multiple snacks because it is what your body needs, have them. Hunger levels will continue to change day to day, so continue to be in tune with how you are feeling and hunger levels throughout the day.

CONTINUING TO LOSE - OPTION 1 - REPEATING THE PROCESS

Let's Talk Option One - Repeating the Process!

Repeating the Process means doing a complete reset of The Program and re-doing the Process over again week to week from the beginning.

Which is an effective option.

The idea being that you are restarting the process with your body now functioning at a more optimal level.

Don't overthink it, it's really just about approaching the second round (or 3rd, 4th, 5th) with Fresh Eyes, and being just as diligent and motivated as you were the first time around.

Keeping in mind each time you repeat the Process, it's key not to assume your body will respond in the same way because your body next time around will be functioning on a whole other level.

Some of you who have more weight to lose, may have to complete another few rounds to reach your goal. Have faith that each time your body will be working more and more in your favour, making the Process easier and easier.

The first time around, you will find yourself more focused on the physical elements of The Program - what you are eating and how your body is responding.

You will find when you repeat the Process, it becomes more of a mental game. So, it is key to approach each new Group with Fresh Eyes.

If this was your first time through The Program and you are considering doing a reset, I would suggest reviewing the Fresh Eyes Post.

You will want to continue repeating the Process until you have reached your goal.

Some of you might reach your goal half way through the second round, or third or maybe even 4th or 5th round.

When you reach your goal, you can continue to follow through on the steps to help solidify your weight and finish The Program, OR start the Maintenance Phase.

You can redo The Program by signing up for the next Group Session or follow along on your own by utilizing the info from this current Group.

You can access any of the information, including all of the Posts, Videos and the Lives, through the Facebook Support Group for the next year and through the Livy Method App.

It is suggested that you follow the days and weeks in order starting with Week 1 (Day 8). Anything that is not included in this Workbook, such as accompanying Videos, can be found in the Support Group by using the Guides or using the Library in the Livy Method App.

Keep in mind, we will not be answering questions in the Group after it ends, but be sure to follow me over on my social media platforms and I will be going Live over on my public Facebook page the week leading up to the next Group to answer any questions.

If your plan is to continue with the next Group, you can continue to lose with Personalizing the Plan until it starts. Or, if you are feeling like the next few weeks are going to be chaotic or busy or you know you will be having a hard time staying focused, there is also the option of implementing Back on Track to bridge the gap.

Back on Track is best used when you go off the rails and indulge. But during stressful or chaotic times, if you feel like you don't have the capacity to focus on your food choices as much as you like in between groups, then BOT can be a good option.

My preference would be for you to continue Personalizing the Plan in preparation for doing a complete reset in the next Group.

For those of you who may be behind in the Group and following on your own timeline:

- Do your best to complete as many weeks as possible before repeating the Process.
- If you are doing The Program on your own, then be sure to complete the full 12 weeks before you start again.
- If your plan is to do the next Group, then keep following along as far as you can and then reset with the new Group.

Repeating the Process is an effective method to continue to lose for many reasons, as each time The Program works just as well, if not better. There is an advantage in knowing what's to come and how to step up your game and capitalize on the Process.

It also gives the option for the body to level up your health and wellness as it challenges the body to address issues and continue to make change.

CONTINUING TO LOSE - OPTION 2 - PERSONALIZING THE PLAN

Let's Talk Option 2 - Personalizing the Plan.

"Personalizing The Plan" is doing all of the things, and making sure to maximize everything you need to do to help keep the body focused on fat loss to get the fat out.

This is the technique you have been using these last 2 weeks and also the method I used for my personal one on one clients. It is very effective.

When Personalizing The Plan, it is assumed you are looking to lose more weight, so you need to be as diligent and as consistent as possible and use all of the tools you have learned along the way to keep the scale moving.

Every minute of every day, you are being in tune to your body's needs to help it focus on, and get into detox and keep it in detox for as long as possible to help the body focus on fat loss.

When Personalizing The Plan, you can still implement Back on Track when you find yourself indulging or going off Plan.

Remember that PTP is checking in at every single meal and snack. It's making the best food choices based on the Guidelines. It's being super in tune to portions, and it's making sure to relentlessly Maximize.

Regardless of which method you choose, keep in mind the scale will still fluctuate and your hunger levels will continue to change day to day.

Be sure to review the Maximizing and the Hunger Posts and remember, although we won't be answering questions, all the information stays in the Facebook Group for you to access for the next year, should you need to review anything.

Being clear about next steps is key, as you don't want to find yourself flip flopping from one technique to another. Set your goal and be clear about your intention.

Continue to work hard and be relentless when it comes to finishing the Process and not only reaching your goal, but solidifying the weight that you have lost.

Personalizing The Plan is an effective method for reaching your goal, so continue to stay focused and visualize the end game. Think of Personalizing The Plan as following a diet specifically designed for you.

After these past few months, you know your body's needs more than anyone and after completing this Process, you are more in tune than ever. Your body is on your side and wants the fat gone just as much as you do.

The benefits of following your Personalized Plan over repeating the Process, is it gives you more flexibility in your day-to-day food choices.

BRIDGING THE GAP BETWEEN GROUPS

Let's talk bridging the gap between the end of this Group & repeating the Process again.

Repeating the Process is an effective way to lose. If that's your plan, I suggest you review the Fresh Eyes Post. It will give you some insight into things to keep in mind each time you repeat the Process.

If you are planning on doing a repeat of The Program on your own, it's a great idea to get a few weeks of Personalizing The Plan under your belt as you want to be as in tune to your body's needs as possible before you jump back into the week to week structure of a reset.

If you are planning on doing the next Group, I would ideally like to see you using the Personalizing The Plan technique until the start date.

If you do find yourself indulging/enjoying/partaking in the weeks in between groups, be sure to use Back on Track as often as you need and then continue on with Personalizing The Plan.

If you find you are at capacity and still want to lose, but know you won't have the same kind of time and energy to give to the Process on your own, you might want to consider using the Back on Track Method to bridge the gap.

Back on Track is ideally reserved for when you go off the rails, but given the added stress and chaos of this year, it could be exactly what you need to help calm the body and enable it to stay more focused on fat loss.

Remember that Personalizing the Plan can also look a lot like the original Food Plan with the added flexibility of skipping or switching up your snacks.

At the end of the day, it's all about intention and what feels best.

TO RECAP:

If you are done losing, you are going to follow the Maintenance Protocol. If you are looking to continue your journey, you are going to:

A: Re-do the program in the next Group

B: Re-do the program on your own using the info in this Group

C: Continue with Personalizing The Plan until you reach your goal and will use BOT for the times you indulge.

If you choose A or B, you are going to Bridge the Gap between this Group and the next by:

A: Personalizing The Plan using Back on Track when needed until you start the next Group

B: Sticking with the original Food Plan (BOT), and working the basics before starting The Program again.

On a final note:

If you are behind in the Group and working through any of the previous weeks, continue to work at your own pace and be sure to reach out if you have any questions.

If you have signed up for the next Group, you can continue with moving forward from where you are at and then reset when the new Group starts.

END OF PROGRAM FAQS

With the program coming to an end, we have compiled a list of some of the most frequently asked questions.

1. **Will we have access to this group when it's done?**

   - Yes! Although we stop posting and answering questions on Sunday December 11, you will still be able to access the group to review the information after we are done.

2. **Will the Winter 2023 Group have its own Support Group?**

   - Yes, each new group has its own separate support group.

3. **Do I need to keep taking the supplements?**

   - If you have reached your goal and you are ready for maintenance you can decide what you want to continue to take for health benefits. Otherwise, you don't need to keep taking them to maintain your weight.

   - If you are still looking to lose you have options, you can take a break from the supplements between groups or keep taking them. There are benefits to both options so it's really personal preference.

   - Same rules apply for the ACV or Lemon water

4. **I'm concerned about gaining weight in between groups. How do I avoid that?**

   - Be sure to review the post on "How not to gain weight back"

   - Be sure to have a plan and be clear on next steps, review the Next Steps Options Posts.

   - Be sure to use BOT when you indulge to the point you feel off and or weight is up.

5. **How do I register for the next Group?**

   - Sign Up Page on our website www.ginalivy.com

6. **Do I need Facebook to sign up for the new Group or can I just use the New App?**

   - The App is to be used alongside the Facebook support group as a companion app.

   - Our stand-alone app will be ready in Winter 2024 so you will need Facebook to follow until then

7. **Where do I download the App?**

   - You can follow the directions sent by email at the time of purchase or download from the Apple App Store or Google Play Store.

   - If you have already downloaded the app, there is no need to download it again

   - For more information about the app, head over to our App Help Guide on our website: https://www.ginalivy.com/appguide

8. **What if I didn't get a code for the New Group or App?**

- Any administrative questions should be sent to through the website www.ginalivy.com or email weightloss@ginalivy.com as they have the resources to help

- Any App specific questions can be directed to techsupport@ginalivy.com

9. **Is there a new PDF Booklet for the Winter 2023 Group?**

- Yes! There will be a new updated version of the PDF Booklet available for the Winter Group

- You can still use the Fall version and then print off any new info from the file section in the Facebook Group.

10. **What if I have feedback about the program I would like to share?**

- We want to hear from you, so please fill out the Survey posted in the group and share your thoughts.

11. **How do I find you in between groups?**

- You can follow Gina over on her social media pages

- Facebook: https://www.facebook.com/ginalivy

- Instagram: https://instagram.com/ginalivy?utm_medium=copy_link

- And if you have reached your weight loss goals, be sure to check out our Weight Loss by Gina: Maintenance and Mindfulness Group on FB! There you can find more information on maintenance, leveling up your life and can receive the same support that you have had during your weight loss journey. Register on www.ginalivy.com/shop.

12. **Will I still be able to listen to the podcasts between groups?**

- Yes, the Weigh In with Gina podcast will be available at any time on all podcast platforms and Gina will also be adding new episodes in between groups.

WLBG RECIPE GUIDE

This section includes just some of the easy and delicious recipe ideas you can make while doing the Program. There will be more recipes and meal ideas posted within the Group.

BREAKFAST RECIPES

BAKED AVOCADOS WITH EGGS, CHORIZO, AND A SIDE OF GUAC

Servings: 2

Prep time: 10 min

Cooking time: 20 min

INGREDIENTS:

- 1 large avocado
- 2 eggs
- 1/2 chorizo sausage
- 1/2 medium tomato
- 1 green onion
- 1/4 lime juiced
- 2 tbsp chopped cilantro
- olive oil
- S&P
- olive oil
- chopped chives for garnish

DIRECTIONS:

13.   Preheat oven to 450F

14.   Remove sausage from the casing. Heat a frying pan over medium high. Add sausage and break it up into small bits using a wooden spatula. Cook until browned all around, 3-5 min. Set aside.

15.   Half the avocado lengthwise and remove the pit. Using a spoon, scoop out the flesh leaving about a 1/2 of the border around*. The hollow area should be large enough to fit an egg. Set the scooped out avocado flesh aside.

16.   Place the avocados into an ovenproof dish, cut side up** Break the eggs into the hollow area and top with cooked chorizo. Bake until the egg whites are set, about 15 min.

17.   While the avocado bakes, chop the tomato, spring onions, and cilantro. Combine the remaining avocado flesh, tomatoes, spring onions, cilantro, lime juice, and olive oil. Salt to taste and mix well. Set aside.

18.   Garnish the avocados with some chopped chives and serve with the guac on the side. Enjoy!

NOTES:

- Try to choose large avocados so the eggs easily fit in. Make the hollows shallow - the eggs will cook through more evenly.

- **If your avocado halves do not stay upright, before you add the eggs, make small nests using strips of tin foil. Roll and squish the foil into a tube and close the two ends together into a ring. Place the avocados in the middle for more stability. Alternatively, you can use small and shallow ovenproof bowls.

BREAKFAST LENTIL WRAPS WITH KALE, AVOCADO AND CHICKPEAS

Servings: 4

Prep time: 15 min + 6-12 hours for soaking the lentils

Cooking time: 30 min

INGREDIENTS:

- 1 cup red lentils
- 2 cups water
- 1 bunch of kale, chopped
- 1 cup canned chickpeas
- 1 avocado, halved and sliced
- 2 tbsp tahini
- 1 lemon
- 1 tbsp honey
- 1 garlic clove
- smoked paprika
- cumin
- sesame seeds
- olive oil
- S&P

DIRECTIONS:

1. Combine the rinsed lentils and water in a medium bowl or other container; loosely cover. Let soak at room temperature overnight.

2. Once soaked, add the entire contents of the bowl including water, and salt to a blender or food processor. Blend on high speed until completely smooth.

3. Over medium high, heat a splash of olive oil in a non-stick pan. Add about 1/4 of the batter into the center. Using a spoon spread the batter to make a circle. Cook until the surface of the tortilla appears dry, about 2-3 min. Flip and cook until nicely browned, about 1 minute. Repeat for the remaining batter.

4.   In a small bowl, combine chickpeas, a splash of olive oil, smoked paprika and cumin. S&P to taste. Mix well until the chickpeas are coated in spices all around. Heat a frying pan over high heat. Transfer the chickpeas and toast, shaking frequently until slightly crispy, 4-6 min. Remove from the pan and set aside.

5.   Splash some olive oil into the pan. Add chopped kale and juice of 1/2 lemon. Saute until bright green and reduced in half, about 2-3 min. Remove from heat and set aside.

6.   Make the sauce: in a small bowl or a mason jar combine tahini, minced garlic, lemon juice and honey. Mix well. Thin with ice cold water as needed, set aside.

7.   Assemble the wraps by layering sauteed kale, chickpeas, and avocado on top of lentil tortillas. Drizzle with tahini sauce and sesame seeds and enjoy!

NOTES:

Red lentil tortillas are a fantastic high protein, plant-based alternative. They are very pliable and are perfect for wraps, tacos, and roll-ups. The tortillas keep well in the fridge for up to a week and are great to make ahead.

GREEN OMELETTE WITH ASPARAGUS, ZUCCHINI AND SCALLIONS

Servings: 1

Prep time: 5 min

Cooking time: 15 min

INGREDIENTS:

- 2 eggs
- 3-4 asparagus stems
- 1/2 zucchini
- 1 spring onion
- 1/4 lemon juiced
- 1 tbsp of feta crumble
- 1 tbsp butter
- microgreens for serving
- balsamic reduction
- S&P

DIRECTIONS:

1. Snap off the woody asparagus ends and quarter the stems. Julienne the zucchini and slice the spring onions finely.

2. In a small nonstick pan, heat 1/2 tbsp of the butter over medium high. When it starts to bubble, add spring onions and sauté for 1-2 min. Add asparagus to the pan and squeeze the lemon juice all over. Saute for another 2-3 minutes, stirring occasionally. Add julienned zucchinis. Salt & pepper to taste. Mix well and set aside.

3. Crack 2 eggs into a small bowl, season with S&P. Using a fork, whisk the eggs until smooth.

4. In a small nonstick pan, heat the rest of the butter over medium high. Add the whisked eggs. Cook until the eggs settle on top, about 1-2 minutes.

5. Transfer the omelette onto a serving plate. Add the cooked veggies on one side. Spread the feta crumble on top. Fold the other half over and drizzle some balsamic over. Serve with microgreens of your choice on a side and enjoy!

NOTES:

Asparagus is a fantastic source of nutrients including fibre, folate and vitamins A, C and K. Its peak season is spring when it's most tender and vibrant! Substitute balsamic for a hot sauce (Sriracha works great) for some heat if desired.

WLBG SPECIAL BLEND CEREAL

Looking for a high protein breakfast to start your day off right that doesn't involve eggs, dairy or gluten? Here's the recipe you've been waiting for!

Prep & Cook time: 20 minutes

Servings: 32

INGREDIENTS

TOASTED QUINOA

- 1 cup quinoa, rinsed well and drained
- 4 cups water
- 1 tbsp olive, avocado, coconut, or grapeseed oil
- 1/2 tsp salt

WLBG SPECIAL BLEND CEREAL

- 1 cup toasted quinoa
- 1 cup chia seeds
- 1 cup raw buckwheat, whole kernels, or groats
- 1 cup hemp hearts/seeds

SUGGESTED TOPPINGS

- Nuts, seeds, and extra hemp hearts
- Coconut, almond, soy milk, or any milk or cream you like
- Unsweetened toasted coconut
- Yogurt
- Nut butter
- Any type of fruit

DIRECTIONS

FOR THE TOASTED QUINOA

1. Rinse quinoa in a mesh sieve over cold running water for about 2 minutes. Let drain.
2. Bring 4 cups of water to a boil and add quinoa. Turn down to a simmer and cook for 10 minutes. Drain well.
3. Turn the oven broiler to high and position a rack in the top third of the oven.

4. Put well drained quinoa back in the pot and mix in olive oil and salt. Spread thinly and evenly on a baking sheet.

5. Broil for 8-10 minutes (times may vary depending on your oven). Watch it carefully and stir halfway through. You will hear it pop and it will start to toast. Keep a very close eye in the last half of broiling. There should be no moisture left so if necessary lower the oven rack and toast a little longer until it is dry and crispy. For extra insurance, turn off the oven and let the quinoa cool down in the oven.

6. When done, let cool completely on the tray. It must be cooled completely before mixing with the other ingredients.

7. Store any extra toasted quinoa in an airtight container in the fridge and use it to top breakfast cereals, yogurt, salads, grilled vegetables etc.

WLBG SPECIAL BLEND CEREAL

1. Mix together all 4 ingredients and keep in an airtight container in the fridge.

2. To make cereal, add 1/4 cup of boiling water to 2 tbsp cereal mix (use more or less water for a thinner or thicker texture). Let stand, covered with a plate, for 3-5 mins or until desired softness is reached. Serve topped with any combination of the suggested toppings above or create your own!

NOTES:

STORAGE: Store in an airtight container in the fridge for up to 1 month.

Extra toasted quinoa is delicious on top of yogurt, other cereals, salads, grilled vegetables, popcorn etc. You will soon be addicted!

LUNCH RECIPES

GARLIC SHRIMP ZOODLES WITH GREEN GODDESS DRESSING

Servings: 2

Prep time: 15 min

Cooking time: 10 min

INGREDIENTS:

- 3 zucchinis
- 20 large shrimp, deveined
- 3 garlic cloves
- 1/2 bunch cilantro
- 1/2 bunch parsley
- 1 shallot
- 1/2 avocado
- 2 tbsp Greek Yogurt
- 1 tbsp lemon juice
- 1 tbsp butter
- olive oil
- S&P
- sesame seeds and chili flakes for garnish

DIRECTIONS:

1. Trim and spiralize the zucchini*

2. In a small bowl, combine deveined shrimp, minced garlic and a splash of olive oil. Salt slightly, mix well and set aside.

3. In a blender or a food processor, combine parley, cilantro, avocado, shallot, Greek Yogurt and lemon juice.** Salt to taste and process until smooth.

4. In a large frying pan, over medium high, heat the butter until it starts to bubble. Add shrimp, cook stirring often, until it turns pink, 2-3 min.

5. Add the zucchini noodles. Toss the noodles with tongs and cook until "al dente" — they should be wilted, but still have a crunch, 4-5 min.

6. Serve the zoodles with a drizzle with the green sauce. Sprinkle it with sesame seeds and chili flakes. Enjoy!

NOTES:

- *Vegetable spiralizer is a fantastic tool to have in a kitchen, however, it is not the only way to make zoodles. You can use a julienne vegetable peeler or a mandolin, as well as a standard vegetable peeler to make wide zoodles or ribbons.

- **You can use any fresh herbs for your green goddess sauce! Not a big fan of cilantro? No problem! Swap for chives, dill, tarragon, spinach... If you enjoy some heat, throw in a Jalapeno or a chili pepper. This sauce keeps well in the fridge for a few days and is great for salads or as a dip.

SPRING BUDDHA BOWL WITH ROASTED BEETS AND TAHINI SAUCE

Servings: 3

Prep time: 15 min

Cooking time: 30 min

INGREDIENTS:

- 1 cup quinoa
- 2-3 small beets
- 2-3 small golden beets
- 2-4 radishes sliced
- 3 cups of microgreens or spring mix greens
- 1/4 cup feta crumble
- 2 tbsp tahini
- 1/2 lemon juiced
- 1 tbsp honey
- 1 garlic clove
- olive oil
- S&P

DIRECTIONS:

1. Preheat oven to 400F

2. Peel and quarter the beets.

3. Add the beets to a large bowl, sprinkle with olive oil and salt to taste. Mix well.

4. Spread the beets evenly on a sheet pan. Roast them until soft on the inside and golden on the outside, about 20-25 min.

5. While the beets roast, cook quinoa according to the packaging.

6. Make the dressing: In a small bowl or a mason jar, combine tahini, minced garlic, lemon juice and honey. Mix well. Thin with ice cold water as needed, set aside.

7. Assemble the bowl: Add about 1/2 cup of cooked quinoa, a handful of roasted beets, micro-greens, and radishes. Sprinkle with crumbled feta. Drizzle the tahini sauce all over and enjoy!

NOTES:

- Early spring beets will usually come with earthy-flavored green tops. Don't throw them away - they taste fantastic when sauteed with some butter, garlic and lemon juice.

- Running quinoa under cold water for a few minutes will help to get rid of any bitterness.

- When thinning tahini sauce, make sure to use ice cold water. Hot water will give tahini chunky texture.

ZA'ATAR CHICKEN WITH SPAGHETTI SQUASH AND BURST TOMATOES

Servings: 3

Prep time: 10 min

Cooking time: 45 min

INGREDIENTS:

- 1 spaghetti squash
- 2 chicken breasts
- 1 cup grape tomatoes
- 2 shallots
- 1/2 lemon juiced
- 1/2 cup of mini bocconcini
- 1 tsp za'atar spice
- basil for garnish
- olive oil
- S&P

DIRECTIONS:

1. Preheat oven to 400F

2. Slice the spaghetti squash in half lengthwise and scoop out the seeds. Drizzle the inside of the squash with olive oil and sprinkle it with salt and pepper. Place the spaghetti squash cut side down on an ovenproof dish. Use a fork to poke holes all around. Roast for 30 to 40 minutes or until lightly browned on the outside.

3. In a bowl, combine chicken with za'atar and lemon juice. Drizzle with olive oil. Mix well until the spices cover the chicken all around.

4. Over high, heat a splash of olive oil on an ovenproof skillet. Sear the chicken until golden brown, about 1 min per side. Add tomatoes and shallots to the skillet and salt to taste. Transfer to the oven alongside with the spaghetti squash and roast until the internal temperature of the chicken is 165°F/75°C, about 20-25 min. Remove from the oven and let it rest for a few minutes, then slice.

5. Once the spaghetti squash is done, remove from the oven and flip it so the cut side is facing up. When it is cool to touch, use a fork to scrape and fluff the strands from the sides of the squash.

6. Serve the squash with the chicken and burst tomatoes. Add halved bocconcini on top, and sprinkle with some chopped basil. Enjoy!

NOTES:

Za'atar Spice is a blend of savory dried herbs like oregano, marjoram or thyme, and toasted earthy spices like cumin and coriander, with sesame seeds, salt and sumac. You can purchase premade spice mix in the grocery store or make up a blend on your own!

Spaghetti Squash can be tricky to halve. If you find it tough to get the knife in, start by making several large slits through the skin with the tip of a sharp knife. This helps the air release as your squash heats up (so your squash doesn't explode when you microwave it). Next, microwave the squash on high for approximately 2-3 minutes to soften the skin, which makes it easier to cut.

DINNER RECIPES

PAN SEARED TROUT WITH WALNUT DILL PESTO

Servings: 2

Prep time: 10 min

Cooking time: 5 min

INGREDIENTS:

- 1 large trout fillet
- 1 small bunch of dill
- 1/2 cup of nuts (pecans or walnuts)
- 4 cups of mixed greens
- 1/2 cup of shredded carrots
- olive oil
- white wine vinegar
- smoked paprika
- cayenne
- turmeric
- garlic powder
- S&P

DIRECTIONS:

1. Season the trout with salt, paprika, cayenne, turmeric and garlic powder. Add a splash of olive oil and completely coat the fillet in seasoning.

2. In a pan, heat a splash of olive oil, over medium high heat.

3. When the oil starts to smoke, place the trout skin side down. Sear for about 1-2 min per side, then remove from heat and set aside.

4. Chop the dill and nuts roughly. In a small bowl combine dill, nuts, olive oil and a splash of white wine vinegar. Mix well.

5. On a large plate or in a bowl, combine 2 cups of mixed greens and 1/4 cup of shredded carrots.

6. Place the trout over the salad and drizzle the pesto all over the fish. Enjoy!

NOTES:

Trout is a fantastic alternative to salmon that is affordable and ultimately equal in nutritional value. You can sub the salad base with arugula, spinach, or any other greens of your choice.

CORIANDER CRUSTED PORK CHOP WITH BEET TURNIP PUREE

Servings: 2

Prep time: 10 min

Cooking time: 50 min

INGREDIENTS:

- 2 pork chops, bone in
- 2 medium turnip
- 1 medium beet
- 1 cup grated parmesan
- 1 cup microgreens
- 2 tbsp chopped thyme
- 2 tbsp coriander seed
- 2 tbsp butter
- S&P
- Olive oil

DIRECTIONS:

1. Preheat oven to 400F

2. Peel and quarter beets and turnips. In a medium pot, place the turnips and beets and cover with cold water. Bring to a boil and reduce to medium heat. Simmer until fork tender, about 30-40 min

3. While the beets and turnips cook, take the mortar and pestle and crush the coriander seeds. Chop the thyme finely. Combine the coriander and thyme and mix well

4. Salt and pepper the pork chops to taste. Press the chops into the herb mixture, coating the meat all around.

5. Heat the olive oil in an ovenproof skillet over medium heat. Sear the pork until nicely browned all around, about 2 minutes per side. Transfer the skillet into the oven and roast until the internal temperature reaches 160F, about 10 min.

6. While the pork is in the oven, drain the cooked beets and turnips and cool slightly. Reserve about 1/2 cup of the water. Transfer the beets and potatoes into the food processor adding the butter and parmesan. S&P to taste. Process until smooth adding the beet turnip water as needed.

7. Plate the puree and place the pork chop on top, Garnish with microgreens and shaved parmesan. Enjoy!

FETA & SPINACH STUFFED CHICKEN WITH ROASTED BALSAMIC TOMATOES

Servings: 3

Prep time: 10 min

Cooking time: 30 min

INGREDIENTS:

- 6 chicken thighs (skin & bone off)
- 6oz block of feta
- 2 cups spinach
- 3-4 vines of grape tomatoes
- 2 medium shallots, quartered
- balsamic vinegar reduction
- olive oil
- pepper

DIRECTIONS:

1. Preheat oven to 400F

2. Peel and quarter the shallots, chop up the spinach and slice the feta block into slices about 2/4 inches thick.

3. Stuff the chicken by unfolding the thigh, placing one slice of feta, and topping with about 1-2 tbsp of chopped spinach. Fold the thigh over and secure with a wooden toothpick so it holds together. Repeat for all of the thighs.

4. Place the stuffed thighs into an ovenproof dish. Place the tomato vines and quartered shallots around the chicken.

5. Brush the chicken and tomatoes with olive oil and season lightly with pepper. Sprinkle with balsamic vinegar reduction.

6. Place in the oven and bake until the chicken is cooked, and some edges are a little brown, about 30 min.

7. Let the chicken cool for a few minutes, then serve on the plate and pour over the juice from the skillet. Enjoy!

NOTES:

- Swap the chicken thighs to breast if desired. Depending on the size, double the stuffing for the breast vs thighs.

- Feta cheese will give the chicken a lot of salty flavor, so the recipe doesn't call for any additional salt.

- This recipe is great to make ahead or for meal prep. Feel free to add any other veggies to the skillet, such as peppers or diced zucchinis.

SCIENCE GUIDE

This section contains more in-depth information and science behind The Livy Method. It is not mandatory reading, but is for those of you who want to dive deeper into the science behind the Program. This is an evolving section and we will continue to add more resources and articles in the future.

THE SET-POINT THEORY

Welcome to the science posts which are designed to help provide some foundational information and understanding of how our bodies function, and how implementing The Livy Method optimises our health, wellness, and mindfulness, by providing an environment where our bodies no longer feel the need to store fat!

We will begin this journey by discussing the Set-Point Theory and other theories of weight loss that might help us explain how The Livy Method works, and why it is different from other diets that involve deprivation and calorie restriction. Let's dive into this!!

THE HISTORY OF DIETING

It may be assumed by some that obesity and dieting is a concern of more recent times. But upon delving deeper into this subject matter, it is interesting to note that the concept of dieting or "slimming" has been around for centuries. The Ancient Greeks and Romans already understood that food and physical exercise influence our health and our weight. The Greek word 'diatia' (from which the word 'diet' is derived) referred to a whole way of living focused on self-control and eating in moderation. Interestingly, the first best selling diet book was written in 1474 by the Italian humanist Bartolomeo Sacchi, aka Il Platina. Advances in printing techniques meant that his *De honesta voluptate e valetudine* was read throughout Europe, and high society became obsessed with his recommendations regarding the relationship between gastronomic pleasure (voluptate) and health (valetudine).

Throughout the ages, humans have been in pursuit of fitting the criteria of what was deemed beautiful or accepted by the society they lived in. For many cultures, and in different eras, being thin has been one of the main measures of beauty. Although this can be problematic for so many different reasons, there is a distinction that needs to be made between weight loss and overall health, as opposed to seeking it to fit societal norms.

Hippocrates, who is considered the founder of medicine born in 460 BC, was one of the first to document the association between weight and health with the statement, "Those by nature overweight, die earlier than the slim". Today we know that obesity-related conditions which include heart disease, stroke, type 2 diabetes, and certain types of cancer, are among the leading causes of preventable, premature death.

Many health issues can be preventable by some degree of weight loss. From the ancient Greeks to current day, many of us have had some struggle with our weight and have likely tried many different diets in order to lose and gain the same weight, many times. There needs to be options for those that are looking to lose weight in a healthy, sustainable way! This is why The Livy Method is designed with overall health in mind, which includes not only a physical focus, but includes the mental, emotional, and for some even their spiritual health. Let's talk more about the impact of obesity on health and why one might consider trying to lose weight.

WHAT ARE SOME HEALTH RISKS OF OVERWEIGHT AND OBESITY?

TYPE 2 DIABETES

Type 2 diabetes is a disease that occurs when your blood glucose (or blood sugar), is too high. Your body cannot make enough insulin (a hormone that helps control the amount of glucose or sugar in your blood), or does not properly use the insulin it makes. Diabetes Canada (2022) reports that Type 2 diabetes is caused by several different risk factors and accounts for 90% of diabetes cases in Canada! According to the NIDDK (National Institute of Diabetes and Digestive and Kidney Diseases, 2018) About 8 out of 10 people with type 2 diabetes are overweight or have obesity. Over time, high blood glucose can lead to issues such as heart disease, stroke, kidney disease, eye problems, nerve damage, and other health problems.

If you are at risk for type 2 diabetes, losing 5 to 7 percent of your body weight and participating in regular physical activity may prevent or delay the onset of type 2 diabetes. (NIDDK, 2018) There is more discussion regarding the precursor to diabetes in the science post Hormones Important to Weight Loss & Digestion Part 1-Insulin, so check it out for more details!

HIGH BLOOD PRESSURE

High blood pressure, also called hypertension, is a condition in which blood flows through your blood vessels with a force greater than normal. High blood pressure can strain your heart, damage blood vessels, and increase your risk of heart attack, stroke, kidney disease, and even death. Being overweight and obese may raise your risk for high blood pressure.

HEART DISEASE

Heart disease is a general term used to describe several problems that may affect your heart, such as those that have suffered a heart attack, heart failure, angina, an abnormal heart rhythm (also called arrhythmia), or sudden cardiac death.

High blood pressure, abnormal levels of blood fats (blood lipids), and high blood glucose levels may increase your risk for heart disease. Blood lipids include HDL cholesterol, LDL cholesterol, and triglycerides. See the science post on The Science of Fat and Fat Loss for a more detailed description of fats in the body!

According to the NIDDK (2018, February) losing 5 to 10 percent of your weight may lower your risk factors for developing heart disease. Weight loss may improve blood pressure, cholesterol levels, and blood flow in the body.

STROKE

Stroke is a condition in which a blockage or the bursting of a blood vessel in your brain or neck, prevents blood flow from getting to the brain. A stroke can damage brain tissue, affecting your ability to speak or move parts of your body. According to the NIDDK (2018, February) High blood pressure is the leading cause of strokes. As discussed above, even a 5-10% reduction in weight can improve blood pressure, which could decrease the risk of stroke.

SLEEP APNEA

Sleep apnea is a sleep disorder in which your breathing can be affected while sleeping. Sleep apnea may present as irregular breathing patterns, or where your breathing stops (apnea) altogether for short periods of time. According to Jonathan Jun, M.D., (Johns Hopkins Medicine, 2022) a pulmonary and sleep medicine specialist at the Johns Hopkins Sleep Disorders Centre, sleep apnea happens when upper airway muscles relax during sleep and pinch off the airway, which prevents you from getting enough air. Your breathing may pause for 10 seconds or more at a time, until your reflexes kick in and you start breathing again. This results in decreased oxygen to the body and vital organs. If left untreated, sleep apnea may raise your risk of other health problems, such as type 2 diabetes and heart disease.

Jun discusses that sleep apnea occurs in about 3 percent of normal weight individuals but affects over 20 percent of people with obesity. In general, sleep apnea affects men more than women. However, sleep apnea rates increase sharply in women after menopause.

There are two kinds of sleep apnea: obstructive sleep apnea and central sleep apnea. Obstructive sleep apnea happens when air can't flow into or out of the nose or mouth, although you're trying to breathe. Central sleep apnea happens when the brain fails to send the right signals to your muscles to make you start breathing. (This type is less common.)

Symptoms of sleep apnea can manifest in the following ways:

- Pauses in breathing, or snoring (both of which may be noticed by a partner). Snoring is the sound caused by the vibration created by airway resistance. Snoring can be caused by the relaxing of the airway as described above, so snoring as an isolated symptom does not mean you have sleep apnea. Also, you may have sleep apnea, without much snoring, so if you suspect sleep apnea may be an issue for you, further testing may be necessary.

- Unexplained fatigue and mood swings due to the prevention of settling into the deep stages of restorative sleep. This may lead to increased tiredness and grogginess resulting in decreased productivity, impacting focus and attention. This can also result in dire consequences if one participates in activities that require attention such as driving a car, or operating machinery.

- Waking up with a dry mouth, as those with sleep apnea tend to breathe with their mouths wide open. This leads to the saliva in their mouths drying out.

- Headaches upon waking, which may be caused by low circulating blood oxygen or high carbon dioxide levels during sleep due to inadequate breathing.

- Although one can have sleep apnea independent of being overweight, evidence suggests a link between sleep apnea and diabetes, as sleep apnea can cause an increase in blood sugar levels.

- For those who are overweight or obese, weight loss is key for treating or avoiding sleep apnea.

People who accumulate fat in the neck, tongue and upper belly are especially vulnerable to getting sleep apnea. This weight reduces the diameter of the throat and pushes against the lungs, contributing to airway collapse during sleep.

METABOLIC SYNDROME

Metabolic syndrome is a group of conditions that put you at risk for heart disease, diabetes, and stroke, and is related to obesity. These conditions include high blood pressure, high blood glucose levels (pre-diabetes and type 2 diabetes), high triglyceride levels in your blood, low levels of HDL cholesterol (the "good" cholesterol) in your blood, and the accumulation of fat around the abdomen.

As discussed in the science post Hormones Important to Weight Loss & Digestion Part 1-Insulin, experts believe obesity, especially too much fat in the abdomen and around the organs (called visceral fat) is a main cause of insulin resistance. Insulin resistance may lead to pre-diabetes and type 2 diabetes. A lack of physical activity may also be a factor.

Insulin resistance is when cells in your muscles, fat, and liver don't respond well to insulin and are not able to easily take up glucose from your blood. As a result, your pancreas increases the production of insulin to help glucose enter your cells, a condition called **hyperinsulinemia**. However, as long as your pancreas can produce enough insulin to overcome your cells' weak response to insulin, your blood glucose levels should stay in the healthy range.

Having a waist measurement of 40 inches or more for men and 35 inches or more for women is linked to insulin resistance. This is true even if your body mass index (BMI) falls within the normal range. However, research has shown that Asian Americans may have an increased risk for insulin resistance even without a high BMI. (The discussion of BMI is used in reference to this study, although the concept of BMI is problematic as a measure of obesity).

Studies have also shown that belly fat produces hormones and other substances that can contribute to chronic, or long-lasting, inflammation in the body. Inflammation may play a role in insulin resistance, type 2 diabetes, and cardiovascular disease. Since excess weight may lead to insulin resistance, this also is a contributing factor in the development of fatty liver disease.

FATTY LIVER DISEASES

Fatty liver diseases are conditions in which fat accumulates in the liver that can, over time, affect liver function and cause liver injury. Fatty liver diseases include non-alcoholic fatty liver disease (NAFLD) and non-alcoholic steatohepatitis (NASH). Fatty liver diseases may lead to severe liver damage, cirrhosis (late-stage scarring or fibrosis of the liver), or even liver failure.

People who drink too much alcohol may also have fat in their liver, but that condition is different from fatty liver disease.

There are 2 types of fatty liver disease. If you just have fat accumulation but no damage to your liver, the disease is called non-alcoholic fatty liver disease (NAFLD). If you have fat accumulation in your liver plus signs of inflammation and liver cell damage, the disease is called non-alcoholic steatohepatitis (NASH). According to Johns Hopkins Medicine, about 10% to 20% of Americans have NAFLD and about 2% to 5% have NASH.

Fatty liver disease is sometimes called a silent liver disease because it can occur without causing any symptoms. Most people with NAFLD live with fat in their liver without ever developing liver damage, whereas a few people develop NASH. Symptoms of Nash may take years to develop, and can potentially cause cirrhosis.

Symptoms from NASH may include severe tiredness, weakness, weight loss, yellowing of the skin or eyes (jaundice), spider like blood vessels on the skin, and long-lasting itching.

NASH that turns into cirrhosis could cause symptoms like fluid retention, internal bleeding, muscle wasting, and confusion. People with cirrhosis over time may develop liver failure and need a liver transplant.

The exact cause of fatty liver disease is unknown, but it is thought that obesity is the most common cause. Obesity in the U.S. has doubled in the last decade, and health care providers are seeing a steady rise in fatty liver disease. Although children and young adults can get fatty liver disease, it is most common in middle age.

Risk factors include:

- Being overweight
- Having high blood fat levels, either triglycerides or LDL ("bad") cholesterol
- Having diabetes or prediabetes
- Having high blood pressure

Fatty liver disease can happen without causing any symptoms. It's usually diagnosed when you have routine blood tests to check your liver. Your health care provider may suspect fatty liver disease with abnormal test results, especially if you are obese.

If you have NAFLD without any other medical problems, making some lifestyle changes can control or reverse the fat buildup in your liver. However, you will want to work alongside your healthcare provider (HCP) as you work through this process.

This may include:

- Losing weight (losing just 3-5% of your weight can decrease the amount of fat in your liver)
- exercise
- Lowering your cholesterol and triglycerides

- Controlling your diabetes
- Avoiding alcohol
- Check out the science post on detox! It has many great suggestions on how to support your liver.

OSTEOARTHRITIS

Osteoarthritis is a common, long-lasting health problem that causes pain, swelling, and reduced motion in your joints. Being overweight or having obesity may raise your risk of getting osteoarthritis by putting extra pressure on your joints and cartilage.

According to the Arthritis Foundation in the US (2022, May), maintaining a healthy weight can ease the pain of arthritis and help your medicines work better. The CDC also reports that 31% of obese Americans have doctor-diagnosed arthritis.

Here are some reasons that the Arthritis Foundation suggest why reaching and maintaining a healthy weight can help ease your arthritis:

REDUCE PRESSURE ON YOUR JOINTS

A key study published in Arthritis & Rheumatism of overweight and obese adults with knee osteo-arthritis (OA) found that **losing one pound of weight resulted in four pounds of pressure being removed from the knees**. In other words, losing just 10 pounds would relieve 40 pounds of pressure from your knees! This is so impactful when you really think about what weight loss means for the joints in your body. Even a small amount of weight loss can make a big difference on your joints.

EASE PAIN

Multiple studies show that losing weight results in arthritis pain relief. A 2018 study published in Arthritis Care and Research went further to find that losing more weight – to an extent -- results in more pain relief. The study of overweight and obese older adults with pain from knee OA, found that greater weight loss resulted in better outcomes than losing a smaller amount of weight. Losing 10–20 percent of starting body weight improved pain, function, and quality of life better than losing just five percent of body weight.

REDUCE INFLAMMATION

The tissue fat itself is an active tissue that creates and releases pro-inflammatory chemicals. By reducing fat stores in the body, your body's overall inflammation will go down. An article published in 2018 explained that obesity can activate and sustain body-wide low-grade inflammation. This inflamma-tion can amplify and aggravate autoimmune disorders, such as rheumatoid arthritis, psoriatic arthritis, lupus and their associated comorbidities (like heart disease).

REDUCE DISEASE ACTIVITY

Losing weight can reduce the overall severity of your arthritis. A 2018 study reviewed the records of

171 RA (rheumatoid arthritis) patients and found that overweight or obese people who lost at least 5 kg (10.2 pounds) were three times as likely to have improved disease activity compared to those who did not lose weight. A smaller 2019 study found that short-term weight loss in obese people with psoriatic arthritis (PsA) yielded "significant positive effects" on disease activity in joints, entheses (an enthesis is the site of attachment of tendon, ligament, fascia, or capsule to bone), and skin.

IMPROVE CHANCE OF REMISSION.

Several studies have shown that being obese reduces your chance of achieving minimal disease activity or remission if you have RA or PsA. A 2017 review article analyzed data from more than 3,000 people with RA and found that obese patients had lower odds of achieving and sustaining remission compared with non-obese people. A 2018 article analysed several studies totaling more than 3,800 patient records. The authors found that obesity "hampered the effects of anti-TNF agents" and showed that the odds of reaching a good response or achieving remission were lower in obese than non-obese patients taking anti-TNF medications. TNF or tumour necrosis factor is a protein that is produced by the body that causes inflammation. In healthy individuals TNF is blocked naturally, but is elevated in the blood of those with rheumatic conditions (rheumatology.org, 2022). These medications help inhibit TNF in order to reduce inflammation.

LOWER URIC ACID LEVELS AND CHANCE OF GOUT ATTACK.

Gout is a common form of inflammatory arthritis that is very painful. It usually affects one joint at a time (often the big toe joint). There are times when symptoms get worse, known as flares, and times when there are no symptoms, known as remission. Repeated bouts of gout can lead to gouty arthritis, a worsening form of arthritis. Gout is caused by a condition known as hyperuricemia, where there is too much uric acid in the body. The body makes uric acid when it breaks down purines, which are found in your body and the foods you eat. When there is too much uric acid in the body, uric acid crystals (monosodium urate) can build up in joints, fluids, and tissues within the body. Hyperuricemia does not always cause gout, and hyperuricemia without gout symptoms does not necessarily need to be treated.

A 2017 analysis of 10 studies found that weight loss was beneficial for obese or overweight people with gout. Overall, people who lost weight had lower serum uric acid levels and fewer gout attacks.

The following make it more likely that you will develop hyperuricemia, which can cause gout:

- Being male

- Being obese

- Having certain health conditions, including: Congestive heart failure, hypertension (high blood pressure), insulin resistance, metabolic syndrome, diabetes, poor kidney function

- Using certain medications, such as diuretics (water pills).

- Drinking alcohol. The risk of gout is greater as alcohol intake goes up.

- Eating or drinking food and drinks high in fructose (a type of sugar).

- Having a diet high in purines, which the body breaks down into uric acid. Purine-rich foods include red meat, organ meat, and some kinds of seafood, such as anchovies, sardines, mussels, scallops, trout, and tuna.

SLOWS CARTILAGE DEGENERATION IN OSTEOARTHRITIS

A 2017 study assessed magnetic resonance images (MRIs) of osteoarthritic knees in 640 overweight or obese people. Participants who lost weight over 4 years showed significantly lower cartilage deterioration. The more weight lost, the lower the rate of disease progression.

GALLBLADDER DISEASES

According to the NIDDK (2017, November) being overweight or having obesity may make you more likely to develop gallstones, especially if you are a woman. Researchers have found that people who have obesity may have higher levels of cholesterol in their bile, which can cause gallstones.

People who have obesity may also have large gallbladders that do not work well. Some studies have shown that people who carry large amounts of fat around their waist may be more likely to develop gallstones than those who carry fat around their hips and thighs.

Losing weight very quickly may raise your chances of forming gallstones. When you don't eat for a long period of time (fasting) or you lose weight too quickly, your liver releases extra cholesterol into the bile. Fast weight loss (associated with very low-calorie diets) can also prevent the gallbladder from emptying properly. Weight-loss surgery may lead to fast weight loss and higher risk of gallstones.

Weight cycling, or losing and regaining weight repeatedly, may also lead to gallstones. The more weight you lose and regain during a cycle, the greater your chances of developing gallstones.

Your chances of developing gallstones may depend on the type of weight-loss treatment you choose. A program like The Livy Method that supports the body, and helps people lose weight in a healthy way, is a good option when trying to lose weight.

Regular physical activity, which will improve your overall health, may also lower your chances of developing gallstones. To improve health or prevent weight gain, aim for at least 150 minutes a week of moderate-intensity physical activity, like brisk walking or fast dancing. Also, muscle-strengthening activity, like lifting weights or using your own body weight (callisthenics) can be beneficial. The science post Issues of Digestion, discusses the gallbladder in further detail and options for those that have had it removed. Check it out for further details!

SOME CANCERS

Cancer is a collection of related diseases. In all types of cancer, some of the body's cells begin to divide without stopping and spread into surrounding tissues. Overweight and obesity may raise your risk of developing certain types of cancers.

KIDNEY DISEASE

Kidney disease is a generic term that means there is damage to the kidneys and they are not able filter blood of wastes like they should. This is a vital process for the body. Obesity raises the risk of diabetes and high blood pressure, the most common causes of kidney disease. Even if you do not have diabetes or high blood pressure, obesity itself may promote kidney disease and quicken its progression.

PREGNANCY PROBLEMS

Overweight and obesity raise the risk of health issues that may occur during pregnancy. Pregnant women who are overweight or obese may have a greater chance of:

- Developing gestational diabetes.
- Having pre-eclampsia, which presents initially as high blood pressure during pregnancy and can cause severe health problems for the mother and baby if left untreated.
- The need for a Caesarean section (C-section) which can come with increased risks, and a longer recovery after giving birth.

Overweight and obesity are also associated with mental health problems such as depression. People who deal with overweight and obesity may also experience the stigma of weight bias from others, including health care providers. This can lead to feelings of rejection, shame, or guilt, further worsening mental health.

THE RISE OF OBESITY IN THE WORLD

According to the World Health Organization (WHO), being overweight or obese is defined as having "abnormal or excessive fat accumulation that presents a risk to health". Although the BMI can be a problematic assessment of obesity, it is still widely used in order to categorise a person's weight. As per the WHO, a body mass index (BMI) over 25 is considered overweight, and over 30 is obese. A report from the global burden of disease describes that this issue has grown to epidemic proportions, with over 4 million people dying each year as a result of being overweight or obese in 2017.

The estimated annual medical costs related to obesity in the United States was nearly $173 billion in 2019. The medical costs for adults who were diagnosed with obesity were $1,861 higher than medical costs for people with a healthy weight.

In the US, the CDC discussed in their most recent report from 2017-2020, that the prevalence of obesity was 41.9%. They also report that from 1999 –2000 through 2017 –March 2020, that the prevalence of obesity had increased from 30.5% to 41.9% and the prevalence of severe obesity increased from 4.7% to 9.2% in this same time frame.

According to the Government of Canada, statistics gathered from the Canadian Risk Factor Atlas (CRFA) using pooled data from the Canadian Community Health Survey, 2015-2018 determined that:

- About 1 in 4 Canadian adults (26.6%) are currently living with obesity.

- Obesity rates in Canadian adults are higher in men compared to women (28.0% versus 24.7%).

In Canada, a health report released on October 20, 2021 from Statistics Canada, found that chronic diseases account for 89% of all deaths and more than $80 billion in annual health care costs. Adopting healthy lifestyle behaviours, such as healthy eating, has the potential to prevent 80% of type 2 diabetes and cardiovascular disease, 40% of cancers, and other chronic diseases. Despite healthy eating recommendations issued by Health Canada, eating habits continue to deteriorate, and overweight prevalence rates continue to increase!

Rates of those that are overweight and obese continue to grow in adults and children. From 1975 to 2016, the prevalence of overweight or obese children and adolescents aged 5–19 years increased more than four times from 4% to 18% globally.

The WHO describes obesity as one side of the double burden of malnutrition and states that today more people are obese than underweight in every region except sub-Saharan Africa and Asia. Once considered a problem only in high-income countries, being overweight and obese is now dramatically on the rise in low- and middle-income countries, particularly in urban settings. The vast majority of overweight or obese children live in developing countries, where the rate of increase has been more than 30% higher than that of developed countries. This can be attributed to the lower cost of calorie dense, but nutrient poor foods that are widely available all over the world. Decreased physical activity is also a factor.

Interestingly in Canada though, the rate of obesity is higher for adults living in rural areas compared with those living in urban areas, regardless if one identifies with being male or female. Living in an urban setting is defined as living in areas with a high-density concentration of population (i.e. areas with a population of at least 1,000 and a population density of at least 400 persons per km^2). Living in a rural setting is defined as all areas outside urban areas, or embedded in urban areas.

- In rural areas, about 1 in 3 Canadian adults are living with obesity (31.4%).

- In urban areas, about 1 in 4 Canadian adults are living with obesity (25.6%)

This means that there are on average 5.8 more cases of obesity per 100 adults living in rural areas compared with urban areas.* **Note: Not all provinces or Territories show higher rates of obesity in rural compared to urban areas.** Check out https://health-infobase.canada.ca/datalab/canadian-risk-factor-atlas-obesity-blog.html?=undefined&wbdisable=true for more details on the Canadian demographics!

OBESITY AFFECTS SOME GROUPS MORE THAN OTHERS

According to the CDC, in the US Non-Hispanic Black adults (49.9%) had the highest age-adjusted prevalence of obesity, followed by Hispanic adults (45.6%), non-Hispanic White adults (41.4%) and non-Hispanic Asian adults (16.1%). The prevalence of obesity was noted to be 39.8% among adults aged 20 to 39 years, 44.3% among adults aged 40 to 59 years, and 41.5% among adults aged 60 and older.

In the *Morbidity and Mortality Weekly Report (MMWR)* it is discussed that the association between obesity and income or educational level is complex and differs by sex and race/ethnicity. It was found that:

- In the US overall, men and women with college degrees had lower obesity prevalence compared with those with less education.

- This same obesity and education pattern occurred among non-Hispanic White, non-Hispanic Black, and Hispanic women, and non-Hispanic White men. However, the differences were not all statistically significant. Although the difference was not statistically significant among non-Hispanic Black men, obesity prevalence increased with increased education.

- No differences in obesity prevalence by education level were noted among non-Hispanic Asian women and men and Hispanic men.

SOCIO-ECONOMIC IMPACTS ON OBESITY

In the MMWR report, it was noted that the prevalence of obesity was lower in the lowest and highest income groups compared with the middle-income group. Researchers observed this same pattern among non-Hispanic White and Hispanic men. However, the prevalence of obesity was higher in the highest income group than in the lowest income group among non-Hispanic Black men. This can be attributed to how socio-economic and culture influence food choices, and lifestyle. In many cases those with more education, tend to have access to healthier food choices, and tend to be more active. Although interestingly in some cultures, greater affluence leads to more indulgent choices and activities leading to obesity (PRB, 2013).

Historically, urbanisation was considered one of the most important drivers of the rise in obesity in industrialised countries. However, in Canada, it has been more recently shown that the urbanisation of rural life has contributed to a larger increase in rural obesity.

This change in the geographic distribution of obesity can be partly explained by the growing economic and social disadvantage that rural communities experience compared to urban cities. In particular, rural communities experience lower education and income, lower availability of healthy and fresh foods at a reasonable cost, less access to public transportation, and lack of supportive environments to promote walkability, sports and recreational activities.

In Canada overall, adult obesity is more prevalent among disadvantaged population groups such as those unemployed or with lower household income and education levels.

Recent global trends show that the prevalence of obesity is rising faster among people living in rural areas than those living in urban areas. When looking at cities in Canada

- The lowest rates of adult obesity were observed in the largest urban census metropolitan areas.

- In general, obesity rates in adults tend to be higher in smaller cities.

- Although adult obesity rates in the territories are among the highest in Canada, there were no urban-rural disparities.

- In Canada overall, adult obesity is more prevalent among disadvantaged population groups such as those unemployed or with lower household income and education levels.

Having access and understanding this data on how obesity rates in rural and urban populations is changing, as well as the socio-economic and cultural demographics, may assist policy-makers and local communities to target policies, programs and services aiming to promote healthy weight appropriately. This is where implementing a program like The Livy Method, and access to healthy food and activity could incite real change!!!

THE LIVY METHOD

To understand weight loss better, it's important to understand the problem of obesity and the impact it is having on society. After looking at these statistics, one thing is very clear, the way we approach our health at a global level needs to change. A big part of this would be having access to real nutritious food, clean water and sanitation, housing, fresh air, and feeling physically and psychologically safe amongst many other things. The other factor is understanding how the issue of obesity impacts our health, along with our food and lifestyle choices.

As you can now see The Livy Method is VERY different from many of the diets and weight loss methods that are out there or you may have experienced. The diet and food industry are a profit driven industry, with a focus on sales and retaining consumers. At WLBG, some of the core missions are to help people change their lives by improving their health, their relationship with food, the quality of food that they eat and the way in which they eat it, and to promote people prioritising and showing up for themselves. This all ultimately leads to weight loss.

However, many question, how does this program work? How can I be losing weight when I am eating more than I ever have? I have always been taught to count macros and/or calories!

These are all great questions and points, so let's dive into this deeper!

THE SET POINT THEORY

According to Healthline (2020, March), set point theory in relation to weight loss states that we have a pre-set weight baseline that is hardwired in our DNA, and specific for our individual bodies. Based on this theory, our weight and how much it changes from that set point might be limited. The theory states that some of us have higher weight set points than others and our bodies fight to stay within these ranges.

Recent studies point to body weight being affected by a combination of factors. Weight can be determined by inherited traits, the environment, and by hormonal, psychological, and genetic elements. Weight can also depend on energy expenditure compared to what kinds of foods and how much has been ingested.

The set point model relies on the concept of a genetic pre-set weight range that's controlled by biological and physiological signals in our bodies (NIDDK, 2011). The body has a regulatory system that keeps you at a steady-state level, or set point. You may have also heard this called homeostasis.

The hypothalamus, a small region of the brain located at the base of the brain, near the pituitary gland, is involved in the integration of signals directed to it from hormones like leptin (from adipose or fat cells), ghrelin (from the digestive system), insulin (the pancreas), along with many other hormones that regulate our hunger and satiety. Your metabolism also constantly adjusts up or down based on a variety of signals. The set point theory also suggests that your weight may go up or down temporarily but will ultimately return to its normal set range. The signalling system we have in place helps to maintain our weight.

The science post <u>Hormones Important to Weight Loss & Digestion Part 2-Hormones of Hunger and Satiety and Timing of Digestion</u>, takes a much deeper dive on how our hormones influence our hunger and satiety, and how The Livy Method helps to support these hormones, which can help influence weight loss and a drop in set point!

*Check out this video to see a detailed breakdown of the important role the hypothalamus plays in our body!

https://www.youtube.com/watch?v=xCXtcoUxJZc

This model is consistent with many of the biological aspects of energy balance, but struggles to explain the significance that environmental, economical and social influences play on obesity, food intake and physical activity. More on this later!

However, why does our weight climb beyond a few pounds if we have a set point?

Some researchers (Jung & Kim, 2013) believe that the reactive signal system stops working efficiently over time and leptin and insulin resistance develop, causing us to gain weight. Although not a human study, Dalvi et al, (2017) found that when mice were fed a mostly high fat diet, it led to inflammation of the hypothalamus. However, a different study in mice that same year, concluded that a diet high in both fat *and* sugar, caused inflammation of the hypothalamus (Gao et al., 2017). The thought is that foods that are high in fat and sugar, like many processed foods available today, lead to not only inflammation in the body, but also in the brain. Because the hypothalamus is so important in regulating, and interpreting the signals involved in hunger, satiety, and metabolism, inflammation can lead to a disruption in the pathway of these signals and even in how fat is stored. This can lead to weight gain.

It is also important to note that adequate sleep is also important to keep our hypothalamus healthy. The anterior region has an important role in regulating our circadian rhythm (which are physical and behavioural changes that occur on a daily cycle). An example of a circadian rhythm is being awake during the day and sleeping at nighttime which is influenced by the presence or absence of light (Seladi-Schulman, J., 2022, Jan 31). Adequate good quality sleep, which has been discussed in most of the science posts, has a great positive impact on many aspects of our weight and health.

Other influences also contribute to weight gain over time. According to the NIDDK (2018, February) weight gain can be influenced by: Family history and genes, race or ethnicity, age, sex, eating and physical activity habits, where you live, work, play, and worship, stress, lack of sleep, medical conditions and medications.

Gradually, according to set point theory, the normal body set point keeps adjusting upward over time if there is any disruption in our signalling system. Many factors influence this system and can lead to weight gain if the balance is interrupted. Factors include: lack of good sleep, poor digestion, lack of nutrition and vitamin/mineral deficiencies, increased stress, inadequate hydration, the development of insulin resistance, lack of movement/exercise, or any health/medical issues.

When we try to lose weight, our body fights to maintain the higher set point weight by slowing down our metabolism. This can ultimately limit weight loss. This is also when strategies such as eating less and/or exercising more begin to backfire, by feeding into that negative feed-back loop that further affects our hormones, stresses our body, and an even further lack of nutrition/vitamins/minerals, causing our bodies to hold onto our fat stores even more. This can also lead to mental and emotional duress as by implementing what we thought would help us lose the weight, actually sets us up for further weight gain and a sense of failure.

THE SETTLING POINT MODEL

However, there is a secondary theory for weight called the "settling point" model that is an enhancement to the set point theory. This concept suggests our weight is influenced by more than just physiological factors. How we navigate our food choices together with our biological traits and our energy balance affects weight shifts over time. This model can help us further understand obesity, especially in its rise, as it incorporates the influence of family/social dynamics of food, how the food itself has changed (food science and big business), environmental (chemicals/obesogens), socio-economic (having access to healthy food or alternatively living a more indulgent lifestyle) and the kind lifestyle you lead (active or inactive).

Overall, there are an abundance of different theories out there as well as groups researching obesity that have widely different views. However, what seems clear is the evidence that our weight is influenced by a complex set of internal and external signals — a combination of environmental and biological factors. The good news? The Livy Method helps us address all of these influences, including giving us the tools to do so!

CAN WE CHANGE OUR SET POINT WEIGHT? ACCORDING TO SET POINT THEORY, YES!

In order to reset our set point to a lower level, set point theory proponents recommend going slowly with weight loss goals. A gradual 10% step-down weight loss approach with persistent maintenance at each stage can help prepare the body to accept the new lower set point! This further corroborates why it is so important to allow our bodies to settle into its new weight and set point and embrace plateaus or stabilising periods as part of successful weight loss. This is also why it is important to allow adequate time for the body to adjust to maintenance by "consolidating your weight in maintenance" as Gina says. This is achieved by continuing with the plan for a few months upon achieving your goal, before reintroducing foods back into your life. Then it's about living your life, eating the foods that make you feel good, and doing so mindfully!

WHAT ABOUT CALORIES IN VS. CALORIES OUT?

According to set point theory, the reason typical diets don't work is that after a time, your body will fight reduced calorie intake by influencing your hunger hormones to leave you in a constant state of hunger and feelings of deprivation. It will then proceed to slow down your metabolism in an attempt to bring you back to your normal set point.

This can lead to binge eating and cycling through various diet programs like so many of us have experienced in the past. Set point theory believes your body and brain are in a struggle to regain a set point weight. However, by following a plan like The Livy Method which focuses on eating and feeding into your hunger signals, and allowing your insulin levels to stabilise over time, your hormone feedback system will improve. The Livy Method also focuses on improving digestive health, hydration, sleep, stress management, eating nutrition rich foods to satisfaction, rather than strict calorie restrictions with large energy burns from exercise. All of these factors will ultimately help lower your set point.

Finally, it is important to stop thinking about food as calories. According to Harvard Medicine (2016, November), looking only at calories, and comparing calorie to calorie, ignores the important fact that our body processes various foods differently. In fact, the calories in more nutrient dense foods with higher fibre and water content, actually changes in how you digest it and retrieve the energy from that food (metabolic effect). An example of this would be when comparing a chocolate bar, and comparing its caloric equivalent in spinach, or nuts. You would feel naturally full on less when eating the spinach and nuts. Also, your body would receive much more nutritional benefit in the form of vitamins, minerals, and hormone stability. The chocolate bar would increase your blood sugar more than the spinach or nuts would, causing your body to release insulin to store the excess glucose. Increased insulin eventually leads to more intake, and thus the negative feedback loop has been stimulated.

Another consideration is that different foods go through different metabolic pathways. Some of these pathways are more efficient than others. According to Healthline (2018, May) the more efficient a metabolic pathway is, the more of the food's energy is used for work and less is dissipated as heat. The metabolic pathways for protein are less efficient than the metabolic pathways for carbs and fat. Protein contains 4 calories per gram, but a large part of these protein calories is lost as heat when it is metabolised by the body.

The thermic effect of food is a measure of how much different foods increase energy expenditure, due to the energy required to digest, absorb and metabolise the nutrients. Sources vary on the exact numbers, but it's clear that protein requires much more energy to metabolise than fat and carbs.

Therefore, to illustrate this when ingesting 100 calories of food, with a thermic effect of 25% for protein and 2% for fat, this would mean that 100 calories of protein would end up as 75 calories available, whereas 100 calories of fat would end up as 98 calories available to be used as energy or to be stored by the body.

Another example of this principle would be in how the body utilises fibre. There are 2 different types of fibre, soluble and insoluble. Both are important for health, digestion, and preventing diseases.

- **Soluble fibre** attracts water and turns to gel during digestion. This slows digestion. Soluble fibre is found in oat bran, barley, nuts, seeds, beans, lentils, peas, and some fruits and vegetables. It is also found in psyllium, a common fibre supplement. Some types of soluble fibre may help lower risk of heart disease.

- **Insoluble fibre** is found in foods such as wheat bran, vegetables, and whole grains. It adds bulk to the stool and appears to help food pass more quickly through the stomach and intestines.

The higher the fibre in foods, not only the better for your health, but less caloric energy is actually extracted from it for storage in the body. An example of this would be corn. Corn on the cob is nutritious, delicious, and high in fibre. In fact, it is very difficult for the body to process, requiring lots of chewing and work for the body to break down to use what it needs. However, if you take this same amount of corn and crush it into a flour and make a tortilla, the body hardly has to work, as it is already ground down and processed. In fact, most of its caloric energy is made available to the body, as opposed to when eating it in its whole form. This means the body will utilise almost all of the calories from the processed form, whereas the body will only use some of the calories in its whole form. Furthermore, its processed form can also impact the hormones in the body very differently. This may lead to an increased release in insulin and other hunger and satiety hormones, that can impact our hunger and satisfaction levels, which may lead us to eating more of it than we need! Hopefully this makes sense when understanding why it is recommended to eat food in its most whole form as much as possible.

REFERENCES

A history of restriction. (n.d). Alimentarium. https://www.alimentarium.org/en/fact-sheet/history-restriction

American College of Rheumatology. (2022, February). *Tumor necrosis factor (TNF) inhibitors.* https://www.rheumatology.org/I-Am-A/Patient-Caregiver/Treatments/TNF-Inhibitors

Aristizabal, J.C., Freidenreich, D.J., Volk, B.M., Kupchak, B.R., Saenz, C., Maresh, C.M., Kraemer, W.J., & Volek, J.S. (2015). Effect of resistance training on resting metabolic rate and its estimation by a dual-energy X-ray absorptiometry metabolic map. *European Journal of Clinical Nutrition, 69*, 831-836. https://doi.org/10.1038/ejcn.2014.216

Beth Israel Deaconess Medical Center. (2017, October 12). *Week one: The science of set point.* https://www.bidmc.org/about-bidmc/wellness-insights/nutrition/week-one-the-science-of-set-point

Centers for Disease Control and Prevention. (2022, May 17). *Adult obesity facts.* https://www.cdc.gov/obesity/data/adult.html

Centers for Disease Control and Prevention. (2022, June 3). *Obesity basics.* https://www.cdc.gov/obesity/basics/index.html

Centers for Disease Control and Prevention. (2022, July 14). *Why it matters.* https://www.cdc.gov/obesity/about-obesity/why-it-matters.html

Centers for Disease Control and Prevention. (2022, July 15). *Consequences of obesity.* https://www.cdc.gov/obesity/basics/consequences.html

Centers for Disease Control and Prevention. (2020, July 27). *Gout.* https://www.cdc.gov/arthritis/basics/gout.html#:~:text=quality%20of%20life%3F-,What%20is%20gout%3F,no%20symptoms%2C%20known%20as%20remission.

Considine, R.V., Sinha, M.K., Heiman, M.L., Kriauciunas, A., Stephens, T.W., Nyce, M.R., Ohannesian, J.P., Marco, C.C., McKee, L.J., Bauer, T.L., & Caro, J.F. (1996). Serum immunoreactive-leptin concentrations in normal-weight and obese humans. *The New England Journal of Medicine, 334*, 292-295. DOI: 10.1056/NEJM199602013340503

Dalvi, P.S., Chalmers, J.A., Luo, V., Han, D.-YD., Wellhauser, L., Liu, Y., Tran, D.Q., Castel, J., Luquet, S., Wheeler, M.B., & Belsham, D.D. (2017). High fat induces acute and chronic inflammation in the hypothalamus: Effect of high-fat diet, palmitate and TNF-⊠ on appetite-regulating NPY neurons. *International Journal of Obesity, 41*, 149-158. https://doi.org/10.1038/ijo.2016.183

Diabetes Canada. (n.d.). *Type 2 diabetes.* https://www.diabetes.ca/about-diabetes/type-2

Dr. Wendi. (2020, September 15). *Hypothalamus and pituitary gland* [Video]. Youtube. https://www.youtube.com/watch?v=xCXtcoUxJZc

Gao, Y., Bielohuby, M., Fleming, T., Grabner, G.F., Foppen, E., Bernhard, W., Guzmán-Ruiz, M., Layritz, C., Legutko, B., Zinser, E., García-Cáceres, C., Buijs, R.M., Woods, S.C., Kalsbeek, A., Seeley, R.J., Nawroth, P.P., Bidlingmaier, M., Tschöp, M.H., & Yi, C.-X. (2017). Dietary sugars, not lipids, drive hypothalamic inflammation. *Molecular Metabolism, 6*(8), 897-908. https://doi.org/10.1016/j.molmet.2017.06.008

Geary, N. (2020). Control-theory models of body-weight regulation and body-weight-regulatory appetite. *Appetite, 144,* 104440. https://doi.org/10.1016/j.appet.2019.104440

Ghoshal, M. (2020, March 19). *What you need to know about set point theory.* Healthline. https://www.healthline.com/health/set-point-theory#summary

Government of Canada. (2020, November 5). Public Health Infobase. *Differences in obesity rates between rural communities and urban cities in Canada.* https://health-infobase.canada.ca/data-lab/canadian-risk-factor-atlas-obesity-blog.html?=undefined&wbdisable=true

Government of Western Australia. (2018, January 25). *Set point theory.* Centre for Clinical Interventions. https://www.cci.health.wa.gov.au/~/media/CCI/Mental%20Health%20Professionals/Eating%20Disorders/Eating%20Disorders%20-%20Information%20Sheets/Eating%20Disorders%20Information%20Sheet%20-%2024%20-%20Set%20Point%20Theory.pdf

Hall, K.D., Ayuketah, A., Brychta, R., Cai, Hongyi., Cassimatis, T., Chen, K.Y., Chung, S.t., Costa, E., Courville, A., Darcey, V., Fletcher, L.A., Forde, C.G., Gharib, A.M., Guo, J., Howard, R., Joseph, P.V., McGehee, S., Ouwerkerk, R., Raisinger, K., … Zhou, M. (2019). Ultra-processed diets cause excess calorie intake and weight gain: An inpatient randomized controlled trial of ad libitum food intake. *Cell Metabolism, 30*(1),67-77.E3. https://doi.org/10.1016/j.cmet.2019.05.008

Harris R. B. (1990). Role of set-point theory in regulation of body weight. *FASEB Journal. 4*(15), 3310–3318. https://doi.org/10.1096/fasebj.4.15.2253845

Heart attack. (n.d). Johns Hopkins Medicine. https://www.hopkinsmedicine.org/health/conditions-and-diseases/heart-attack

Hjorth, M.F., Roager, H.M., Larsen, T.M., Poulsenn, S.K., Licht, T.R., Bahl, M.I., Zohar, Y., & Astrup, A. (2018). Pre-treatment microbial prevotella-to-bacteroides ratio, determines body fat loss success during a 6-month randomized controlled diet intervention. *International Journal of Obesity, 42,* 580-583. https://doi.org/10.1038/ijo.2017.220

Houle, B. (2013, December 3). *How obesity relates to socioeconomic status.* Population Reference Bureau. https://www.prb.org/resources/

how-obesity-relates-to-socioeconomic-status/#:~:text=They%20found%20that%20obesity%20rose,less%20likely%20to%20be%20obese.

Jung, C. H., & Kim, M. S. (2013). Molecular mechanisms of central leptin resistance in obesity. *Archives of Pharmacal Research, 36*(2), 201–207. https://doi.org/10.1007/s12272-013-0020-y

Kearns, C.E., Schmidt, L.A., & Glantz, S.A. (2016). Sugar industry and coronary heart disease research: A historical analysis of internal industry documents. *JAMA Internal Medicine, 176*(11), 1680–1685. doi:10.1001/jamainternmed.2016.5394

Liu, S., Munasinghe, L.L., Ohinmaa, A., & Veugelers, P.J. (2020). Added, free and total sugar content and consumption of foods and beverages in Canada. *Health Reports, 31*(10), 14-24. https://www.doi.org/10.25318/82-003-x202001000002-eng

Mayo Clinic Staff. (2021, February 6). *Cirrhosis.* Mayo Clinic. https://www.mayoclinic.org/diseases-conditions/cirrhosis/symptoms-causes/syc-20351487#:~:text=Cirrhosis%20is%20a%20late%20stage,it%20tries%20to%20repair%20itself

Müller, M. J., Bosy-Westphal, A., & Heymsfield, S. B. (2010). Is there evidence for a set point that regulates human body weight?. *F1000 medicine reports, 2,* 59. https://doi.org/10.3410/M2-59

Müller, M.J., Geisler, C., Heymsfield, S.B., & Bosy-Westphal A. (2018). Recent advances in understanding body weight homeostasis in humans [version 1; peer review: 4 approved]. *F1000Research, 7*[F1000 Faculty Rev]1025 https://doi.org/10.12688/f1000research.14151.1

National Institute of Diabetes and Digestive and Kidney Diseases. (2018, February). *Factors affecting weight & health.* https://www.niddk.nih.gov/health-information/weight-management/adult-overweight-obesity/factors-affecting-weight-health

National Institute of Diabetes and Digestive and Kidney Diseases. (2018, February). *Health risks of overweight & obesity.* https://www.niddk.nih.gov/health-information/weight-management/adult-overweight-obesity/health-risks?dkrd=/health-information/weight-management/health-risks-overweight

National Institute of Diabetes and Digestive and Kidney Diseases. (2021, September). *Overweight & obesity statistics.* https://www.niddk.nih.gov/health-information/health-statistics/overweight-obesity

Nonalcoholic fatty liver disease. (n.d). Johns Hopkins Medicine. https://www.hopkinsmedicine.org/health/conditions-and-diseases/nonalcoholic-fatty-liver-disease

Pesta, D.H., & Samuel, V.T. (2014). A high-protein diet for reducing body fat: Mechanisms and possible caveats. *Nutrition & Metabolism, 11*(1), 53. https://doi.org/10.1186/1743-7075-11-53

Petty, R.E. (2016). Structure and function. In R.E. Petty, R.M. Laxer, C.B. Lindsley & L.R Wedderburn (Eds.), *Textbook of pediatric rheumatology (7th ed., pp.* 5-13.e2). W.B. Saunders. https://doi.org/10.1016/B978-0-323-24145-8.00002-8

Pugle, M. (2022, January 27). *How your body tries to prevent you from losing too much weight.* Healthline.https://www.healthline.com/health-news/how-your-body-tries-to-prevent-you-from-losing-too-much-weight

SANESolution bibliography table of contents. (n.d.). SANESolution. https://sanesolution.com/sanesolution-bibliography/

Sarwan, G., & Rehman, A. (2022, June 5). Management of weight loss plateau. In *StatPearls.* StatPearls Publishing. https://www.ncbi.nlm.nih.gov/books/NBK576400/

Schoeller, D.A., Cella, L.K, Sinha, M.K., & Caro, J.F. (1997). Entrainment of the diurnal rhythm of plasma leptin to meal timing. *The Journal of Clinical Investigation, 100*(7), 1882-1887. https://doi.org/10.1172/JCI119717

Seladi-Schulman, J. (2022, January 31). *Hypothalamus overview.* Healthline. https://www.healthline.com/human-body-maps/hypothalamus

Soluble vs. insoluble fiber. (n.d). MedlinePlus. https://medlineplus.gov/ency/article/002136.htm#:~:text=Insoluble%20fiber%20is%20found%20in,through%20the%20stomach%20and%20intestines.

Stunkard, A.J., Harris, J.R., Pedersen, N.L., & McClearn, G.E. (1990). The body-mass index of twins who have been reared apart. *The New England Journal of Medicine, 322,* 1483-1487. DOI: 10.1056/NEJM199005243222102

The dangers of uncontrolled sleep apnea. (n.d). Johns Hopkins Medicine. https://www.hopkinsmedicine.org/health/wellness-and-prevention/the-dangers-of-uncontrolled-sleep-apnea

Wdowik, M. (2017, November 6). The long, strange history of dieting fads. *The Conversation.* https://theconversation.com/the-long-strange-history-of-dieting-fads-82294

World Health Organization. (n.d). *Obesity.* https://www.who.int/health-topics/obesity#tab=tab_1

THE BASICS OF DIGESTION

The goal of these posts is to help provide some foundational information and create an understanding of how our bodies function. We will also discuss how implementing The Livy Method optimizes our health, wellness, and mindfulness, by providing an environment where our bodies no longer feel the need to store fat!

Our plan is to take a deeper dive into some topics, but we are going to start by providing and building onto some of the basics.

Many of you reported coming into this program with digestive issues, or wanting to know more about how your body may respond to the plan with issues like IBS, Crohn's disease, GERD (Gastric-Esophageal Reflux), missing your gallbladder, gastric bypass or other modifications. So, we are going to break this all down for you in our series about the digestive system!

WHY IS DIGESTION SO IMPORTANT?

Digestion is the complex process where our body breaks down the food and liquids that we eat in the form of carbohydrates, proteins and fats, into smaller components and nutrients, which the body uses for energy, growth, and cell repair. If there are any impairments in this process, there can be an impact in how our body is able to absorb and utilize the nutrients, vitamins, and minerals that we need to maintain optimal health! This is why with The Livy Method, there is a huge emphasis on improving digestive health, eating nutritious food, and making all meals and snacks as nutrient dense as possible.

THE CEPHALIC PHASE:

Many of us don't realize this, but digestion actually starts in our brain! When we think about, see, smell, touch, or taste food, our hormones become activated. We begin to secrete **saliva** in our mouths and our stomachs begin to secrete gastric juices. In fact, this phase is responsible for the secretion of up to 50% of our gastric and digestive hormone secretions, in order to aid in the processing of what we eat (Zafra, M.A., Molina, F., & Puerto, A., 2006)!

This is where our mindfulness should really start, in order to take full advantage of the optimal digestion of our foods. We can do this by checking in with ourselves to see what ingredients appeal to us most, taking the time to prepare our foods thoughtfully, and using all our senses in the food preparation process. Be in the moment and enjoy it!

This is also the time we can really dive into the first two mindfulness questions of eating: Are you feeling hungry? How is this portion for me?

THE EATING PHASE:

The next phase of digestion continues to the mouth with the ingestion of food. This is where we begin to chew our foods and saliva continues to flood into our mouths. The action of chewing with our teeth helps to break down the foods we are eating into smaller bits for our body to process, mixing with enzymes contained in our saliva. **"Enzymes" are special proteins we have in our body that help speed up certain chemical reactions, and are involved in helping to build certain substances or break them down (like in the case of digestion).**

Although we have multiple glands that produce saliva and enzymes, the **parotid gland** is most responsible for producing **amylase (the enzymes that help break down carbohydrates into glucose).** Our saliva also provides lubrication to help our food to travel down our digestive tract. The most important part of this phase is the act of chewing, as it allows for good mixing of the broken-down food with the saliva and enzymes. It also does some good work of breaking down the food before it enters our stomach. The big takeaway here is, the better we are able to chew our food, the better our bodies are able to process it!

This is where we can really tune into the third set of mindfulness questions; Are you getting full? Is this food satisfying you? How would you feel if you took a few more bites? How would you feel if you stop eating now? Do you feel any physical effects of eating? Doing this allows us to chew our foods from our meals and snacks as they were meant to be chewed, instead of rushing through the process.

This is really important when we are eating those 4-5 token bites when we aren't hungry, in order to get the digestive process going. Which is why it is recommended to chew, chew, chew, chew, chew, chew, chew, chew with every bite while having our token bites!

THE PROCESS OF DIGESTION

ESOPHAGUS & STOMACH

When we swallow the food we have chewed (which is now called a "**bolus**"), it passes through our throat via the **pharynx** to the **esophagus**. The esophagus is a smooth muscular tube that is attached from our throat to our stomach that uses involuntary muscular contractions to propel the bolus to our stomach. This process is called **peristalsis.**

Once the food enters into the stomach, the cells in the stomach lining begin to secrete gastric juices that are rich in **HCl (Hydro-Chloric Acid).** This increases the acidic environment of the stomach and activates **pepsin, the enzyme responsible for breaking down protein into amino acids.** Amino acids are then able to be used by the body as building blocks for vital processes such as building proteins, hormones, and neurotransmitters.

This acidic environment is also important for our immunity/defense system, as it creates an inhospitable environment for bacteria and other pathogens to grow, thus keeping us healthy!

The stomach begins to churn and contract, and that food we worked so hard to break down by chewing, forms a semi-liquid form of partially digested food called "**chyme**".

THE SMALL INTESTINE, THE LIVER, THE GALLBLADDER, AND THE PANCREAS

The stomach stores the contents of the chyme, and it is slowly emptied into the small intestine. The small intestine is divided into three different segments, known as the **duodenum, the jejunum** and the **ileum**.

The chyme first enters our **duodenum (the first part of our small intestine)** at a rate of about two teaspoons per minute. The duodenum receives enzymes from a variety of organs also involved in the digestive process; **the liver, the gallbladder, and the pancreas**.

The liver is a large organ located above the stomach in the upper abdomen. The liver produces bile which is stored in the gallbladder, stores nutrients, and helps remove toxins from the body.

When we eat fatty foods, the gallbladder (a small pouch) is stimulated to secrete **bile** via the **bile ducts** to the small intestine, which helps to emulsify the fats and makes it easier for **lipases (enzymes that break down fat)** to do their job!

The pancreas which is located in the upper part of the abdomen, behind the stomach, secretes what is known as "**pancreatic juice.**" This juice contains a substance called **bicarbonate (which helps to neutralize the high acidity of the incoming food)** and pancreatic enzymes. These pancreatic enzymes include **protease (which breaks down protein)** as well as amylase and lipase which have been discussed earlier. The pancreas also produces chemicals that help regulate blood sugar levels, which affect how much energy the body has available to use. One of these is the infamous **insulin**, which we will discuss in more detail in our series.

The small intestine also secretes its own enzymes for digestion known as **peptidases, sucrase, lactase** and **maltase**. These enzymes contribute mostly to the **hydrolysis of polysaccharides**, meaning they use water to break down these longer chain carbohydrate molecules into simpler sugars like glucose.

Once our food has been broken down into the basic building blocks of glucose, amino acids, vitamins, minerals, and fatty acids, they are ready to be absorbed into our bloodstream which carries the nutrients to cells throughout the body! The small intestine is where most of digestion and absorption take place. The chyme moves in rhythmic movements along the intestines to allow for the mixing of fluids, and for a longer period of time for digestion to take place. The walls of the intestines are lined with fingerlike projections called villi, which are then lined further with even tinier fingerlike projections called microvilli. These allow for an incredibly expansive surface area for all of this absorption to take place, providing your body with those super important nutrients and energy!!!

THE LARGE INTESTINE

The last phase of digestion is the movement of the remaining undigested food into the large intestine (otherwise known as the **colon**) into the formation of stool or poop. The colon is primarily responsible for the reabsorption of water and the last bit of nutrients from this final stage of processing food, the content that remains forms stools which we poop out through our **rectum** via the **anus**.

The colon also contains our gut flora which is composed of trillions of microbes known as the **microbiome**. This is definitely a hot topic around here with our members, and a topic we will be looking further into down the road. These bacteria help to ferment the indigestible food and produce vitamins such as Vitamin K and B vitamins that are reabsorbed by the colon. But that's not all, an estimated 80% of our immune system is found in our gut (Wiertsema SP, Van Bergenhenegouwen J, Garssen J, Knippels, 2021). Having a healthy digestive system, which includes a good balance of our healthy gut flora, ensures a healthier immune system and better nutrient absorption. This is why the Livy Method recommends taking a good quality probiotic, along with a prebiotic (if needed), to help feed those good microbes. Eating the high fibre, nutrient rich foods on plan not only gives our body what it needs, but is also vital in supporting our gut flora.

For a comprehensive video looking at digestion, check out this video:

https://www.youtube.com/watch?v=X3TAROotFfM

THE LAST QUESTION IN MINDFULNESS

This sums up the topic of the basics of digestion, and brings us to the fourth series of questions in mindfulness when eating. Do you feel full and if so, what is your definition of full? How do you know when you have eaten enough? How do you feel physically? Meaning, is it a physically full belly feeling, or is it more of an insulin rush or a tired feeling? Or is it that you just eat everything on your plate because it's there kind of thing? Or maybe you feel like you could eat more?

As you can see, establishing mindfulness around your eating not only helps you connect and become more in tune with your body, but additionally promotes optimal digestion! Hope this helps!

Now that we understand the basics of digestion, check out our post where we discuss issues with digestion!

REFERENCES

Anatomy of the digestive system. (2017). BarCharts, Inc.

Azzouz, L.L., & Sharma, S. (2021). *Physiology, large intestine*. StatPearls Publishing. https://www.ncbi.nlm.nih.gov/books/NBK507857/

Boland, M. (2016). Human digestion - a processing perspective. *Journal of the Science of Food and Agriculture*, *96*(7), 2275–2283. https://doi.org/10.1002/jsfa.7601

Granger, N.D., Morris, J. D., Kvietys, P. R., & Granger, J. P. (2018). *Physiology and Pathophysiology of Digestion*. Morgan & Claypool Life Science Publishers.

McClements, D.J. (2019). *Future foods: How modern science is transforming the way we eat. Copernicus Publications.* https://doi.org/10.1007/978-3-030-12995-8

Morris, J.D., Granger, D. N., Granger, J. P., & Kvietys, P. R. (2018). *Physiology and Pathophysiology of Digestion: Part 2*. Biota Publishing.

Prados, A. (2022, February, 2). *Four science-backed ways of taking care of your gut microbiota*. Gut Microbiota for Health. https://www.gutmicrobiotaforhealth.com/four-science-backed-ways-of-taking-care-of-your-gut-microbiota

Schwenke, T. (2020, May 3). *Human digestive system - How it works!* [Video]. Youtube. https://www.youtube.com/watch?v=X3TAROotFfM

Sethi, S., & Jewell, T. (2019, February 1). *What causes dysbiosis and how is it treated?* Healthline. https://www.healthline.com/health/digestive-health/dysbiosis

Your digestive system & how it works. (2017, December). National Institute of Diabetes and Digestive and Kidney Diseases. Retrieved March 30, 2022, from https://www.niddk.nih.gov/health-information/digestive-diseases/digestive-system-how-it-works

Wiertsema SP, van Bergenhenegouwen J, Garssen J, Knippels LMJ. The Interplay between the Gut Microbiome and the Immune System in the Context of Infectious Diseases throughout Life and the Role of Nutrition in Optimizing Treatment Strategies. *Nutrients*. 2021 Mar 9;13(3):886. doi: 10.3390/nu13030886. PMID: 33803407; PMCID: PMC8001875.().

Zafra, M.A., Molina, F., & Puerto, A. (2006). The neural/cephalic phase reflexes in the physiology of nutrition. *Neuroscience and Biobehavioral Reviews*, 30(7), 1032–1044. https://doi.org/10.1016/j.neubiorev.2006.03.005

THE PSYCHOLOGY OF EFFORT

The science posts are where we are providing some foundational information and understanding of how our bodies function, and how implementing The Livy Method optimizes our health, wellness, and mindfulness, by providing an environment where our bodies no longer feel the need to store fat!

In this post we are initiating the conversation about the concept of the psychology of "effort", and how effort can impact our weight loss journey and process. So, to better understand more about the psychological concept of effort and the kind of impact it has, let's take a deeper dive into effort! We will also discuss the concept of setting goals, the formation of habits (which will help in forming more positive ones in order to help with weight loss), and how to navigate through psychological roadblocks that may impact weight loss.

For so many of us, the journey behind weight loss can be a daunting and overwhelming process. Many of us have been on the hamster wheel of dieting and trying to lose weight for many years or have tried more diets than we can count. And yet here we are again, some of us at our wits end, unsure that The Livy Method will work. For many of us, this is our last attempt before giving up and accepting our current reality as our future.

HOW IS THE LIVY METHOD DIFFERENT?

With this method, there is a completely different emphasis on how we should be treating our bodies as well as our mindsets. We are changing our focus to supporting our bodies by giving our bodies what they need, establishing good nutrition, and on lifestyle changes that complement the weight loss process. We are also challenging ourselves in a more cerebral and emotional way, by purposefully implementing tweaks that address issues we may have consciously or subconsciously. The Livy Method post and video is an excellent resource, discussing how this process is different from the other diets that are out there or what we have experienced in the past!

However, this method is not a quick fix and may require some amount of effort in order to attain success! Although many members come into this process with gusto, ready to do all it takes, many can also be challenged as time evolves and their level of success may not be reflected by their perceived effort. Everybody is different, with different histories, physiologies and health issues they may be working through, varying mental/emotional experiences, stresses, financial situations, as well as life challenges. To be straight up, some people may need a lot of help and time before their body may be willing to make changes or start to drop weight on the scale. Some may really struggle with the time and energy it may take to work through this.

This raises the question, what happens when one's effort does not match their success on the scale? Many people use the scale to judge their level of achievement, yet discount any possible **NSVs (non-scale victories)** that they may have experienced or are experiencing. They may also not be realistic about the time that may be required to get their bodies healthy before they will begin to drop any weight.

Effort is a very interesting and complicated concept, as one may perceive they are exerting much more effort than they truly are, thus expecting a bigger return than they may be experiencing. In fact, they may be seeing themselves at their finish line in their minds, yet not putting in the actual level of effort required, thus feeling frustration with their current experience as reflected on the scale. Effort is subjective and irreflective of outcome. Let's delve deeper into the concept of Effort.

EFFORT DEFINED

Effort refers to the "subjective intensification of mental and/or physical activity in the service of meeting some goal" (Inzlicht, M., Shenhav, A., & Olivola, C. Y., 2018). Although related, effort is not the same as motivation, "which is a force that drives behavior by determining both a direction (e.g., goal) and the intensity or vigor with which this direction is pursued". Effort refers to the intensity of behavior but does not refer to any specific goal.

Effort is an "intentional process and application, therefore it corresponds with what a person is actively doing and not to what is passively happening to them. Effort is distinguishable from demand or difficulty, as effort corresponds to the intensity of mental or physical work that someone applies to achieve some outcome. Although effort typically involves demand (with people working harder when the task is more difficult), this relationship breaks down when incentives are too low or when demands are too high. Finally, it is important to distinguish effort from associated mental constructs, such as boredom." (Inzlicht, M., Shenhav, A., & Olivola, C. Y., 2018)

Effort can also be "visible to others and is difficult to fake, making it plain to observers whether someone is exerting themselves or not. The fact that effort is easily recognized in self and others gives it important signaling functions; for example, communicating dedication, intention, and commitment." (Inzlicht, M., Shenhav, A., & Olivola, C. Y., 2018)

THE PARADOX OF EFFORT

Effort, whether it is mental or physical, is a common occurrence in daily life and is encountered every time we need to push ourselves. We regularly face activities that require us to exert some level of energy to achieve a goal or task, whether it is forcing ourselves to get up for work, or exercise at the end of the day.

Effort is often associated with something that can feel difficult and averse and as a result, people tend to avoid effort, including the effort that comes from merely thinking things through. In fact, people often develop strategies that allow them to avoid situations that require more work or effort.

However, in contrast to this, while people will work hard to obtain something of value, working hard can also make those same things more valuable. In fact, effort can even be experienced as valuable or rewarding in its own right. People may readily apply more effort for better outcomes, and view those outcomes as more rewarding if more (not less) effort was used to attain them! In the example of weight loss, a person may see more value in the work they put in to achieve their weight loss goal, than in the actual weight loss itself!

COGNITIVE DISSONANCE THEORY AND EFFORT JUSTIFICATION

According to cognitive dissonance theory and its research, the more effort one exerts, the more valuable one perceives the reward associated with that effort (Harmon-Jones, E., Clark, D., Paul, K., & Harmon-Jones, C., 2020). This effect has been referred to as effort justification. Thus, cognitive dissonance theory would suggest that increasing the attractiveness of a reward would encourage greater effort, however we need to be clear on the effort we are really exerting. In the Livy Method members sometimes feel that the reward (e.g. weight loss) is not reflective of their effort. However, the Livy Method 20 questions assessment will help members to rate the effort they are truly exerting, and thus identify where they can level up. Basically, you may tell yourself that you are doing all the things, although in reality you may not be. While following the Livy Method may be challenging and unpleasant for some, being realistic about the effort you are applying (through the 20 questions) will help reduce the cognitive dissonance and stress when you think you are doing everything, but in reality there are ways we can always level up.

According to cognitive dissonance theory, when perceived effort does not match your results; "I should be at my goal" is in contradiction with the cognition, "I am not seeing the weight loss I had expected to see on the scale." The dissonance can be reduced by examining if "I am maximizing each aspect of the 20 questions and doing all the things." The variables of critical importance in dissonance theory are psychological (subjective) (e.g., the perception of effort). Because one may be perceiving themselves as exerting maximum effort, although they still have a long road ahead of them. They may be elevating the effort they are putting into the weight loss process, yet, in reality could be doing so much more.

Dissonance theory research suggests that people use effort justification when they perceive their goal cannot be predicted with certainty, and so they use how much effort they perceive they are exerting as a justification for obtaining the reward. This causes cognitive dissonance when the reward (in our case weight loss) is not immediately apparent.

Check out this video that explains the theory of cognitive dissonance in more detail!

https://www.youtube.com/watch?v=9Y17YaZRRvY

Check out this video that explains effort justification in more detail!

https://www.youtube.com/watch?v=PEGEJ21kASQ

WHAT IS BEING VALUED, EFFORT ITSELF OR THE PRODUCT OF EFFORT?

There is evidence that people hold greater value to goods and outcomes (e.g., group membership, furniture, coffee mugs, etc.) that they worked for and required effort, compared with identical goods and outcomes that they obtained without effort (e.g., by chance, as windfalls). Therefore, it can be assumed that those that achieved weight loss by following the plan and putting in a good effort to do so, will see the outcome of the process as more valuable.

People tend to associate effort with reward and will sometimes select objects or activities precisely because they require effort (e.g., mountain climbing, marathons). Effort adds value to the products achieved, but effort itself also has value. The value of effort is not only accessed concurrently with, or immediately following effort exertion, but is also in anticipation of such expenditure, suggesting that we already have an intuitive understanding of effort's potential positive value.

From examining the literature around effort, it can be seen that putting real effort into The Livy Method is putting in real effort into yourself. That effort alone may have value to you, even if it is difficult. Recognizing the scale and NSVs accomplished, will also increase the value you achieve from this process. However, it is important to see things from an accurate lens and to be real. Recognize where you could truly put in more effort. Be honest when answering the 20 questions so you can see where you can level up and maximize your efforts!

Now that we have discussed the importance of effort, let's talk about setting goals to put forth your effort into action!

SETTING GOALS REWIRES YOUR BRAIN'S EFFECTIVENESS

Goal setting can be very powerful and can motivate people to accomplish tasks they might not have thought they could.

A study in Behavioral and Cognitive Neuroscience Reviews showed that people that set goals are generally more "together" than everyone else (Top Stack, 2019, November). This is because goal setting rewires our brains to make the component parts work more effectively. This study showed that when you set a goal, multiple parts of the brain are suddenly engaged: The amygdala, which is the brain's emotional center, evaluates the goal for how important it is to you. The frontal lobe, which is the brain's logical problem-solving portion, defines the goal and digests it. Both the amygdala and the frontal lobe then work together to push you toward the completion of the goal. As the brain moves you into situations to help you achieve your goal, the organ changes to help you optimize behaviors and tasks.

Another study, in the Journal of Applied Psychology reports that people who established an ambitious goal usually achieved it. The study suggested that ambitious goals stimulate the brain more, motivating the person to accomplish the impossible. The study found that the higher the goal that was set, the more likely one would achieve it. The Psychological Bulletin said 90% of the studies showed that more challenging goals led to higher performance. More manageable goals, "do your best" goals, or no goals did not have the same effect on the brain, or the person's ability to achieve their goals. Researchers report that "goal setting is most likely to improve task performance when the goals are specific and sufficiently challenging" (Top Stack, 2019, November). Also, decades of research on achievement suggests that successful people reach their goals not simply because of who they are, but more often because of what they do.

Interestingly, these studies suggest brain rewiring occurs when the individual sets the goal themselves. However, the brain does not seem to change if the goal is set by someone else. When we apply this to the Livy Method it calls attention to the importance of regularly checking in on your "why" – it is only you who can decide your "why".

So, for those looking for success while following the Livy Method, let's talk more about the process of goal setting!

1. Get specific. When you set yourself a goal, try to be as specific as possible. "Lose 5 pounds" is a better goal than "lose some weight," because it gives you a clear idea of what success looks like. Knowing exactly what you want to achieve keeps you motivated until you get there. Also, think about the specific actions recommended by The Livy Method that need to be taken to reach your goal. Just stating you will "sleep more" is too vague, be clear and precise. "I'll be in bed by 10pm on weeknights, and sleep between 7-8 hours" is a specific goal.

2. Seize the moment to act on your goals. For example, increasing your activity or exercise is part of maximizing. Achieving your goal means organizing this activity into your calendar, especially as many of us live busy lives! Be as specific as possible (e.g., " on Monday, Wednesday, or Friday, I'll work out for 45 minutes before work."). Studies show that this kind of planning will help your brain to detect and seize the opportunity when it arises, increasing your chances of success by roughly 300% (Grant, H., 2011, February).

3. Know exactly how you are progressing. Achieving any goal also requires honest and regular monitoring of your progress. If you do not know how well you are doing, you are not able to adjust your behavior or strategies accordingly. While following The Livy Method, check your progress daily by using the APP to document your weight, water, activity, sleep, meals, snacks, and journal. This will keep your head in the game as you are maintaining accountability and seeing your daily weight progress will help keep you focused.

4. Be a realistic optimist. Believing in your ability to succeed is enormously helpful for creating and sustaining your motivation. However, do not underestimate how difficult it may be to reach your goal. Most goals worth achieving require time, planning, effort, and persistence. Studies show that people that assume that things will happen easily and with little effort, will have more difficulty achieving their goal as they may be unprepared for the journey ahead.

5. Have grit. Grit is a willingness to commit to long-term goals, and to persist in the face of difficulty. Grit is a good determiner of who will be successful in the long term. Everyone has the potential for grit!! By putting in the effort, planning, persistence, and strategies needed to succeed, will not only help you see yourself and your goals more accurately, but also do wonders for your grit.

6. Make sure your choices are in line with your goals. We make multiple choices and decisions every day. When you are choosing what to eat, take a minute to think through – is this in line with my goals? Will this help advance my journey to finally and forever? Think through what choice you are making and be comfortable with the decision you make.

FOCUS ON WHAT YOU HAVE ACHIEVED

On the days when you feel frustrated with yourself for not meeting your goals, try taking a closer look at the things you have achieved. Revisiting what you have accomplished in the process so far can help you keep things in perspective. This is a good time to examine your "why" of wanting to lose weight or to get healthier by participating in the program. It is also important to look deeper at all the non-scale victories you have experienced!

KNOW YOUR LIMITS

Even with the best intentions and the willingness to put in maximum effort, you may not find it possible to improve every situation or meet every expectation. Although effort can get you closer to fulfilling your weight loss goal, you might need additional resources you just don't have access to, like the financial limitations of purchasing supplements, or may be overwhelmed with stress, or at capacity. You are a human being with normal physical and emotional limitations. If you find yourself not meeting an expectation you have set, acknowledge that you did your best and offer yourself compassion instead of blame. You will get there!

SHARE YOUR EXPECTATIONS

Discuss your goals and needs with the supporters in your life. By sharing your needs with those in your immediate circle, you are actively communicating what will help you be successful. This will help ensure your success in meeting your goals, but also allows those that care about you to support and be there for you!

KEEP A FLEXIBLE MINDSET

The more flexible you are with your goals, the better you will be able to accommodate life's unpredictability. The path to weight loss as we know is not a straight one. Just do the best you can and roll with the punches!

The last thing that will be discussed along with effort, goal setting, and expectations, is the formation of habits. Oftentimes it is certain habits that have led us to the path of weight gain or yo-yo dieting. However, The Livy Method is about real change, and implementing healthier life habits. Let's examine how long we may expect to incite real change into our lives.

HOW LONG DOES IT TAKE TO FORM A NEW HABIT?

According to a 2009 study published in the European Journal of Social Psychology, "it takes 18 to 254 days for a person to form a new habit." (Legg, T.J., & Frothingham, S., 2019, October) The study also concluded that, on average, it takes 66 days for a new behavior to become automatic, ultimately depending on the habit in question.

- Certain habits take longer to form. As demonstrated in the study, many participants found it easier to adopt the habit of drinking a glass of water at breakfast, than to do 50 sit-ups after their morning coffee.

- Some people are better suited to forming habits than others, as some gravitate towards a consistent routine, whereas others do not.

HOW THE MYTH OF "21 DAYS" CAME ABOUT

Many people subscribe to the belief that it takes 21 days to create a new habit. This concept can be traced back to "Psycho-Cybernetics," a book published in 1960 by Dr. Maxwell Maltz. Dr. Maltz identified this number as an observable metric in both himself and his patients and wrote, "these, and many other commonly observed phenomena, tend to show that it requires a minimum of about 21 days for an old mental image to dissolve and a new one to gel." As the book became more popular, this situational observation has become accepted as fact.

THE PSYCHOLOGY OF FORMING A HABIT

According to a 2012 study published in the British Journal of General Practice, habits are "actions that are triggered automatically in response to contextual cues that have been associated with their performance." (Legg, T.J., & Frothingham, S., 2019, October) For example, when you get into your car, you automatically put on the seat belt. You do not think about doing it or why you do it, you just do it. Your brain likes habits because they are efficient, and when you automate common actions, you free up mental resources for other tasks.

WHY IT CAN BE DIFFICULT TO BREAK A HABIT

According to the National Institutes of Health (NIH), pleasure-based habits are particularly difficult to break, because enjoyable behavior prompts your brain to release dopamine (Legg, T.J., & Frothingham, S., 2019, October). Dopamine is the reward that strengthens the habit and creates the craving to do it again. As discussed in the post on hormones, sugar also stimulates our dopamine response, eventually leading to a dulled response. We often seek more of these types of foods to stimulate the dopamine release. This may also account for snacking at night. You may enjoy some chips as you unwind for the night, while watching television. This will start to stimulate the dopamine reward center, reinforcing the habit of snacking while watching television. These types of habits may have a negative impact on the success of following The Livy Method.

HOW TO CHANGE A HABIT

Dr. Nora Volkow, director of the NIH's National Institute on Drug Abuse, suggests that the first step is to become more aware of your habits so you can develop strategies to change them. One strategy

Volkow suggests is to identify the places, people, or activities that are connected in your mind to certain habits, and then adjust your behavior toward those things.

For example, if you like to eat chips, you can avoid buying chips until you feel more comfortable being around them without wanting to impulsively eat them. This can help you achieve your goal of avoiding them as you start your weight loss journey until your habit has changed.

Another strategy is to replace a bad habit with a good one. For example, instead of snacking on these same potato chips at night when watching TV, consider swapping them out for a nice warm cup of tea. Over time, you will change your association of watching tv with eating chips, creating a new routine with healthier habits when unwinding in the evenings.

In summation, it can take anywhere from 18 to 254 days for a person to form a new habit, and an average of 66 days for a new behavior to become automatic. Everyone is different, as well as their life circumstances, reinforcing why this time frame may be so different for everyone. Some habits are easier to form than others, and some people may find it easier to develop new behaviors than others. Just know that the only timeline that matters is the one that works best for you. If you maximize all your efforts, have the confidence that you WILL achieve your goals.

REFERENCES

Axsom, D., & Cooper, J. (1985). Cognitive dissonance and psychotherapy: The role of effort justification in inducing weight loss. *Journal of Experimental Psychology,* 21(2), 149-160. https://doi.org/10.1016/0022-1031(85)90012-5

Berkman, E. T. (2018). The neuroscience of goals and behavior change. Consulting P*sychology Journal,* 70(1), 28–44. https://doi.org/10.1037/cpb0000094

Cherry, K., & Morin, A. (2020, July 22). *Self efficacy and why believing in yourself matters*. Verywell Mind. https://www.verywellmind.com/what-is-self-efficacy-2795954

Frey, M., & Goldman, R. (2021, June 28). *How to overcome 5 psychological blocks to weight loss*. Verywell Fit. https://www.verywellfit.com/overcome-emotional-stress-to-lose-weight-3495947

Grant, H. (2011, February 25). *Nine things successful people do differently*. Harvard Business Review. https://hbr.org/2011/02/nine-things-successful-people

Harmon-Jones, E., Clark, D., Paul, K., & Harmon-Jones, C. (2020). The effect of perceived effort on reward valuation: Taking the reward positivity (RewP) to dissonance theory. *Frontiers in Human Neuroscience*, 14(157).https://doi.org/10.3389/fnhum.2020.00157

Inzlicht, M., Shenhav, A., & Olivola, C. Y. (2018). The effort paradox: Effort is both costly and valued. *Trends in Cognitive Sciences*, 22(4), 337–349. https://doi.org/10.1016/j.tics.2018.01.007

Knight, R. (2014, December 29). *Make your work resolutions stick.* Harvard Business Review. https://hbr.org/2014/12/make-your-work-resolutions-stick

Krueger, J., & Perina, K. (2021, May 15). *Effort and value: Is the hard work worth it?* Psychology Today. https://www.psychologytoday.com/ca/blog/one-among-many/202105/effort-and-value

Legg, T.J., & Frothingham, S. (2019, October 24). *How long does it take for a new behavior to become automatic?* Healthline. https://www.healthline.com/health/how-long-does-it-take-to-form-a-habit

Legg, T.J., & Raypole, C. (2020, November 30). *Dreaming too big? 12 tips for understanding and reframing unrealistic expectations.* Healthline. https://www.healthline.com/health/mental-health/unrealistic-expectations

Maich, K.H. (2013). Reducing cognitive dissonance through effort justification: Evidence from past studies and daily experience. *Western Undergraduate Psychology Journal*, 1 (1). https://ojs.lib.uwo.ca/index.php/wupj/article/download/1659/1038

Teixeira, P.J., Silva, M.N., Mata, J., Palmeir, A.L., & Markland, D. (2012). Motivation, self-determination, and long-term weight control. I*nternational Journal of Behavioral Nutrition and Physical Activity*, 9, 22. https://doi.org/10.1186/1479-5868-9-22

Top Stack. (2019, November 29). *Learn how goal setting affects your brain.* https://topstackgroup.com/learn-how-goal-setting-affects-your-brain/

DETOX

Welcome back to the science posts where the goal is to help provide some foundational information and create an understanding of how our bodies function. We will also discuss how implementing The Livy Method optimizes our health, wellness, and mindfulness, by providing an environment where our bodies no longer feel the need to store fat!

In this post we are starting the conversation about the concept of detoxification, otherwise known as detox, and how it relates to The Livy Method. To better understand what detoxification is and the relevance of how it impacts the weight loss process, let's take a deeper dive into the concept of detoxification, and what that actually means!

WHAT IS DETOXIFICATION?

Detoxification, or detox, has become pretty popular in the discussion of health in mainstream media over the years. However, this is not a new concept at all!! In fact, people have been trying to relieve their bodies of "toxins" for thousands of years. A toxin is defined "as a substance that is synthesized by a plant species, an animal, or by microorganisms, that is harmful to another organism". However, toxins can also include chemicals like pesticides, pollution, plastics, as well by consuming processed food which can include artificial ingredients, colours, and preservatives from the foods that we eat!

Some examples of traditional "detox" practices that have existed for centuries include bloodletting, enemas, sweat lodges, fasting, and drinking detoxification teas and tonics. Many of these practices were even used as medical treatments up until the early 20th century, however you still hear about many of these detox practices today. Those promoting these diets and products often imply and claim that by following their specific diet or by using their special products, your body will be rid of "toxins", thereby improving health and promoting weight loss.

A typical detox diet may involve a period of fasting, followed by a strict diet of fruit, vegetables, fruit and/or vegetable juices, and water. Sometimes a detox also includes herbs, laxatives, diuretics, teas, supplements, and colon cleanses or enemas.

These claim to:

- Rest your organs by fasting
- Stimulate your liver to help it rid of toxins
- Promote toxin elimination through stool, urine, and sweat
- Improve circulation
- Provide your body with healthy nutrients that it needs to help detox
- Change the PH of your body making it more alkaline in nature

These diets also claim to help with various health problems including obesity, digestive issues, autoimmune diseases, inflammation, allergies, bloating, and chronic fatigue.

However, human research on detox diets is lacking, and the handful of studies that exist are significantly flawed. In fact, popular detox diets rarely identify the specific toxins they aim to remove or the mechanism by which they supposedly eliminate them. There is also little evidence that supports the use of these diets for toxin elimination or sustainable weight loss.

The other concern is the potential for harm. Although some countries have strict regulations of supplements and products that are made available to consumers, many dietary supplements and detox products are not as strictly regulated in other countries. In fact, in the U.S, The FDA (The Food and Drug Administration) often finds "detoxifying" weight loss products contain dangerous drugs and chemicals not advertised on the packaging. These are listed on the FDA website. While some detox teas for example may contain natural tea ingredients like tea leaves, others could contain toxic or allergy-triggering substances, including drugs and medications! The other issue is that with today's technology, we are able to acquire these products for purchase online with just the click of a button. With the ease of online shopping, we are able to purchase pretty much any product from any country, so it can really be difficult to know what is in the products we buy.

Check out this link from the FDA showing the list for supplement advisories

https://www.fda.gov/food/dietary-supplement-products-ingredients/dietary-supplement-ingredient-advisory-list#updates

Check out this list for Weight Loss and Detox tainted products

https://www.fda.gov/drugs/medication-health-fraud/tainted-weight-loss-products

For Canadians, check out the Natural Health Products Database

http://webprod.hc-sc.gc.ca/nhpid-bdipsn/atReq.do?atid=whats.quoi&lang=eng

This is the main page for Canadian consumers and those in the industry

https://www.canada.ca/en/health-canada/services/drugs-health-products/natural-non-prescription.html

IS THERE ANYTHING WE CAN DO TO FACILITATE DETOX?

Now it's time for the good news! Your body is very well-equipped to eliminate toxins on its own without the extra help from special diets or expensive supplements and products. Your body has a very self-sufficient and comprehensive way of eliminating toxins that involves the liver, kidneys, digestive system, skin, and lungs. However, it is only when these organs are healthy, that they can effectively eliminate unwanted substances.

Furthermore, you **can** enhance your body's natural detoxification system. In fact, by following The Livy Method, you are setting your body up for success in supporting your body's own detoxification pathways.

In order to understand the concept of detox, let's discuss some of the common misconceptions reviewed by Healthline, how our body naturally detoxifies itself, and how by following The Livy Method we can enhance and support our body's own detoxification system.

CAN WE TARGET THE ELIMINATION OF TOXINS?

As discussed above, detox diets rarely identify the specific toxins they aim to remove. According to Healthline, the mechanisms by which they work are also unclear. In fact, there is little to no evidence that detox diets can remove any toxins from your body.

Furthermore, your body is capable of cleansing itself by utilizing the liver as the primary detoxification organ, and through the elimination of stool, urine, breath, and sweat.

The liver initiates this process by transforming the toxic substances to a less harmful form, then ensures that the substance is eliminated from the body by way of the lungs, skin, kidneys and/or digestive system.

However, there are a few chemicals that may not be as easily removed by these processes, which can include persistent organic pollutants (POPs), phthalates, bisphenol A (BPA) found in plastics, and heavy metals.

These materials tend to accumulate in fat tissue or blood, and can take years for your body to eliminate. However, as we have gained an increased awareness about the harm that these compounds cause, many of these materials have been removed or limited in commercial products produced today. That being said, there is little evidence that detox diets help eliminate any of these compounds.

HOW EFFECTIVE ARE THESE DIETS?

Some people report feeling more focused and energetic during and after detox diets.

However, this improvement in well-being may simply be due to the elimination of processed foods, alcohol, and other unhealthy substances from their diets. They may also be receiving the nutrients, vitamins, and minerals that they were lacking before, thus resulting in feeling better.

EFFECTS ON WEIGHT LOSS

Very few scientific studies have investigated how detox diets impact weight loss. While some people may lose a lot of weight quickly, this effect is likely due the loss of fluid and carbohydrate stores rather than fat. This weight is usually regained fairly quickly once one resumes their previous lifestyle. If a detox diet involves severe calorie restriction, it may allow for weight loss, but will unlikely be sustainable in keeping the weight off in the long term. In fact, this is a major factor in creating an environment that promotes the body to store fat.

DETOX DIETS, SHORT-TERM FASTING, AND STRESS

According to Healthline (Bjarnadottir, A. 2019, January), several varieties of detox diets may have effects similar to those of short-term or intermittent fasting. Short-term fasting may improve various disease markers in some people, including improved leptin and insulin sensitivity.

However, these effects do not apply to everyone. Studies in women show that both a 48-hour fast and a 3-week period of reduced calorie intake may increase stress hormone levels. Crash diets can be a stressful experience, as they involve resisting temptations and feeling extreme hunger, ultimately affecting the hormones involved in hunger and satiety as discussed in the science post on hormones! These diets often lead to over indulgence from the deprivation involved, and stimulate/increase the hunger hormones and negative feedback loops that these diets perpetuate.

SEVERE CALORIE RESTRICTION

Several detox diets recommend fasting or severe calorie restriction. Short-term fasting and limited calorie intake can result in fatigue, irritability, and other physical symptoms.

Long-term fasting can result in energy, vitamin, and mineral deficiencies, as well as electrolyte imbalances and major health consequences, even death.

Furthermore, colon cleansing methods which are sometimes recommended during detoxes, can cause dehydration, cramping, bloating, nausea, vomiting, and the flushing out of the important bacterial microbiome that lives in the colon and is crucial to the digestive process.

OVERDOSING

Some detox diets may pose the risk of overdosing on supplements, laxatives, diuretics, and even water. There is a lack of regulation and monitoring in the detox industry, and many detox foods and supplements may not have any scientific basis on how their product is produced or manufactured.

In the worst and most insidious cases, the ingredient labels of detox products may be inaccurate. This can increase your risk of overdosing, potentially resulting in serious, and even fatal effects.

If you decide that you want to go down the path of a detox because it is something you choose to do, be sure to seek advice from a regulated health care professional, or Naturopathic Doctor that can oversee and monitor your health during the process!

SO, AFTER ALL THIS, HOW DOES THE BODY DETOX?

THE LIVER

The liver is such an amazing organ and does so much for our bodies! As discussed in the previous science posts, it has an important role in the digestive process and in storing and releasing energy in the form of glucose to the body! Let's discuss this amazing organ in more detail!

The liver is your body's largest solid organ. On average, it weighs around 3 pounds in adulthood and is roughly the size of a football. This organ is vital to the body's metabolic, detoxification, and immune system functions. Without a functioning liver, a person cannot survive.

The liver's position is held most prominently in the right upper region of the abdomen, just below the diaphragm. A portion of the liver is located in the left upper abdomen as well. The liver has two main segments, also called lobes. Each lobe is further divided into eight segments. Each segment has an estimated 1,000 lobules, also called small lobes. Each of the lobules has a small tube, a duct that flows into other ducts that join to become the common hepatic duct. This meets the cystic duct and then becomes the common bile duct.

Compared to the rest of the body, the liver has a significant amount of blood flowing through it, an estimated 13% of the body's blood is in the liver at any given time.

According to Johns Hopkins Medicine, the liver's major functions are in the metabolic processes of the body, but is also involved in many life-sustaining processes, which include:

- creating immune system factors that can help the body fight against infection or pathogens in the body

- producing proteins in conjunction with vitamin K (that is produced largely in the colon) that are important in the blood clotting process, and an important part of healing

- the liver is also one of the organs that help break down old or damaged blood cells and eliminate them from the body

From a digestive and metabolic standpoint, the liver produces an estimated 800 to 1,000 milliliters (ml) of bile each day. This yellow, brownish, or olive green liquid, is collected in small ducts and then passed on to the main bile duct which carries the bile to a part of the small intestine called the duodenum. The small intestine uses the bile to further help with the breakdown and absorption of fats. Any extra bile is stored in the gallbladder to be used later.

In the metabolism of carbohydrates, the liver helps to ensure that the level of sugar in your blood (blood glucose) maintains stability. As discussed in the science post on insulin, if your blood sugar levels increase, for example after a meal, the liver removes sugar from blood supplied by the portal vein and stores it in the form of glycogen. If the blood sugar levels drop or are too low, the liver breaks down glycogen and releases sugar into the blood to be used by the body as needed.

In addition to glycogen, the liver also stores fat-soluble vitamins and minerals such as copper and iron, and releases them into the blood when needed.

The liver also plays an important role in the metabolism of proteins. The liver cells change the amino acids in the foods we eat so that they can be used to produce energy, or make carbohydrates or fats for the body. A substance called ammonia is a by-product of this process which can be toxic to the body in large amounts. In order to prevent the ammonia from increasing to "toxic" levels, the liver cells convert the ammonia to a much less toxic substance called urea which is released into the blood. Urea is then transported to the kidneys and passes out of the body through urine.

The liver also controls the synthesis and removal of cholesterol in the body, which has a crucial role in the production of hormones.

LET'S TALK ABOUT THE LIVER AND DETOXIFICATION

The liver has a primary role in storing and releasing energy, but let's break down the vital role it plays in helping us eliminate toxins from our body.

The liver begins the process of making toxins less harmful to the body and removing them from the bloodstream, by receiving blood with nutrients from the digestive organs via a vein known as the hepatic portal vein. The hepatocytes (cells of the liver), accept and filter this blood. They act as little sorting centers, determining which nutrients should be processed, what should be stored, what should be eliminated via the stool, and what should be diverted back to the blood. In fact, as a last resort, the liver will even store toxins itself to protect the rest of the body!!

The liver filters toxins that enter or are produced by the body through an area called the sinusoid channels, which are lined with immune cells called Kupffer cells. These Kupffer cells engulf the "toxin", digest, and excrete it. This process is called phagocytosis.

As many chemicals are relatively "new", it may take thousands of years from an evolutionary standpoint before our body properly adapts to them. The main takeaway here is, if the liver cannot figure out what to do with a substance, it may simply store the substance(s), often in fat tissue, in other organs, or in the liver itself. This is potentially damaging to any of the tissues or organs involved in this process.

Check out these following videos for more information on how the liver functions and the detoxification process works.

https://www.youtube.com/watch?app=desktop&v=wbh3SjzydnQ

https://www.khanacademy.org/science/in-in-class-11-biology-india/
x9d1157914247c627:digestion-and-absorption/x9d1157914247c627:digestive-glands/v/liver

For a deeper dive on the removal of xenobiotics (substances that are foreign to the body or to an ecological system), check out this informative video https://www.youtube.com/watch?v=zkS7PZUE27g&t=425s

So now, let's break down detox even further. The detoxification of substances that require elimination or results in storage in the body is thought to take place in three phases.

PHASE I

Two of the key phases of detox, Phase I and II, occur in the liver.

The first phase of detoxification occurs mostly in the liver and helps to transform potentially harmful lipid soluble (substances that dissolve in fat) molecules, into less harmful substances that will be easier for the body to excrete. This must occur prior to proceeding to phase II of detoxification.

In Phase I, a group of enzymes called cytochrome p450 enables the transformation of dangerous substances into less harmful substances through the chemical processes of oxidation (oxidation is a process in which a chemical substance changes because of the addition of oxygen), reduction (when a chemical substance loses an oxygen), hydration (when a chemical substance mixes with water), dehalogenation (a process when harmful compounds known as halogens are removed and converted to a more stable product), and hydrolysis (a reaction where water is used to break down a substance further).

These chemical changes require the activity of cytochrome p450 enzymes, as well as a variety of nutrients, to both support the activity of enzymes, and neutralize harmful molecules known as free radicals formed as a result of these processes. If free radicals are not neutralized, they can result in inflammation in the body. Many nutrients play a key role in phase I and the neutralizing of free radicals, including a variety of B vitamins, amino acids, vitamin C, zinc, vitamin A, and flavonoids.

Genetic issues, liver damage, nutrient deficiencies, and certain toxins can all impair the activity of p450 enzymes, reducing the ability of the liver to detoxify. Exposure to certain chemicals increases phase I activity, leading to a high production of phase I end products. If these products are not converted by phase II, they can be harmful to cellular DNA and RNA, and may be linked to diseases such as Parkinson's and cancer.

PHASE II

In phase II, the focus is on a process called conjugation. In conjugation, there is the addition of a chemical group to the by-product that was produced in phase I, making it water soluble and subsequently less harmful. Once the substance becomes water soluble, it can be excreted through the kidneys and intestines in the form of urine and bile.

There are many processes of conjugation. These include glutathionylation, methylation, glucuronidation, sulfation, and acetylation. Each of these processes involves the addition of a different substance to a phase I end-product, requiring specific nutrients, mostly amino acids, which must be obtained from our diet. Without these specific nutrients, phase II detoxification can be impaired. If phase II detoxification becomes impaired, an accumulation of phase I products occurs, resulting in inflammation and tissue damage in the body.

However, if phase I and II occur effectively, toxins can be eliminated by the kidneys and bowels via urine and stool. Although the liver is thought of as our primary detoxification organ, it requires a large variety of nutrients that must first be absorbed via the digestive system, in order to function optimally. Ironically though, the digestive system is also the initial site of exposure to ingested toxins. Due to these factors, it is recognized that there is an additional third phase of detoxification which occurs primarily in the digestive system.

PHASE III

The third phase of detoxification refers to a highly concentrated anti-porter (transport) system of proteins in the body. There are many anti-porters being researched, particularly P-glycoprotein, an anti-porter in the small intestine that moves toxins from cells into the gut. Another important protein known as blood-brain protein, is located in the kidneys, the blood brain barrier, and the liver. This transport system ensures the movement of harmful compounds out of the cell and into the detoxification organs.

A healthy diet and microbiome are key to the success of phase III, whereas digestive inflammation leads to the impairment of it. If phase III is compromised, an accumulation of toxins within the cell occurs. Errors in P-glycoprotein expression have been linked to Alzheimer's disease, and suspected to play a role in stress management and inflammatory bowel disease.

Due to the importance of these three phases, inefficient detoxification in any of the three phases can be detrimental.

Because of the constant stress placed on our detoxification systems, following a plan like The Livy Method which consistently supports these three phases can greatly help to also support our detoxification system and help keep us healthy! Let's talk more about strategies to best support our body in detox.

LIMIT ALCOHOL

More than 90% of alcohol is metabolized in your liver. Liver enzymes convert alcohol to a substance called acetaldehyde, a known cancer-causing chemical. Recognizing acetaldehyde as a toxin, your liver converts it to a harmless substance called acetate, which is later eliminated from your body.

Excessive drinking can severely damage liver function by causing fat buildup, inflammation, and scarring. When this happens, your liver cannot function properly and perform its necessary tasks, including filtering waste and other toxins from your body. Therefore, limiting alcohol can keep the liver healthy, thus supporting the body in detox.

FOCUS ON SLEEP

Ensuring adequate and quality sleep each night can help to support your body's health and natural detoxification system.

Sleeping allows your brain to reorganize and recharge itself, as well as remove toxic waste byproducts that have accumulated throughout the day. A waste product that the body produces is a protein called beta-amyloid, which contributes to the development of Alzheimer's disease. With sleep deprivation, your body does not have time to perform these functions, thus toxins can build up, affecting several aspects of health.

Poor sleep has been linked to health issues such as stress, anxiety, high blood pressure, heart disease, type 2 diabetes, and obesity. It is suggested to get at least seven to nine hours of good quality sleep per night, on a regular basis to promote good health and a healthy detoxification system. This is a foundational recommendation of The Livy Method!

DRINK ENOUGH WATER

Water and adequate hydration have a huge impact on how the body functions. Water regulates your body temperature, lubricates joints, aids digestion and nutrient absorption, and detoxifies your body by removing waste products.

Your body's cells must continuously be repaired to function optimally and break down nutrients for your body to use as energy. However, these processes release waste in the form of urea and carbon dioxide, which cause harm if able to build up in your blood.

Water allows for transport of these waste products, efficiently removing them through urination, breathing, or sweating. By increasing your water intake, your body reduces the secretion of the antidiuretic hormone and increases urination, eliminating more water and waste products. Thus, proper hydration is very important for detoxification of the body and to keep us healthy!

REDUCE YOUR INTAKE OF SUGAR AND PROCESSED FOODS

Sugar and processed foods are thought to be one of the root causes of today's public health crises. The increased consumption of sugary and highly processed foods has been linked to obesity and other chronic diseases, such as heart disease, cancer, and diabetes.

These diseases hinder your body's ability to naturally detoxify itself by harming organs that play an important role in the process, such as your liver and kidneys. For example, the high consumption of sugary beverages can cause **fatty liver disease**, a condition that negatively impacts liver function as discussed in the science posts on digestion. By following a healthful plan like The Livy Method during the weight loss process and in maintenance, by focusing on the foods that make you feel good, you can keep your body's detoxification system healthy in the long term.

However, with the onset of a diet and lifestyle change when initiating a program like The Livy Method, many people can experience symptoms from these changes. These changes are described in the program as detox.

SYMPTOMS OF DETOX

One of the common reactions to a healthier lifestyle/diet change is the onset of headaches.

Detox headaches are often caused by your body's reaction to missing an item, such as sugar or caffeine, that was habitually present. This may result in:

- a reduction in circulating hormones
- toxins such as chemical food additives or drugs leaching into your circulation to be eliminated
- a release of energy from tension and stress

However, headaches may also be a result of low sodium. Be sure to be mindful of adding in good salts like pink Himalayan, Celtic, and Sea Salts to your diet throughout the day! The low sodium post is a great one to refer to if you have any questions about this.

Along with headaches, other symptoms of detox may include:

- fatigue
- irritability
- hunger pangs
- rashes/breakouts
- diarrhea

These symptoms may be called various names including healing reactions, cleansing reactions, detox symptoms, and healing crises.

EAT ANTIOXIDANT RICH FOODS

Antioxidants protect your cells against damage caused by molecules called free radicals. Oxidative stress is a condition caused by excessive production of free radicals. Your body naturally produces these molecules in everyday cellular processes, such as digestion. However, alcohol, tobacco smoke, a poor diet, and exposure to pollutants, can also produce excessive free radicals in the body. By causing damage to your body's cells, these molecules have been implicated in a number of conditions, such as dementia, heart disease, liver disease, asthma, and certain types of cancer.

However, eating a diet rich in antioxidants can help your body fight oxidative stress caused by excess free radicals and other toxins that increase your risk of disease. Examples of antioxidants include vitamin A, vitamin C, vitamin E, selenium, lycopene, lutein, and zeaxanthin. Foods like berries, fruits, nuts, cocoa, vegetables, spices, and beverages like coffee and green tea, have some of the highest amounts of antioxidants.

EAT MORE CRUCIFEROUS VEGETABLES, LEGUMES, NUTS/SEEDS, AND LEAFY GREENS

Cruciferous vegetables and leafy greens are not only high in fiber and dense with nutrients, vitamins and minerals, but help the body engage in and support each phase of the detoxification pathway. They also support the microbiome and organs involved in detoxification! A review in the Journal of Nutrition and Metabolism notes clinical evidence of the effects from cruciferous vegetables, allium vegetables (such as garlic, onions, leeks, chives, scallions, and shallots), apiaceous vegetables (such as carrots, parsnips, celery, parsley), grapefruit, fish oil, foods that contain daidzein (found in abundance in legumes, especially in soybeans, but are present in many other vegetables, fruits, nuts, peas, lentils, and seeds), and eating food high in antioxidants have a profoundly positive nutritional impact on the detoxification process (Hodges, R. E., & Minich, D. M., 2015). The Livy Method recommends eating lots of vegetables, many of which include cruciferous vegetables (there is even a post about them), leafy greens, legumes, nuts, and seeds which will all support your body in detox!

EAT FOODS HIGH IN PREBIOTICS AND CONSIDER PROBIOTICS

Gut health is important for keeping your detoxification system healthy. Your intestinal cells have a detoxification and excretion system that protects your gut and body from harmful toxins, such as chemicals. Good gut health starts with prebiotics, a type of fiber that feeds the good bacteria in your gut called probiotics. With prebiotics, your good bacteria are able to produce nutrients called short-chain fatty acids that are beneficial for health.

The "good" bacteria in your gut can become unbalanced with "bad" bacteria from the use of antibiotics, poor dental hygiene, and a diet of poor quality.

Consequently, this unhealthy shift in bacteria can weaken your immune and detoxification system, increasing your risk of disease and inflammation. Eating foods rich in prebiotics can keep your immune and detoxification systems healthy. Good food sources of prebiotics include tomatoes, artichokes, bananas, asparagus, onions, garlic, and oats.

Take a good prebiotic, as well as a probiotic, both of which are recommended supplements of The Livy Method.

GET ACTIVE

Regular exercise is associated with a longer life and a reduced risk of many conditions and diseases, including type 2 diabetes, heart disease, high blood pressure, and certain cancers which have been discussed in previous science posts.

While there are several mechanisms behind the health benefits of exercise, reduced inflammation is a key factor. While some inflammation is necessary for recovering from infection or healing wounds, too much of it weakens your body's systems and promotes disease.

By reducing inflammation, exercise can help your body's systems including its detoxification system, function properly and protect against disease.

When maximizing The Livy Method, incorporating exercise will help the body support the detoxification system.

CAN I SWEAT OUT TOXINS THAT ARE IN MY BODY?

With some forms of exercise your body works up a sweat that helps to cool your body down. You may have also heard that sitting in a sauna, hot tub, or going to a hot yoga class will help your body sweat out toxins. However, your sweat is 99% water, and the rest of the 1% is composed of: electrolytes and minerals like sodium, potassium, calcium, and magnesium (It is important to replace them after periods of heavy sweating!); small amounts of pheromones, which are chemicals that act like hormones outside of your body; bacteria that grow in the sweat that you release and can cause body odor; and tiny amounts of toxins. Trace amounts of metals and other chemicals can be present in your sweat, but your kidneys and liver do most of the work when it comes to getting rid of toxins in the body. Therefore, what you eat has a bigger impact when it comes to eliminating toxins in the body. That being said, saunas, hot yoga, hot tubs, and warm baths can be very relaxing with other health benefits, so can still have a positive impact on your health. However, if you have health issues such as cardiovascular disease, issues with blood pressure, or are pregnant, consult with your health care provider before using these types of heat-based therapies.

OTHER HELPFUL DETOX TIPS

Although no current evidence supports the use of detox diets for removing toxins from your body, certain dietary changes and lifestyle practices may help reduce toxin load and support your body's detoxification system.

- **Eat sulfur-containing foods**

  Food high in sulfur, such as onions, broccoli, and garlic, enhance excretion of heavy metals like cadmium.

- **Try out chlorella**

  Chlorella is a type of algae that has many nutritional benefits, and may enhance the elimination of toxins like heavy metals, according to animal studies.

- **Flavor dishes with cilantro**

Cilantro enhances excretion of certain toxins, such as heavy metals like lead, and chemicals, including phthalates and insecticides.

- **Support glutathione**

  Eating sulfur-rich foods like eggs, broccoli, and garlic helps enhance the function of glutathione, a major antioxidant produced by your body that is heavily involved in detoxification.

- **Avoid the use of plastic and aluminum for heating and storing food**

  Use stainless steel or glass containers over plastic ones for foods and beverages. Avoid heating foods in plastic containers, and if using plastic containers, opt for ones featuring the BPA-free and phthalate-free labels.

- **Switch to natural cleaning products**

  Choosing natural cleaning products like vinegar and baking soda over commercial cleaning agents can reduce your exposure to potentially toxic chemicals.

- **Choose natural body care**

  Using natural deodorants, makeups, moisturizers, shampoos, and other personal care products can also reduce your exposure to chemicals. While promising, many of these effects have only been shown in animal studies. Therefore, studies in humans are needed to confirm these findings.

Hopefully you learned a bit more about the detox process and how by focusing on better nutrition, sleeping well, exercise, and positive lifestyle changes, will not only limit your exposure to chemicals, but help your body process them out optimally!

REFERENCES

https://www.sciencedirect.com/topics/earth-and-planetary-sciences/toxin

https://www.sciencedirect.com/topics/medicine-and-dentistry/detoxication

https://www.sciencedirect.com/topics/agricultural-and-biological-sciences/daidzein#:~:text=Daidzein%20and%20genistein%20are%20in,peas%2C%20lentils%2C%20and%20seeds.

Balingit, A., & Nall, R. (2022, January 24). *The liver.* Healthline. https://www.healthline.com/human-body-maps/liver#keep-liver-healthy

Bjarnadottir, A. (2019, January 10). *Do detox diets and cleanses really work?* Healthline. https://www.healthline.com/nutrition/detox-diets-101#methods

Collins. (n.d.). Oxidation. In *Collinsdictionary.com dictionary.* Retrieved March 30, 2022, from https://www.collinsdictionary.com/us/dictionary/english/

oxidation#:~:text=(Pharmaceutical%3A%20Physiology)-,Oxidation%20 is%20a%20process%20in%20which%20a%20chemical%20substance%20 changes,involves%20the%20oxidation%20of%20magnesium.

Detoxification. (n.d.). The Hepatitis C Trust. Retrieved March 30, 2022, from http://hepctrust. org.uk/information/liver/detoxification#:~:text=The%20liver%20filters%20toxins%20 through,body%20properly%20adapts%20to%20them.

Detoxes and cleanses: What you need to know. (2019, September). National Center for Complementary and Integrative Health. Retrieved March 30, 2022, from https://www.nccih.nih.gov/health/ detoxes-and-cleanses-what-you-need-to-know

Dietary supplement ingredient advisory list. (2021, October 29). U.S. Food & Drug Administration. Retrieved March 30, 2022, from https://www.fda.gov/food/ dietary-supplement-products-ingredients/dietary-supplement-ingredient-advisory-list#updates

Han, S., & Frothingham, S. (2018, July 17). *Dealing with a detox headache.* Healthline. https://www. healthline.com/health/detox-headache

Higdon, J., Drake, V. J., Delage, B., & Traka, M. (2017, April). *Cruciferous vegetables.* Oregon State University. https://lpi.oregonstate.edu/mic/food-beverages/cruciferous-vegetables

Higdon, J., Drake, V. J., & McCann, S. (2021, March). *Lignans.* Oregon State University. https://lpi. oregonstate.edu/mic/dietary-factors/phytochemicals/lignans

Hodges, R. E., & Minich, D. M. (2015). Modulation of metabolic detoxification pathways using foods and food-derived components: A scientific review with clinical application. *Journal of Nutrition and Metabolism, 2015,* 760689. https://doi.org/10.1155/2015/760689

Institute for Quality and Efficiency in Health Care (IQWiG). (2016, August 19). *How does the liver work?* https://www.ncbi.nlm.nih.gov/books/NBK279393/

Jackson, E., Shoemaker, R., Larian, N., & Cassis, L. (2017). Adipose tissue as a site of toxin accumulation. *Comprehensive Physiology, 7*(4), 1085–1135. https://doi.org/10.1002/cphy.c160038

Jung, J.S., Kim, W.L., Park, B.H., Lee, S.O., & Chae, S.W. (2020). Effect of toxic trace element detoxification, body fat reduction following four-week intake of the wellnessup diet: a three-arm, randomized clinical trial. *Nutrition & Metabolism, 17, 47.* https://doi. org/10.1155/2015/760689

Kuczma, M. (n.d.). *Understanding the 3 phases of detoxification. Integrative Naturopathic Medical Centre.* https://integrative.ca/blog/3-phases-detoxification

Lang, A., & Rose-Francis, K. (2022, February 11). *What are obesogens, and should we be concerned? Healthline.* https://www.healthline.com/nutrition/what-are-obesogens

Liver: Anatomy and functions. (n.d.). Johns Hopkins Medicine. Retrieved March 30, 2022, from https://www.hopkinsmedicine.org/health/conditions-and-diseases/liver-anatomy-and-functions

Loconti, C., & Begum, J. (2021, December 1). *What to know about sweating.* WebMD. https://www.webmd.com/skin-problems-and-treatments/what-to-know-about-sweating

Narayan, R. [Khanacademymedicine]. (2014, May 15). *Liver | Gastrointestinal system physiology | NCLEX-RN* [Video]. Youtube. https://www.youtube.com/watch?v=rDjWrNRKfvg

Natural health products. (2022, March 22). Government of Canada. Retrieved March 30, 2022, from https://www.canada.ca/en/health-canada/services/drugs-health-products/natural-non-prescription.html

Natural health products ingredients database. (2022, March 25). Health Canada. Retrieved March 30, 2022, from http://webprod.hc-sc.gc.ca/nhpid-bdipsn/atReq.do?atid=whats.quoi&lang=eng

Ninja Nerd. (2018, June 11). *Gastrointestinal | Biotransformation of drugs and toxins* [Video]. Youtube. https://www.youtube.com/watch?v=zkS7PZUE27g&t=425s

Organ systems: Detoxification. (n.d.). Texas A&M College of Veterinary Medicine & Biomedical Sciences. Retrieved March 30, 2022, from https://vetmed.tamu.edu/peer/detoxification/

Peterson, S., Lampe, J. W., Bammler, T. K., Gross-Steinmeyer, K., & Eaton, D. L. (2006). Apiaceous vegetable constituents inhibit human cytochrome P-450 1A2 (hCYP1A2) activity and hCYP1A2-mediated mutagenicity of aflatoxin B1. *Food and Chemical Toxicology, 44*(9), 1474–1484. https://doi.org/10.1016/j.fct.2006.04.010

Petre, A. (2018, October 3). *Lycopene: health benefits and top food sources.* Healthline. https://www.healthline.com/nutrition/lycopene#cancer

Salehi, B., Mishra, A. P., Nigam, M., Sener, B., Kilic, M., Sharifi-Rad, M., Fokou, P., Martins, N., & Sharifi-Rad, J. (2018). Resveratrol: A double-edged sword in health benefits. *Biomedicines, 6*(3), 91. https://doi.org/10.3390/biomedicines6030091

Seitz, A., & Seitz, D. (2021, June 14). *The truth about the lemon water detox.* Healthline. https://www.healthline.com/health/lemon-water-detox-the-truth

Tainted weight loss products. (2022, March 22). U.S. Food & Drug Administration. Retrieved March 30, 2022, from https://www.fda.gov/drugs/medication-health-fraud/tainted-weight-loss-products

TED. (2021, July 8). *A cleanse won't detox your body but here's what will | Body stuff with dr. jen gunter* [Video]. Youtube. https://www.youtube.com/watch?v=DESCcjSQSKY

TED-Ed. (2014, November 25). *What does the liver do? - Emma bryce* [Video]. Youtube. https://www.youtube.com/watch?app=desktop&v=wbh3SjzydnQ

U.S. Food and Drug Administration. (2013, January 29). *Being fooled by empty diet promises* [Video]. Youtube. https://www.youtube.com/watch?v=wcdO6dDnUKE

Van De Wall, G. (2019, March 10). *Full body detox: 9 ways to rejuvenate your body.* Healthline. https://www.healthline.com/nutrition/how-to-detox-your-body

Woreta, T. (n.d.). *Detoxing your liver: Fact versus fiction.* Johns Hopkins Medicine. https://www.hopkinsmedicine.org/health/wellness-and-prevention/detoxing-your-liver-fact-versus-fiction

Zeratsky, K. (2020, April 18). *Do detox diets offer any health benefits?* Mayo Clinic. https://www.mayoclinic.org/healthy-lifestyle/nutrition-and-healthy-eating/expert-answers/detox-diets/faq-20058040

THE MIGRATING MOTOR COMPLEX (MMC) AND HUNGER

We are continuing the conversation on digestion (who knew there was so much to discuss!!!) The goal of these posts is to help provide some foundational information and create an understanding of how our bodies function. We will also discuss how implementing The Livy Method optimizes our health, wellness, and mindfulness, by providing an environment where our bodies no longer feel the need to store fat!

YOUR STOMACH IS "GROWLING", IS THIS A SIGN THAT YOU ARE HUNGRY AND NEED TO EAT?

Many of us growing up have learned to associate our stomach "growling" or noises coming from our abdomen, with hunger and the need to eat! In fact, many of us feel the immediate need to take action and eat as soon as we receive these signals from our bodies. But does this mean we are hungry and we should eat? This is one of the most common questions that our members have when they begin the journey of the Livy Method as they initiate the process of becoming more in tune with their bodies.

So, why do our stomachs and abdomens make these noises, and how do we distinguish some of the things that our body does (like our stomach churning, rumbling and growling) with the actual need to eat? Is it because we are hungry?

HUNGER

The feeling of "hunger" is fairly complex and can be affected by many things. Hunger can be influenced by physical/physiological, emotional, social, economic and mental factors, and can be a difficult thing to gauge at times.

In fact, many of us have lost touch with our hunger signals at a young age or never really become in tune with them in the first place. We may have become so detached from understanding or recognizing these cues because of the influence of our family, social/economic factors, years of dieting and cycles of deprivation, over training and exercise, and eating when we are not hungry because we are following a set number of calories or macros determined by others in the diet industry. It's no wonder that we do not even know where to start!

But not to worry!! These signals are still there, and an imperative part of The Livy Method process is reconnecting our members with these very important signals that their body provides to them!!

HOW CAN YOU GET BACK IN TOUCH WITH YOUR HUNGER SIGNALS?

JOURNALING AND SELF-REFLECTION

The Livy Method recommends journaling as a complementary process to the program as it can have a great benefit to the overall weight loss process. Also, as mentioned in the science post Issues with Digestion, can help identify any foods that have an impact on your digestion, as well as identify potential intolerances.

Journaling your feels/emotions and highlighting external factors such as stress, exercise/activity, and boredom can give you great insight into how your feelings, patterns, or behaviours, may influence your eating when not necessarily hungry. Using the traditional pen to paper process, or using the WLBG APP is a great way to do this!

If you are the type of person that needs a more **quantitative (quantitative data refers to any information that can be quantified, counted or measured, and given a numerical value)** way of understanding things, the use of a measurement tool such as a **hunger scale** may be of benefit to you!

A **hunger scale** is a tool that can help you learn how to identify the difference between actual physical hunger and the "feeling" of hunger that may be brought on by emotions like stress, boredom, sadness, or happiness.

Checking in and asking yourself the first two Mindfulness questions is a great way to assess this; but let's take this a step further by using a hunger scale.

Check out an example of a great hunger scale from Alberta Health Services! There are also additional questions and considerations that can help clarify the concept of eating to satisfaction.

https://www.albertahealthservices.ca/assets/info/nutrition/if-nfs-hunger-and-fullness-signals. pdf?fbclid=IwAR2m9j2uy8XsnUdcUQxAI6DX5T9fUMJDVErkWKVEhS-rsYw_E2h4WJ9KaVI

BEFORE YOU EAT, ASK YOURSELF IF YOU ARE HUNGRY?

When serving or portioning out your food and before you eat ask yourself; How is this portion for me? How would I feel if I ate all of this?

When you start feeling like you want something to eat, rate your hunger on a scale of 1 to 10, with 1 being overwhelmingly hungry and 10 being so full you feel sick. A rating of 5 or 6 means you are comfortable, neither too hungry nor too full. When you feel hungry even though you recently ate, check to see if what you are feeling is really a craving brought on by something psychological or emotional. The goal is to bring awareness to your changing hunger levels. For example, sometimes you are really hungry but then when you eat, you feel full fast. Other times you are not hungry at all, but when you start to eat, you feel hungry. Both are completely normal to experience!

You may not get a really strong response or any answer from your body at first, but trust that once you begin this process of talking to yourself and taking the time to listen, your body will start to talk back!

WHILE EATING YOUR FOOD, PAY ATTENTION TO HOW YOU FEEL AND ASK YOURSELF:

Are you getting full, is this food satisfying you? How would you feel if you took a few more bites? How would you feel if you stop eating now? Do you feel any physical effects of eating? On the scale of 1-10 how are you feeling and where do you fall on that hunger scale?

WHEN YOU ARE DONE EATING, ASK YOURSELF HOW YOU FEEL:

Do you feel full and if so, what is your definition of full? How do you know when you have eaten enough? How do you feel physically; energetic, comfortable, tired? Are you just eating everything on your plate because it is there? Or maybe you feel like you could eat more? Again, you can rate how you feel on the scale from 1-10 to see where you fall with the goal being about a 5 or a 6!

In terms of journaling and using the scale as a tool to assess satisfaction, reflecting on when and what you eat, as well as what you were doing and feeling before you started eating can be really insightful in helping to identify psychological triggers for eating when you are not hungry. This may also help to identify habitual patterns of eating when you are not truly hungry. An example of this is wanting to eat a late-night snack while watching television, because this is a nightly ritual that you indulge in on evenings.

Here are a few more tips for assessing hunger devised by the University of Michigan Medicine (Healthwise Staff 2020, September 23), that very much align with the philosophy of The Livy Method:

- Try not to let your hunger drop to a 1 or 2 on the hunger scale. When you get that hungry, you are likely to eat faster, make poorer food choices, and keep eating past the "satisfied" point.

- On the other hand, let yourself feel **some** hunger between meals. Mild hunger is a good thing. After all, it›s a sign that you are not overeating. Teach yourself to appreciate hunger pangs as a natural part of life, and as a sign that you are a healthy eater.

- Give cravings 10 minutes. When you suddenly feel the need to eat, tell yourself that you will wait 10 minutes. If it was only a craving, you will have forgotten about it by then, and the urge will be gone. If 10 minutes goes by and you still have the urge to eat, you may be starting to get hungry. Also keep in mind, if you are craving something sweet, you may need more water, and if you are craving something salty, you may need more fat or salt!

- Don't eat more now because you think you might not have time to eat later. Eat what your body needs now, and worry about later, later.

- Does leaving food on your plate bother you? Take smaller servings. Save leftovers for another meal. Share plates with someone. Ask yourself what is more important—a few bites of "wasted" food, or your health? This aligns with the Ginaism, "your body is not a garbage can"! This is truly a very impactful statement when framing leaving food on your plate!

- When you eat, make your food the main attraction. Sit down at the table with your family. Do not eat in front of the TV. Do not read while you eat. Give your attention to what you are putting in your mouth, how it tastes, and how your body reacts to what and how much you are eating.

Hopefully you found these tips helpful!

OK so after tuning in, you have determined that you are not "feeling" hungry and still have time before you could eat your next meal or snack. However, your stomach is rumbling...Should you still eat?

This is a great question, so let's take a deeper dive into answering this!

GASTRO INTESTINAL (GI) INNERVATION AND FUNCTION

As discussed in The Basics of Digestion, our digestive system, from our esophagus to our anus, is made up of a special type of muscle called smooth muscle. Smooth muscle, which like other muscles in our body, contracts and relaxes. However, this mostly occurs automatically in our bodies without our conscious thought, although we do have some control over some aspects of it, such as the act of eating or having a bowel movement.

See this video for more detail about smooth muscle!

https://www.youtube.com/watch?v=yh4bUdnU2MQ

Our digestive system is controlled by our central nervous system (CNS), and something called the enteric nervous system (ENS). These systems control our digestive processes primarily motility (a term used to describe the contraction of the muscles that mix and propel [move forward] the contents in the GI tract), the secretion of hormones and enzymes important to hunger, satiety and digestion, the absorption of nutrients in digestion, and regulates blood flow to the digestive system. Our digestive system is often referred to as the "second brain" (containing as many neurons as the spinal cord!) because of the amazing capabilities it has to perform many of these functions without consulting the brain! However, that being said, our digestive system is still influenced by the **SNS (sympathetic nervous system) and the (PSNS) parasympathetic nervous system** as we had discussed in the article Issues With Digestion.

Check out this great short video about the ENS!

https://www.youtube.com/watch?v=lGdauJ9Fcdc

Normal gastrointestinal motility results from the coordinated contractions of the smooth muscle in the digestive system. There are 2 fundamental patterns of movement conducted by the digestive system, **propulsion** and **segmentation contractions**.

Propulsion is when the broken-down food (bolus) is propelled in a forward motion along the length of the digestive tube for the purposes of digestion and elimination (bowel movement). This movement is accomplished by **peristalsis**. In peristalsis, the smooth muscle contracts in a "ring" like form in front of the bolus (mouth side), propelling the bolus in the direction of the anus. The muscles on the opposite side of the bolus relax to allow the bolus to pass, and occur until the bolus is broken down, absorbed and eliminated from the body.

Check out this video to see what peristalsis looks like!

https://www.youtube.com/watch?v=kVjeNZA5pi4

As discussed in the last few posts, the majority of absorption occurs in the small intestine. For the purpose of optimal absorption, a movement involving **mixing** and a movement called **segmentation**, facilitates the combining of the ingested food with the secretions and enzymes needed for breaking down the carbohydrates, proteins and fats. These macronutrients are broken down into the smaller components needed to support body function, as well as allow for the extended time needed for absorption via the wall of the small intestine.

In segmentation, the muscular rings of the smooth muscle alternate between a state of contraction and relaxation of the muscles along the wall of the intestines, which promote the effective mixing of its contents. This movement is not meant to propel the contents forward. Segmentation's primary role is for mixing and allowing the time needed for optimal absorption of nutrients, vitamins, and minerals at the bowel wall.

Check out this video to see how segmentation facilitates absorption!

https://www.youtube.com/watch?v=ATXMxRPRPfU

SO, WHAT HAPPENS WHEN THE FOOD WE HAVE EATEN IS DIGESTED?

The migrating motor complex (MMC) also known as the migrating motility complex

The MMC is a distinct pattern of muscular activity observed in gastrointestinal smooth muscle during the periods between eating, after most of the food that has been ingested has been digested.

The MMC is often referred to as the "housekeeper" of the digestive system. These muscular contractions facilitate the movement or "sweeping" of any residual undigested material through the digestive system.

Although the majority of our bacterial gut flora live in our colon or large intestine (which aid in digestion and promote the production of B vitamins and vitamin K), there is a small proportion of bacteria that do live in our small intestine. An important part of the MMC and its movement of undigested foods through our digestive tract is to prevent the proliferation or growth of these bacteria, which can lead to something called **SIBO or small intestine bacterial overgrowth.** So, the big takeaway here is that the MMC has a very important role in keeping us healthy and preventing the overgrowth of bacteria in our digestive system!

The MMC also stimulates peristalsis, which is important in moving food through our digestive system and out of our bodies (by the way of bowel movements) but interestingly, the MMC is stimulated and **only functions when we are not eating!**

The MMC is thought to be controlled by the CNS and elicited by the hormone **motilin**. The MMC is elicited when the body is in a "non-fed" state in a cycle that recurs every 1.5 to 2 hours, and consists of four distinct phases or stages. When the body is ready to stimulate the MMC to initiate its "housekeeping" of the digestive tract, motilin is released from the upper portion of the small intestine. However, all that one needs to do to halt this process, is to initiate eating again.

Stage 1 is initiated by a quiet period with minimal muscular activity. There is only the occasional contraction occurring in the digestive system, lasting approximately 45-60 minutes.

Stage 2 is about 30 minutes in duration. In this stage, peristalsis increases in intensity and occurrence. Peristalsis starts in the stomach and is directed towards the small intestine.

Stage 3 is about 5 to 15 minutes in duration and is initiated by the occurrence of rapid evenly spaced peristaltic contractions. The **pylorus** (lower part of the stomach connecting to the duodenum of the small intestine) remains open during these peristaltic contractions, allowing indigestible materials to pass into the small intestine. This is in contrast to what occurs during the ingestion of food.

After the completion of stage 3, there is a short period of time that elapses before these stages all begin again. This transition period is stage 4!

Interestingly, while the MMC is activated, there is an increase in gastric, biliary, and pancreatic secretions seen with this contractile activity, which also likely assists in controlling the bacterial population in the upper segments of the digestive system.

MYTH BUSTER- A growling stomach does not necessarily mean hunger it is likely the MMC in action.

As you can see, a "growling" stomach, even after a meal, does not mean you are hungry! This is the stimulation of your very important MMC doing its very important job of cleaning out your digestive tract and keeping you healthy!

The Livy Method and how it promotes an optimal functioning MMC

1. A healthy digestive system promotes a healthy MMC! The focus of The Livy Method is to improve and optimize digestion and absorption, and although the MMC is engaged in the periods we are not eating, they both go hand in hand.

2. Although we are eating fairly frequently at least 6 times a day, we still have up to 3.5 hours in between meals and snacks that allows for the MMC to engage. Because we are not eating to the point of being over-full, and likely eating smaller amounts when eating to satisfaction, we are more likely to stimulate the MMC earlier than we might have in the past! Also, this is a means to an end in the pursuit of weight loss and change. Eventually, as we complete maintenance, we will not necessarily be eating this often unless it's what our body needs!

3. The recommendation of eating our dinner earlier in the evening and to minimize late night snacking is also in line with optimizing the role of the MMC. The body can focus on rest and repair, and allow the MMC a good period of time overnight to do its thing!

4. The Livy Method promotes prioritizing restful sleep, selfcare and stress management techniques that reduce cortisol levels and helps keep hormones in homeostasis, preventing us from "stressing" our digestive system or impairing the function of the MMC!

The following are a couple of videos that discuss digestion and the MMC in greater detail if you are interested!

https://www.youtube.com/watch?v=3Bl1wknR1lc

This is a great video on motility. Discussion of the MMC starts at about 10:35 min of the video if you choose to skip ahead.

https://www.coursera.org/lecture/physiology/helpUrl-nUnNY

Hopefully, this post has given you more insight into the amazing MMC, the importance of digestion and how the foods we choose impact our health, the concept of hunger, and how using the tools and strategies discussed may help in assessing your hunger better!

REFERENCES

https://www.sciencedirect.com/.../migrating-motor-complex

Al-Missri, M., & Jialal, I. (2021, September 28). *Physiology, motilin.* StatPearls Publishing. https://www.ncbi.nlm.nih.gov/books/NBK545309/…

Betts, G.J., Young, K.A., Wise, J.A., Johnson, E., Poe, B., Kruse, D.H., Korol, O., Johnson, J.E., Womble, M., & DeSaix, P. (2019, May 29). *Anatomy and physiology.* Openstax. https://opentextbc.ca/anatomyandph.../chapter/smooth-muscle/

Cabrey, J., & Jakoi, E. (n.d.). *Motility* [Video]. Coursera. https://www.coursera.org/lecture/physiology/helpUrl-nUnNY

Costa, M., Brookes, S.J.H., & Henning, G.W. (2000). Anatomy and physiology of the enteric nervous system. *Gut, 47*(4), iv15-iv19. http://dx.doi.org/10.1136/gut.47.suppl_4.iv15

Deloose, E., & Tack, J. (2016). Redefining the functional roles of the gastrointestinal migrating motor complex and motilin in small bacterial overgrowth and hunger signaling. *American Journal of Physiology, 310*(4), 228-233. https://doi.org/10.1152/ajpgi.00212.2015

Deloose, E., Janssen, P., Depoortere, I., & Tack, J. (2012). The migrating motor complex: control mechanisms and its role in health and disease. *Nature Reviews:Gastroenterology & Hepatology*, 9(5), 271–285. https://doi.org/10.1038/nrgastro.2012.57

Electrophysiology of gastrointestinal smooth muscle. (n.d.). Vivo Pathophysiology. Retrieved March 30, 2022, from http://www.vivo.colostate.edu/.../basics/slowwaves.html

Gastrointestinal motility and smooth muscle. (n.d.). Vivo Pathophysiology. Retrieved March 30, 2022, from http://www.vivo.colostate.edu/.../basics/gi_motility.html

Gastrointestinal transit: How long does it take? (n.d.). Vivo Pathophysiology. Retrieved March 30, 2022, from http://www.vivo.colostate.edu/.../dig.../basics/transit.html

Gorard, D.A., Vesselinova-Jenkins, C.K., Libby, G.W., & Farthing, M. (1995). Migrating motor complex and sleep in health and irritable bowel syndrome. *Digestive Diseases and Sciences*, 40(11), 2383–2389. https://doi.org/10.1007/BF02063242

Grundy, D., & Brookes, S. (2011). Neural control of gastrointestinal function. *Colloquium Series on Integrated Systems Physiology: From Molecule to Function, 3*(9), 1-134. (https://doi.org/10.4199/C00048ED1V01Y201111ISP030)

Healthwise Staff. (2020, September 23). *Healthy eating: Recognizing your hunger signals.* University of Michigan Health: Michigan Medicine. https://www.uofmhealth.org/health-library/zx3292

How long does it take to digest food: Breaking down digestion speed. (2021, April 19). Cleveland Clinic. Retrieved March 30, 2022, from https://health.clevelandclinic.org/how-long-does-it-take.../

Hunger and fullness signals. (2021, March). Alberta Health Services. Retrieved March 30, 2022, from https://www.albertahealthservices.ca/.../if-nfs-hunger…

Nao. (2017, March 21). Why does my tummy rumble? *Dr. How's Science Wows.* http://sciencewows.ie/blog/tag/migrating-motor-complex/

Takahashi, T. (2012). Mechanism of interdigestive migrating motor complex. *Journal of Neurogastroenterology and Motility, 18*(3), 246-257. https://doi.org/10.5056/jnm.2012.18.3.246

The migrating motor complex. (n.d.). Vivo Pathophysiology. Retrieved March 30, 2022, from http://www.vivo.colostate.edu/.../stomach/mmcomplex.html

Tomomasa, T., Morikawa, A., Sandler, R. H., Mansy, H. A., Koneko, H., Masahiko, T., Hyman, P. E., & Itoh, Z. (1999). Gastrointestinal sounds and migrating motor complex in fasted humans. *The American Journal of Gastroenterology*, 94(2), 374–381. https://doi.org/10.1111/j.1572-0241.1999.00862.x

HORMONES IMPORTANT TO WEIGHT LOSS & DIGESTION PART 1: INSULIN

Welcome back to our science posts where the goal is to help provide some foundational information and create an understanding of how our bodies function. We will also discuss how implementing The Livy Method optimizes our health, wellness, and mindfulness, by providing an environment where our bodies no longer feel the need to store fat!

Insulin, we have heard this word discussed throughout the program as an important part of The Livy Method process. We are encouraged to eat high quality foods, support our bodies with supplements if we can, approach eating to the point where we feel satisfied, incorporate some exercise or activity to move our bodies, manage our stress levels, and prioritize having good, restful sleep. All of these things will help not only improve our health, wellness, and promote weight loss, but will also help to naturally lower our insulin levels.

So, what exactly is insulin, and what exactly is its role in the body?

INSULIN

Insulin is a very important hormone in digestion, and has a huge role in helping to process and store the energy provided from the food that we eat! It is composed of 51 amino acids and for this reason is called a peptide hormone (hormones that are composed of small chains of amino acids). It plays an important part in glucose regulation, cell growth, and metabolism.

Insulin was previously believed to be solely produced by special cells in the pancreas called beta cells; however, recent evidence has shown that low concentrations are also found in certain neurons of the central nervous system!

As we have discussed in previous articles, the pancreas plays a principal part in digestion by producing hormones and enzymes that are crucial to the digestive process. However, this amazing organ also has a critical role in using and storing the energy (in the form of glucose) that it had just helped to break down and process, from the foods that we just ate!

So, let's back up this conversation a bit further. Let's recap the basics of digestion and then discuss how the foods we eat are processed for their energy.

SHORT RECAP ON DIGESTION

All parts of our body need energy to work, and this energy comes from the food we eat. As discussed, our bodies begin the digestive process when we think about and use our senses when preparing our food. When we ingest it, it begins mixing in with the saliva and enzymes in our mouths through the process of chewing. Then, the food bolus enters the stomach by way of the esophagus, and begins mixing with fluids (containing acids and enzymes) in the stomach. As the stomach churns and mixes, the food is processed and broken down further, resulting in reducing the carbohydrates we eat (sugars and starches) to their simplest form, a sugar called glucose. Proteins are broken down into amino acids and fat is broken down into fatty acids to be used by the body.

Glucose is the main energy source for our body's cells, and what keeps us functioning at all times whether it is when we are active and moving, resting and sleeping, it keeps our heart beating and lungs breathing. It is what allows all the organs and cells in our bodies to do what they need to do to keep us alive!

So, let's break it down even further, let's take a deeper look at what glucose actually is.

WHAT IS GLUCOSE?

Glucose is the simplest form of carbohydrates and only has one sugar molecule, which is called a **monosaccharide**. Other monosaccharides that may sound familiar include fructose, galactose, and ribose, which the body also processes or may produce for energy. To understand the differences, let's look at all these in more detail!

GLUCOSE

Glucose comes from the Greek word for "sweet" (Watson, S., & DerSarkissian, C. 2020, June 13). As discussed, glucose is a type of sugar you get from the foods you eat, and is what your body uses for energy. You may have heard the terms blood glucose or blood sugar, which are often used to describe the amount of glucose measured in your blood as it travels through your bloodstream to your cells. This can be quantified in a lab blood test, and results can be measured in that moment in time as a blood sugar, as a "fasted" blood sugar (taking your blood sugar after not eating or drinking for 8-12 hours), and as an A1C [which measures the percentage of hemoglobin (a protein in your red blood cells) that are coated in sugar, and can analyze your average blood sugar for the last 3 months].

Glucose is the most common monosaccharide found in nature. Some plants store glucose in linked chains. These chains are called starch. Common starch-containing foods include corn, potatoes, rice, and wheat. Glucose monosaccharides are also found naturally in some foods. The most concentrated whole food source of glucose monosaccharides are honey, followed by dried fruits such as dates, apricots, raisins, currants, cranberries, prunes and figs.

Most of the cells in your body use glucose along with amino acids (the building blocks of protein) and fats for energy. However, glucose is the main source of fuel for your brain. Nerve cells and chemical messengers located there need it to help them process information, and having access to glucose is very important for overall brain function. Your brain uses about 60% of the glucose that our bodies use. However, glucose does not always have to come immediately from foods and beverages. Glucose is also generated by the body to ensure that we always have the amount that is needed. One way that this is achieved is by breaking down something called glycogen, in order to free up the glucose it contains.

Glycogen is released by an important hormone called glucagon. When the body does not need to use glucose for energy, it is stored in the liver and muscles by insulin. This stored form of glucose is made up of many connected glucose molecules and is the glycogen. When the body needs a quick boost of energy or is not getting glucose from food, glycogen is broken down to release glucose into the bloodstream to be used as fuel for the cells. Your body can store enough glycogen in order to keep you fueled for about a day.

The body can also produce glucose through a process called gluconeogenesis. This process occurs when the body (mainly the liver, followed by the kidneys, and to a lesser extent the small intestine) makes glucose from non-carbohydrate sources which include lactate (what our bodies produce during exercise), glycerol (is produced when fats are digested, can be used for energy or stored in adipose tissue) and amino acids. Gluconeogenesis occurs when glycogen stores become low and glucose consumption is too low or nonexistent, such as during periods of starvation or prolonged fasting. Although the body has enough glycogen stored in the muscles and liver to last about a day, after about 14 hours in a fasted state it will begin to increase its percentage of gluconeogenesis, generating energy in increased ratios as time goes on (Chourpiliadis, C., & Mohiuddin, 2021).

One very important consideration is that skeletal muscle (composed of amino acids) can be used as a source when generating glucose through this pathway. This can lead to muscle wasting and loss over time, which can have a major impact on the body!

An additional alternative form of energy that can be generated if needed, is the formation of ketone bodies from our fat reserves. Ketone bodies can serve as a fuel source if glucose levels are too low in the body. Ketones serve as fuel in times of prolonged starvation, carbohydrate deprivation, or when patients suffer from uncontrolled diabetes and cannot utilize most of the circulating glucose. In these scenarios, fat stores are liberated, generating ketone bodies that are sent to the body and brain for energy.

This brings us to the conversation about the famous Keto diet that has been popularized in recent years. There seems to be a lot of compelling research arguing the benefits of using Keto as a means for weight loss. However, a recent study out of George Washington University School of Medicine examined available literature looking at the Keto diet (Crosby, L., Davis, B., Joshi, S., Jardine, M., Paul, J., Neola, M., & Barnard, N.D, 2021). They found that the diet was especially unsafe for pregnant women, women who may become pregnant, and those with kidney disease. They concluded that keto could also lead to long-term health complications, such as cancer, heart disease, and Alzheimer's Disease for most people. The rationale behind this was that this diet includes foods like meats, fish, nuts, and fibrous vegetables while eliminating most fruits, grains, beans, and starchy vegetables resulting in low vitamins, minerals, micro-nutrients and fiber intake. As we know from our last few Science Posts, these are all very important components of improving our overall digestion, microbiome and health! This study further corroborates the evidence that The Livy Method, which includes the food listed above, while minimizing added sugar, sets up our bodies for the best success!

If you want to go even further down the rabbit hole of understanding glucose at the chemical level, check out this video that discusses the structure of glucose in a more simplified way!

https://www.khanacademy.org/science/biology/macromolecules/carbohydrates-and-sugars/v/molecular-structure-of-glucose

GALACTOSE

The main dietary source of galactose comes in the form of lactose. Lactose is derived from milk and yogurt, and then digested and processed by the body, and broken down into the simpler forms of galactose and glucose. Interestingly, foods containing small amounts of free galactose include low-lactose or lactose-free milk, certain yogurts, cheeses, creams, ice cream, and other foods artificially sweetened with galactose. Plain natural foods like fruits, vegetables, nuts, grains, fresh meats, eggs, and milk, usually contain less than 0.3 g galactose per serving.

Galactose is not an essential nutrient! This means that you do not need to get it from food to be healthy, as galactose can be synthesized from glucose in our bodies if we need it. This is why we are able function just fine if we need to limit dairy, such as with those that live a vegan lifestyle, those with lactose intolerance or issues processing galactose like the genetic issue **galactosemia**.

Galactose, like glucose, is absorbed in the small intestine and carried by special proteins called "transport proteins" in the lining of the small intestine. From here, most of the absorbed galactose enters the liver where it is mainly converted to glucose, which is then either incorporated into glycogen or used for energy. Interestingly galactose ingestion, like fructose ingestion (as you will see below), results in lower blood glucose and insulin levels than glucose ingestion.

A common question that many members have when learning about the food plan, is how come they can have something like milk as part of their fluid intake? The thought being, will it increase our blood sugars like juice? It is a liquid, do our bodies not have to work as hard to break it down like food? This is a great question, and one that can be answered in 2 ways!

Milk, although easier to digest, does not raise our insulin levels the way a sugary drink would because of its absorption pathway in the liver (as it contains lactose which is broken down into galactose and glucose). Glucose (which is found in that sugary drink) would more likely be transported directly from the small intestine to the bloodstream increasing blood sugar. Insulin would be released in order to process and store that sugar (do not worry, we are getting to the discussion of insulin in due time, but all this is vital to understanding the role of insulin)! Interestingly, glucose can be absorbed at the wall of the small intestine as well as the liver. The second reason that drinking milk may not increase blood sugar levels, is that it contains protein and fat, that helps slow down our gastric emptying time, which also slows the processing of the blood sugar by the body. However, all this being said, it is still important to remember that most of our fluid intake should still come in the form of water!!

RIBOSE

Ribose is a type of monosaccharide that is made by our bodies from glucose. **It is an essential component of adenosine triphosphate (ATP) which supplies energy to our cells, (RNA) ribose nucleic acids and (DNA) deoxyribose nucleic acids.** DNA is known as the information molecule and stores all the genetic material of a cell. It also contains instructions for the synthesis of other molecules, like proteins. While RNA's function is to carry out the instructions that are encoded in DNA.

Ribose can be found in both plants and animals, including: mushrooms, beef and poultry, cheddar cheese and cream cheese, milk, eggs, caviar, anchovies, herring, sardines, and yogurt. However, it is found in these foods in very small quantities.

FRUCTOSE

Fructose is a fairly sweet, naturally occurring sugar. It comes from most fruits, and even some vegetables.

Pure fructose is also much sweeter than other types of sugar. As a result, people can use less fructose than other sugars in cooking to achieve the same sweetness. The most significant sources of fructose in today's diet include: table sugar (which is called **sucrose**, made from sugar cane or beets, is composed of 50% glucose and 50% fructose), honey, agave nectar, fruit juices, palm sugar and **(HFCS)** high fructose corn syrup (HFCS is a highly processed, inexpensive substitute for cane sugar that was introduced in the 1970s, and is made from corn. It is used to sweeten a variety of processed foods, including soda, candy, baked goods, and cereals).

After we ingest food, the stomach and small intestine go right to work in breaking the food down into its simplest form of glucose, which is absorbed and then released into the bloodstream. Once in the bloodstream, glucose can be used immediately by the cells for energy, or stored in our bodies to be used later. However, glucose and fructose are metabolized very differently by the body. Before it can be used by the body, fructose needs to be converted into glucose, which is conducted by the liver. While every cell in the body can use glucose, the liver is the only organ that can metabolize fructose when ingested in significant amounts!

HOW HAS FRUCTOSE CHANGED?

Before the mass production of refined sugar, humans rarely consumed fructose in high amounts. But as food science has developed over the years, our food has greatly changed from its very simple former self (that is a whole other science article!!!)

While most whole fruits and some vegetables contain fructose, they provide relatively low amounts. Some examples of vegetables that include fructose are artichokes, asparagus, broccoli, leeks, mushrooms, okra, onions, peas, red peppers, shallots and tomatoes.

Unlike glucose, fructose causes a low rise in blood sugar levels. Therefore, some health professionals recommend fructose as a "safe" sweetener for people with type 2 diabetes.

However, here is the crux. Many others are worried that excessive fructose intake may in fact contribute to several metabolic disorders. There is quite the debate in the scientific community around this!

When people eat a diet that is high in calories and high in fructose, the liver is thought to become overloaded and starts turning the fructose into fat. Many scientists believe that excess fructose consumption may be a key driver in many of the most serious diseases today (Gunnars, K., 2018, April 23). These include obesity, type II diabetes, insulin resistance, heart disease, and even cancer. However, more human evidence is needed. Although, researchers debate the extent to which fructose contributes to these disorders, there is a considerable mounting body of evidence justifying the concerns.

THE HARMFUL EFFECTS OF EXCESS FRUCTOSE

According to (Gunnars, K., 2018, April 23), eating a lot of fructose in the form of added sugars may:

- Impair the composition of your blood lipids. Fructose may raise the levels of **VLDL (very-low-density lipoprotein)** cholesterol, leading to the accumulation of fat around the organs. It may potentially cause heart disease, as it may alter how the body breaks down fats and carbohydrates, and lead to **atherosclerosis** (the build-up of plaque in the arteries which can block blood flow to the heart and other vital organs).

- Increase blood levels of **uric acid**, leading to **gout** (a common and complex form of arthritis, characterized by sudden and severe attacks of pain, swelling, redness, and tenderness in one or more joints, most often in the big toe) and high blood pressure. Uric acid is a chemical created when the body breaks down substances called purines. Purines are normally produced in the body and are also found in some foods and drinks. Foods with high content of purines include liver, anchovies, mackerel, dried beans, peas, and beer. Generally, uric acid dissolves in blood and travels to the kidneys. It is processed by the kidneys and is passed out in urine. If your body produces too much uric acid or does not remove enough of it, you can get sick. A high level of uric acid in the blood is called **hyperuricemia**

- Cause deposition of fat in the liver, potentially leading to non-alcoholic fatty liver disease as discussed above.

- Cause **insulin resistance**, which can lead to obesity and type II diabetes. Some studies found that excess amounts of dietary fructose seemed to cause inflammation that could lead to insulin resistance. We will go into more detail about insulin resistance later!

- Fructose does not appear to suppress appetite as much as glucose does. As a result, it might promote overeating. When a person consumes glucose, the chemical structure of that compound triggers the pancreas to release insulin, a hormone that allows cells to use glucose for energy. Fructose does not appear to trigger insulin release or the release of hormones such as leptin which tells the brain that a person is full. It also does not inhibit hormones that tell an individual's body that they are hungry. As a result, fructose may lead to weight gain because it may contribute to overeating. Look out for more information on leptin next week as we discuss the hormones involved in hunger and satiety!

Again, to clarify, not all of this can be proven in controlled studies. However, the evidence is still there, and over time with more human studies conducted, this will likely become more evident.

SO, DO I NEED TO GIVE UP ALL FOODS THAT CONTAIN FRUCTOSE?

The important takeaway here is to realize that all of this does not apply to foods that have naturally occurring fructose, like whole fruits, vegetables, some whole grains, and even having a little bit of good quality sugars like cane sugar, honey or maple syrup. Essentially all healthy carbohydrates that are recommended on The Livy Method food plan!

Fruits, veggies, and heavier carbohydrates like quinoa, darker rices, potatoes and squashes, although containing fructose, are real food packed with nutrition, water and lots of fiber. These foods give your body what it needs, and allow you to feel satisfied with less. This makes them hard to overeat and you would have to eat very large amounts to reach harmful levels of fructose.

Hopefully this helps with the understanding of how our bodies process carbohydrates in order to utilize them for energy! The old adage, you are what you eat really holds true and hopefully as we are progressing through the program, eating better quality carbohydrates, you can all feel the difference this is making.

Here is a good video that briefly describes the monosaccharides in more detail

https://www.youtube.com/watch?v=q5q8NXSDV0s

For those that want to look at the chemical structures of these sugars in more detail, check out this video!

https://www.youtube.com/watch?v=p0soyMv8-Xo

WHAT ABOUT PROTEIN AND FAT? DOES OUR BODY ALSO CONVERT THESE INTO GLUCOSE FOR ENERGY IF WE NEED IT?

Great question, and the answer is yes it does! Fats are used for energy after they are broken into fatty acids and glycerol and protein can also be used for energy, but its primary role is to help with making hormones, muscle, and other proteins.

NOW WE ARE READY TO TALK ABOUT INSULIN!!!

Now that we have reviewed the basics of glucose and the various pathways that the body uses to utilize the different simple sugars, protein, and fat for energy, let's talk about how the body stores this energy.

When a person consumes glucose, the chemical structure of the compound triggers the pancreas to release **insulin**, a hormone that allows cells to use glucose for energy.

THE PANCREAS

To recap our discussion from the science post on The Basics of Digestion, the pancreas is an organ which is located behind your stomach in the upper left part (quadrant) of your abdomen, surrounded by other organs of digestion including the small intestine, liver, gallbladder and spleen. Although the pancreas has an important role in digestion by secreting pancreatic juice rich in digestive enzymes, it also has the critical role of regulating blood sugar!

The body is designed to keep the level of glucose in your blood constant. The human pancreas contains one to two million pancreatic **islets (also called endocrine pancreas cells and islet of Langerhans cells)** housing different endocrine cells, primarily insulin-secreting beta cells, glucagon-producing alpha cells, and somatostatin-secreting delta cells (which serve to block the secretion of both insulin and glucagon from adjacent cells). Interestingly, although islets compose only 1–2% of the human pancreas, they receive up to 10% of the total pancreatic blood supply (Rahman, M. S., Hossain, K. S., Das, S., Kundu, S., Adegoke, E. O., Rahman, M. A., Hannan, M. A., Uddin, M. J., & Pang, M. G.,2021).

The beta cells in your pancreas monitor your blood sugar level every few seconds. When your blood glucose rises after you eat, the beta cells release insulin into your bloodstream. Insulin acts like a key, unlocking muscle, fat, and liver cells, so that glucose can penetrate them. Once inside, the cells convert glucose into energy to use right then, or store it to use later.

As glucose moves from the bloodstream into the cells, blood sugar levels start to drop. The beta cells in the pancreas can tell this is happening, so they slow down the amount of insulin they are making. At the same time, the pancreas slows down the amount of insulin that it is releasing into the bloodstream. When this happens, the amount of glucose going into the cells also slows down. Interestingly, insulin also helps our bodies store fat and protein.

After you have not eaten for a few hours your blood glucose level drops, and your pancreas stops producing insulin. Alpha cells in the pancreas begin to produce glucagon, signaling the liver to break down stored glycogen and turn it back into glucose. This glucose then travels to your bloodstream to replenish your supply until you are able to eat again. Although, as discussed earlier, your liver can also make its own glucose using a combination of waste products, amino acids, and fats.

The big takeaway here is that by following The Livy Method as designed, you are providing your body with a steady supply of energy over the day from healthy nutrient rich sources. As you are eating to satisfaction, you are no longer overeating to the state of being full, which would stimulate your beta cells to secrete a larger amount of insulin to process and store all that glucose being digested! Smaller amounts of food over time means smaller amounts of insulin being produced, feeling more satisfied with less, decreasing stress on the body!

Here is a great video that discusses the role of the pancreas.

https://www.youtube.com/watch?v=NZ4zcrTzUjA

Here is a video that discusses glucagon and its role in glucose release.

https://www.youtube.com/watch?v=9dq3dtudQHM

Here is a great video that discusses the role of insulin in a little more detail.

https://www.youtube.com/watch?v=fPguYEDlQEQ

ISSUES WITH INSULIN

Without enough insulin, glucose cannot move into the cells and the blood glucose level remains elevated. This condition is called hyperglycemia. Prolonged hyperglycemia can damage the blood vessels that carry oxygen-rich blood to your organs, and can increase your risk for heart disease, heart attack, stroke, kidney disease, nerve damage, and an eye disease called retinopathy.

WHAT CAUSES HYPERGLYCEMIA?

Typically, hyperglycemia is a symptom and can be caused when there is an issue with the body's cells not responding to insulin (**insulin resistance**), or there is an issue with the beta cells not producing adequate insulin (**prediabetes and diabetes**).

Other hormones that can raise the blood sugar level include epinephrine (also called adrenaline) and cortisol which are released by the adrenal glands, and growth hormone which is released by the pituitary gland. This is again why it is vitally important to manage stress levels, as chronic stress can have an impact on blood sugar levels.

WHAT IS INSULIN RESISTANCE?

Insulin resistance is when cells in your muscles, fat, and liver do not respond well to insulin and are not able to easily take up glucose from your blood. As a result, your pancreas increases the production of insulin to help glucose enter your cells, a condition called **hyperinsulinemia**. However, as long as your pancreas can produce enough insulin to overcome your cells' weak response to insulin, your blood glucose levels should stay in the healthy range.

WHAT IS PREDIABETES?

Prediabetes means your blood glucose levels are elevated, but elevated enough to be diagnosed as diabetes. Prediabetes usually occurs in people who already have some insulin resistance or whose beta cells in the pancreas are not making enough insulin to keep blood glucose in the normal range. Without enough insulin, extra glucose stays in your bloodstream rather than entering your cells. Over time, you are at increased risk for developing type 2 diabetes.

WHAT CAUSES INSULIN RESISTANCE AND PREDIABETES?

According to the National Institute of Diabetes and Digestive and Kidney Diseases, researchers do not fully understand what causes insulin resistance and prediabetes, but they speculate excess weight and lack of physical activity are major factors.

EXCESS WEIGHT

Many experts believe obesity, and especially visceral fat (the accumulation of fat in the abdomen and around the organs) are the main cause of insulin resistance. Having a waist measurement of 40 inches or more for men and 35 inches or more for women is linked to insulin resistance. This is true even if your body mass index (BMI) falls within the normal range. However, research has shown that Asian Americans may have an increased risk for insulin resistance even without a high BMI. (The discussion of BMI is used in reference to this study, although the concept of BMI is problematic as a measure of obesity).

Studies have also shown that belly fat produces hormones and other substances that can contribute to chronic or long-lasting inflammation in the body. Inflammation may play a role in insulin resistance, type 2 diabetes, and cardiovascular disease. Since excess weight may lead to insulin resistance, this also is a contributing factor in the development of fatty liver disease.

PHYSICAL INACTIVITY

Not getting enough physical activity is linked to insulin resistance and prediabetes. Regular physical activity causes changes in your body that help with glucose regulation. When you participate in moderate exercise that increases your heart rate and breathing, your muscles use more glucose from the body. Over time, this can lower your blood sugar levels and also allows the insulin in your body to work better. You will also receive these benefits for hours after your activity or workout.

However, very intense or strenuous exercise can cause the body to produce more stress hormones, which can lead to an increase in blood sugar as well as stress on the body. This can also help explain one of the reasons why overexercise is not a good weight loss tool!

As you can see by following The Livy Method, and incorporating the food plan and eating nutrient rich foods, including heavier carbs when needed, eating to satisfaction, incorporating stress management strategies, with a focus on getting quality sleep, you can greatly improve your state of health and wellness. By losing weight and following The Livy Method which can decrease abdominal visceral fat over time, health issues can be reversed! Many of our Livy Losers have shared their amazing health related NSVs, and are great reads to tap into motivation if you need to! Finally, incorporating exercise will also help with blood sugar regulation and can be a great stress reliever too! So, if you are feeling it, move that body!!!

REFERENCES

https://www.sciencedirect.com/topics/agricultural-and-biological-sciences/galactose

All about your A1C. (2021, August 10). Centers for Disease Control and Prevention. Retrieved March 30, 2022, from https://www.cdc.gov/diabetes/managing/managing-blood-sugar/a1c.html

Betts, G.J., Young, K.A., Wise, J.A., Johnson, E., Poe, B., Kruse, D.H., Korol, O., Johnson, J.E., Womble, M., & DeSaix, P. (2019, May 29). *Anatomy and physiology.* Openstax. https://open-textbc.ca/anatomyandphysiologyopenstax/chapter/lipid-metabolism/

Biologydictionary.net Editors. (2021, January 09). *Dna vs rna.* Biology dictionary. https://biologydictionary.net/dna-vs-rna/

Brown, S. (2021, August 18). *Study: Keto diet may lead to long-term health risks.* Verywell Health. https://www.verywellhealth.com/keto-diet-long-term-risks-5197991

Bryant, E. (2020, September 15). *How high fructose intake may trigger fatty liver disease.* National Institutes of Health. https://www.nih.gov/news-events/nih-research-matters/how-high-fructose-intake-may-trigger-fatty-liver-disease#:~:text=Studies%20suggest%20that%20high%20fructose,%2Dalcoholic%20steatohepatitis%20(NASH).

Chourpiliadis, C., & Mohiuddin. (2021). *Biochemistry, gluconeogenesis.* StatPearls Publishing. https://www.ncbi.nlm.nih.gov/books/NBK544346/

Cleveland Clinic. (2021, March 1). *What is fructose intolerance? How to cope when your stomach says no to fruit.* Cleveland Clinic. https://health.clevelandclinic.org/what-is-fructose-intolerance/#:~:text=Common%20high%2Dfructose%20foods%20include,pepper%2C%20shallots%20and%20tomato%20products.

Crosby, L., Davis, B., Joshi, S., Jardine, M., Paul, J., Neola, M., & Barnard, N.D. (2021). Ketogenic diets and chronic disease: Weighing the benefits against the risks. *Frontiers in Nutrition, 8,* 702802.https://doi.org/10.3389/fnut.2021.702802

Diabetes tests. (2021, August 10). Centers for Disease Control and Prevention. Retrieved March 30, 2022, from https://www.cdc.gov/diabetes/basics/getting-tested.html#:~:text=Fasting%20Blood%20Sugar%20Test,higher%20indicates%20you%20have%20diabetes.

Frank, J. (2020, September 28). *What are purines?* Arthritis - health. https://www.arthritis-health.com/types/gout/what-are-purines

Greenlaw, E. & Martin, L. J. (2013, January 18). *Exercises to lower your blood sugar.* WebMD. https://www.webmd.com/healthy-aging/features/exercise-lower-blood-sugar#:~:text=When%20you%20do%20moderate%20exercise,in%20your%20body%20work%20better.

Gunnnars, K. (2018, April 23). *Is fructose bad for you? The surprising truth.* Healthline. https://www.healthline.com/nutrition/why-is-fructose-bad-for-you

Healthwise Staff. (2020, August 31). *Carbohydrates, proteins, fats, and blood sugar.* University of Michigan Health: Michigan Medicine. https://www.uofmhealth.org/health-library/uq1238abc#:~:text=Protein%20can%20also%20be%20used,%2C%20muscle%2C%20and%20other%20proteins.&text=Broken%20down%20into%20glucose%2C%20used%20to%20supply%20energy%20to%20cells.

Higdon, J., Drake, V.J., Delage, B., & Liu, S. (2016, March). *Glycemic index and glycemic load.* Oregon State University. https://lpi.oregonstate.edu/mic/food-beverages/glycemic-index-glycemic-load

How our bodies turn food into energy. (n.d.). Kaiser Permanente. Retrieved Month Date, Year, from https://healthy.kaiserpermanente.org/colorado/health-wellness/healtharticle.how-our-bodies-turn-food-into-energy#:~:text=Our%20bodies%20digest%20the%20food,type%20of%20sugar%2C%20called%20glucose.

Islet cell. (n.d.). National Cancer Institute. Retrieved March 30, 2022, from https://www.cancer.gov/publications/dictionaries/cancer-terms/def/islet-cell

Khan Academy. (2015, July 10). *Molecular structure of glucose | Macromolecules | Biology.* [Video]. Youtube. https://www.youtube.com/watch?v=-Aj5BTnz-v0

Kitchin, B. (2009, July 24). *High fructose fracas.* The University of Alabama at Birmingham. https://www.uab.edu/shp/nutritiontrends/nutrition-know-how/consumer-concerns/high-fructose-fracas

Macrophage. (2013, May 31). *Insulin 2: What is glucagon?* [Video]. Youtube. https://www.youtube.com/watch?v=9dq3dtudQHM

Macrophage. (2013, June 10). *Insulin 1: What does insulin do, and why do we need it?* [Video]. Youtube. https://www.youtube.com/watch?v=fPguYEDlQEQ

Marengo, K., & Dix, M. (2021, April 1). *How is protein digested?* Healthline. https://www.healthline.com/health/protein-digestion

Mayo Clinic Staff. (2020, August 25). *Glycemic index diet: What's behind the claims.* Mayo Clinic. https://www.mayoclinic.org/healthy-lifestyle/nutrition-and-healthy-eating/in-depth/glycemic-index-diet/art-20048478

McMillen, M., & Ratini, M. (2021, February 5). *Ribose.* WebMD. https://www.webmd.com/vitamins-and-supplements/ribose-uses-and-risks#:~:text= Ribose%20(d%2Dribose)%20is,supplies%20energy%20to%20our%20cells.

MedlinePlus. (2022, March 21). *Uric acid - blood.* https://medlineplus.gov/ency/article/003476. htm#:~:text=Uric%20acid%20is%20a%20chemical,beans%20and%20peas%2C%20and%20 beer.

MedlinePlus. (2020, August 18). *Galactosemia.* https://medlineplus.gov/genetics/condition/ galactosemia/

MedlinePlus. (2019, February 27). *Vldl cholesterol.* https://medlineplus.gov/vldlcholesterol.html

Nakrani, M.N., Wineland, R.H., & Anjum, F. (2021). *Physiology, glucose metabolism.* StatPearls Publishing. https://www.ncbi.nlm.nih.gov/books/NBK560599/

NutrientsReview. (n.d.). *Galactose.* https://www.nutrientsreview.com/carbs/monosaccharides-galac-tose.html

Pointer, K., & Luo, E.K. (2017, March 24). *Everything you need to know about glucose.* Healthline. https://www.healthline.com/health/glucose

Pereira, R. M., Botezelli, J. D., da Cruz Rodrigues, K. C., Mekary, R. A., Cintra, D. E., Pauli, J. R., da Silva, A., Ropelle, E. R., & de Moura, L. P. (2017). Fructose consumption in the devel-opment of obesity and the effects of different protocols of physical exercise on the hepatic metabolism. *Nutrients, 9*(4), 405. https://doi.org/10.3390/nu9040405

Rahman, M. S., Hossain, K. S., Das, S., Kundu, S., Adegoke, E. O., Rahman, M. A., Hannan, M. A., Uddin, M. J., & Pang, M. G. (2021). Role of insulin in health and disease: An update. *Inter-national Journal of Molecular Sciences, 22*(12), 6403. https://doi.org/10.3390/ijms22126403

Ribose. (2020, August 10). LibreTexts. Retrieved March 30, 2022, from https://chem.libretexts.org/@ go/page/392

Richter, A., & Nall, R. (2021, December 16). *Is fructose bad for you?* Medical News Today. https:// www.medicalnewstoday.com/articles/323818#summary

Skrovan, S. (2017, August 14). *Manufacturers reformulate with sugar as con-sumers sour on corn syrup.* Food Dive. https://www.fooddive.com/news/ manufacturers-reformulate-with-sugar-as-consumers-sour-on-corn-syrup/449233/

Sollid, K. (2021, May 24). *What is glucose?* Food Insight. https://foodinsight.org/what-is-glucose/

ThePancreasPatient. (2013, September 6). *The role and anatomy of the pancreas* [Video]. Youtube. https://www.youtube.com/watch?v=NZ4zcrTzUjA

The Organic Chemistry Tutor. (2019, October 14. *Monosaccharides - Glucose, fructose, galactose, & ribose - Carbohydrates.* [Video]. Youtube. https://www.youtube.com/watch?v=p0soyMv8-Xo

Utiger, R. D. (2011, February 7). *somatostatin*. Encyclopedia Britannica. https://www.britannica.com/science/somatostatin

Watson, S., & DerSarkissian, C. (2020, June 13). *What is glucose?* WebMD. https://www.webmd.com/diabetes/glucose-diabetes

Weatherspoon, D., & Whelan, C. (2018, September 17). *Everything you need to know about fasting before a blood test.* Healthline. https://www.healthline.com/health/fasting-before-blood-test

What is diabetes? (2021, December 16). Centers for Disease Control and Prevention. Retrieved March 30, 2022, from https://www.cdc.gov/diabetes/basics/diabetes.html#:~:text=Diabetes%20is%20a%20chronic%20(long,your%20pancreas%20to%20release%20insulin

Whats Up Dude. (2016, October 16). *What are simple carbohydrates - Monosaccharides - Glucose - Fructose - Disaccharides* [Video]. Youtube. https://www.youtube.com/watch?v=q5q8NXSDV0s

ISSUES WITH DIGESTION

In the post The Basics of Digestion, we discussed digestion fundamentals with a few important take-aways. To recap, we discussed the importance of:

1. The cephalic phase of eating- In this phase, we engage with our brain-gut connection by creating a ritual around thoughtfully preparing our foods, using our senses and focusing on the first two mindfulness questions. We are allowing for adequate time for the stimulation of our saliva and gastric juices which contain digestive enzymes to flood our mouth and stomach, getting our bodies primed and ready for digestion. This sets us up for the optimal absorption of the nutrients we are eating!

2. Chewing our food- In this phase we are ingesting our food and chewing it as best as we can, breaking it down into the smallest pieces possible. This allows for the best mixing of our food with saliva and enzymes which can facilitate optimal digestion. This is the perfect time to engage in the third set of mindfulness questions to see how we are feeling while eating as in the cephalic phase, we want to take our time with this process for it to be the most beneficial!

This brings us to this follow up post that begins the conversation around digestive issues. Now that we have a better understanding of how digestion works, let's take a deeper look at how The Livy Method can best support those who may have concerns or healing needed for their digestive issues.

Because there are so many possible digestive issues, this article will focus on the most common issues that most people have. These articles do not take the place of your doctor or health care provider (HCP). If you have more in-depth issues or concerns, it is very important to consult with your HCP and communicate any questions or concerns with them!

HYPOCHLORHYDRIA, OTHERWISE KNOWN AS THE LOW PRODUCTION OF THE STOMACH ACID HCL (HYDROCHLORIC ACID)

As we discussed in The Basics of Digestion, during the cephalic phase, once our chewed foods enter our stomach, **parietal cells** that are contained in the lining of our stomach begin to release hydrochloric acid. This occurs in order to create an acidic environment to activate the digestive enzyme called pepsin. This begins the process of converting proteins into amino acids to enable utilization by the body. This acidic environment also protects our bodies from bacteria and pathogens that may have been ingested. However, to do this effectively, the **PH ("Potential for Hydrogen" which is a scale from 1-14 that measures how acidic or alkaline a substance is)** must be extremely low or acidic, measuring between **1.5-2** on the PH scale. Now that is acidic!!!!

However, some people have issues producing enough stomach acid for a variety of reasons which can have a major impact on their digestion!

AGE

As we age our production of HCL decreases, becoming more common in those over 65. This can have an impact on how those who are aging digest their foods.

CHRONIC STRESS

Stressful events activate our brain and stimulate our **sympathetic nervous system (SNS)** which is also known as the "fight or flight" response in our bodies. This response is meant to be short-term and is activated to deal with whatever emergency has arisen. When the emergency is over, our bodies are meant to settle back down to our normal **parasympathetic nervous system (PSNS)** state, otherwise known as the "rest and digest" state. When our SNS is activated, we release cortisol which many of us know as the "stress hormone," in order to fight the emergency. From the perspective of digestion, the SNS decreases blood flow to the digestive system, including the stomach, so it can focus on providing good blood flow to the heart, lungs, and brain! This decreased blood flow ultimately leads to lower HCl levels and a decrease in mucous production (which lines and protects the stomach), which has the potential to injure the fragile lining of the gut. Damage to this lining may cause inflammation, ulcers, and impact nutrient absorption. As you can see, if our bodies are in a chronic or prolonged state of stress, there can be a great impact on our digestive system!

POOR DIET LOW IN NUTRIENTS & LIFESTYLE FACTORS

B vitamins and minerals, such as iron and zinc, are responsible for the production of HCL in our bodies. Having a diet low in these nutrients can affect our production of HCL. Lifestyle factors such as smoking and drinking can also decrease our absorption of these vitamins and minerals, impacting how much HCL we are producing.

HELICOBACTER PYLORI (H. PYLORI) INFECTION

H. Pylori is one of the most common bacterial infections in the world, being said to affect up to 67% of the global population. (Bernstein, S., & Khatri, M., 2020, December 7) H. pylori colonizes and lives in the stomach lining of the stomach, and is thought to be transmitted by the ingestion of food, water, and/or shared food, water, and utensils. It can also be contracted through contact with saliva or other bodily fluids of infected people. H. pylori is more common in countries or communities that lack clean water or good sewage systems.

The stomach lining is responsible for producing HCL and mucous, but also protects the stomach itself from the HCL it produces. Any compromise in the tissue of the stomach can lead to something called **"gastritis" or inflammation of the stomach**, leading to the stomach becoming inflamed, ulcers (sores), and/or bleeding of the tissue. This affects the cells that secrete the HCL potentially causing a decreased production of this stomach acid, causing hypochlorhydria, as well as the potential for the decreased ability to digest the foods eaten.

Most cases of those colonized with H. pylori are **asymptomatic (show no symptoms)** but may lead to the emergence of symptoms showing later in life, develop into stomach or duodenal ulcers, or result in gastric cancer for 1-3% of those colonized. The good news is that with good hygiene, the likelihood of acquiring H. Pylori is greatly reduced, and is easily diagnosed and treatable with antibiotics and medications!

LONG TERM USE OF ANTACID MEDICATIONS AND OTHER MEDICATIONS

Sometimes those with hypochlorhydria, experience symptoms that are similar to acid reflux or **GERD (gastroesophageal reflux disease)** and take medications to suppress those symptoms. A specific kind of antacid that people take are called **proton pump inhibitors (PPIs).** PPIs target the production of stomach acid by suppressing the parietal cells in the stomach from producing HCL. However, these cells also produce something called **intrinsic factor (IF)** that helps the small intestine absorb vitamin B12. Long term use of these PPIs may potentially cause a deficiency in B12 absorption. Vitamin B12 is an important component in helping our body produce **red blood cells** and if deficient in this vitamin over time, can lead to a condition called **pernicious anemia**. The big takeaway here is that those who think they have acid reflux or GERD, may actually be affected by having low gastric acid. If there is not enough gastric acid in our stomach, the food is not able to be broken down in the way it was meant to and spends a prolonged amount of time there. This allows the food to ferment and begin to release gases which cause our stomachs to feel bloated, causes burping and creates an acidic feeling in our stomachs. However, if you have been on PPIs for a long time, it is very important to have a discussion and consult your HCP about your medications before discontinuing them, or if you have any questions or concerns about your symptoms! This is a very individualized process and can have different impacts for different individuals.

Gastric bypass and other gastric surgeries

Finally, the last cause of hypochlorhydria is in the case of those that have a history of gastric bypass surgery or other surgeries of the stomach. In these cases, the stomach does not function in the way it had prior to the surgery. This can be a fairly large topic, but the big takeaway is that following The Livy Method as described in the summary can help support the digestive system as optimally as possible. You may have to be mindful of certain foods that can cause symptoms for you! This is very individual and is different for everyone!

SYMPTOMS OF HYPOCHLORHYDRIA

Here are some signs that you may not be producing enough stomach acid. They usually show up a few hours after you have eaten and may include:

Feeling like you want to eat even when you are not hungry, feeling too full after regular meals, indigestion, gas or flatulence, bloating, constipation, diarrhea, soreness or burning in your mouth, stomach upset and cramps, undigested food in stool, nausea, and heartburn.

ACID REFLUX AND GASTROESOPHAGEAL REFLUX DISEASE

In normal digestion, after chewing and swallowing your food, the food travels down the esophagus via muscular contractions called peristalsis. This "bolus" enters the stomach via the **LES** or **lower esophageal sphincter**, a muscular ring which opens to allow food into your stomach. Once the food or bolus enters, the LES closes to stop food and acidic stomach juices from flowing back into the esophagus.

What Is GERD?

Gastroesophageal reflux disease or GERD, is a chronic digestive disorder that occurs when stomach contents, which includes the acidic digestive juices, backs up from the stomach via the LES into the esophagus resulting in heartburn or acid indigestion. This occurs when the LES is weak or relaxes when it should not. Interestingly, an acidic environment triggers the closure of the LES, so in some cases, acid reflux occurs when there is incidence of hypochlorhydria! While it is common for people to experience acid reflux and heartburn once in a while, having symptoms that affect your daily life or occur at least twice each week could be a sign of GERD.

RISK FACTORS FOR GERD

HAVING WEIGHT TO LOSE

Having extra weight and fat on our body, especially in the abdominal region, can increase the pressure on our stomach causing the LES to open and cause reflux. This can also make our bodies less efficient at emptying the stomach contents into our small intestine.

PREGNANCY

Heartburn is common in pregnancy and can get worse as the pregnancy progresses. Hormones that support pregnancy can cause the digestive system to slow down. Peristalsis decreases and as the baby grows, the pressure on the stomach increases and can cause reflux.

DELAYED EMPTYING OF THE STOMACH (GASTROPARESIS)

Some people have a medical condition called **gastroparesis** that causes a delay in gastric emptying time. To recap, our stomach and intestines have strong involuntary muscular contractions that propel food through the digestive tract. Gastroparesis is a condition that affects the normal spontaneous movement of these muscles, otherwise known as motility, in the stomach. The stomach's motility is slowed down or does not function, preventing the stomach from emptying properly. What this means is there can be a delay in the movement of the contents of the stomach to the small intestine, resulting in reflux. This can be an isolated issue, or precipitated by other medical conditions like diabetes.

LIFESTYLE FACTORS SUCH AS SMOKING, CERTAIN FOODS AND DRINKS INCLUDING CHOCOLATE, MINT, FRIED FOODS, COFFEE, AND ALCOHOL

The nicotine from tobacco, chocolate, mint and alcohol can actually relax the LES causing reflux. Some people find fried foods, coffee, acidic or spicy foods can make symptoms of GERD worse.

LARGE MEALS

Eating a large meal can cause an increase in abdominal pressure on the stomach resulting in reflux.

EATING TOO SOON BEFORE BED

After eating, wait 2 to 3 hours before lying down. When you are lying down, the contents of your stomach can push against the LES resulting in reflux, whereas sitting up allows gravity to promote the proper movement and flow of food down the digestive tract. Also, as we are preparing for bed, and the production and secretion of melatonin increases in our bodies as it gets darker, our bodies will want to focus on rest and repair as opposed to digestion. In fact, our digestion naturally slows due to the release of these hormones, and is an important part of something called our "**circadian rhythm**"! This is why it is recommended to finish our meals earlier in the evening, minimizing late evening snacking, as it promotes the optimal environment for digestion!

HYPERCHLORHYDRIA

Some people's bodies naturally have an overproduction of gastric HCL. It may not be an issue for some, but for others it may cause issues with reflux.

MEDICATIONS

Some prescription medications, over the counter medications, and supplements may cause GERD. Consult your HCP or pharmacist to discuss your medications if you have questions.

GERD SYMPTOMS

The most common symptom of GERD is heartburn (acid indigestion). It is described as a burning chest pain that starts behind your breastbone and moves upward to your neck and throat. Many people describe that it feels like food is coming back into the mouth, leaving an acid, sour or bitter taste, lasting as long as 2 hours. Besides pain you may also have nausea, bad breath, trouble breathing, difficulty swallowing, vomiting, the wearing away of tooth enamel, or the feeling of a lump in your throat. If you have acid reflux at night, you may also have a lingering cough, laryngitis that comes on suddenly or gets worse, or issues with sleep. If you have concerns with any of these symptoms, follow up with your HCP!

Check out this video for more details!

https://www.youtube.com/watch?v=TdK0jRFpWPQ

LIVING WITHOUT A GALLBLADDER

Many of our members are coming into this program without a gallbladder, and are concerned that they will have issues following the plan, or with weight loss because of this.

To recap from last week, the liver is a large organ located above the stomach in the upper abdomen. The liver produces bile which is stored in the gallbladder, stores glucose and nutrients and also helps remove toxins from the body.

When we eat fatty foods the gallbladder (a small pouch) is stimulated to secrete **bile** via the **bile ducts** to the small intestine, which helps to emulsify the fats making it easier for **lipases (enzymes that break down fat)** to do their job!

The good news is that your body can still function well without a gallbladder! Although it acts as a storage area for your bile, the liver amazingly adapts to this change in your body and will still produce bile! However, it does this by producing it in continuous drips delivering it directly into the small intestine. This means that your body is still capable of producing bile for the emulsification of fats.

Some people have no issues without having a gallbladder. However, others may have to monitor foods that may cause them digestive discomfort like gas, bloating and diarrhea, limit the ingestion of fried fatty foods, or limit large meals. But as discussed below, The Livy Method supports those without a gallbladder really well!!!

INFLAMMATORY BOWEL DISEASE (IBD) AND INFLAMMATORY BOWEL SYNDROME (IBS)

Inflammatory bowel disease (IBD) is a general term used to describe disorders that involve chronic inflammation of the digestive tract. The 2 major types of IBD include:

ULCERATIVE COLITIS

This condition involves inflammation and sores (ulcers) along the superficial (top layer) lining of the large intestine (colon) and rectum.

CROHN'S DISEASE

This type of IBD is characterized by inflammation of the lining of the digestive tract, which can involve the deeper layers of the digestive tract, involve any part of the small or large intestine, and may be continuous or involve multiple segments of the small or large intestine.

Those with ulcerative colitis and Crohn's disease have symptoms of diarrhea, rectal bleeding, abdominal pain, fatigue and weight loss.

IRRITABLE BOWEL SYNDROME (IBS)

Irritable bowel syndrome, or IBS, is a group of symptoms that affect your digestive system. It's a common but uncomfortable gastrointestinal disorder. Those with IBS have symptoms of excessive gas, abdominal pain, and cramps.

IBS is a type of **functional** gastrointestinal (GI) disorder. A functional disorder or issue is when a person has symptoms of a condition, but the condition itself is unable to be identified or diagnosed by medical testing methods. These conditions, also called disorders of the gut-brain interaction, can affect how the gut and brain work together. When one is affected by IBS, the IBS can cause the digestive tract to be easily stimulated, affecting peristalsis (contraction of the digestive smooth muscle). This overstimulation can result in abdominal pain, diarrhea and constipation. People with IBS may have a lower pain tolerance, and research has also suggested that people with IBS may have bacterial overgrowth in the GI tract which may also contribute to their symptoms. (Cleveland Clinic, 2020, September 24).

Check out this video for more information!

https://www.webmd.com/ibd-crohns-disease/video/video-ibd-complications

HOW THE LIVY METHOD HELPS SUPPORT THE BODY

The Livy method by the very nature of its design helps to support the body in digestion and improve our overall health! Here is a summary of how the program best supports all aspects of your digestive health.

1. Chew, chew, chew, chew and take smaller bites when eating to stimulate your saliva and digestive enzymes, while focusing on your practice of mindfulness. This can eliminate symptoms associated with low stomach acid and can help maintain an appropriate level of HCL in your stomach.

2. The Livy Method recommends eating nutrient rich foods loaded with lots of veggies, leafy greens, some fruit, and grains, which are high in vitamins, minerals, and fiber. These recommended foods can help increase your stomach acid levels, heal the digestive system, promote vitamin absorption, and promote the growth of healthy gut flora. It is also recommended to decrease the ingestion of processed foods, deep fried foods, and foods high in sugars which can cause inflammation in the stomach, decrease acid activity, and trigger acid reflux symptoms. Adding in fermented vegetables and fluids such as kimchi, sauerkraut, kefir, and pickles can also naturally improve your stomach acid levels. These foods also have probiotic effects that can help improve digestion, fight harmful bacteria, and reduce inflammation caused by low stomach acid.

3. Raw apple cider vinegar with the mother is a fermented liquid made from crushed apples, bacteria, and yeast. ACV is rich in protein and enzymes and is bacterial in nature, which can help break down food and improve gut health. Like lemon juice, raw apple cider vinegar can help increase stomach acid levels because of its acidic properties, introducing more acid into the digestive tract when ingested. Both lemon juice and ACV are a 2 on the PH scale!

There is definitely a rabbit hole one can enter when looking at the benefits of using ACV or lemon water! There is limited evidence on its use as something to help stimulate bile production and the diet industry's proclamation of it being a fat burner and insulin stabilizer. However, it can be a great way to start the day in a positive way, by cleansing our palate and setting us up for success!! It's much like a physical action led intention which is a great addition to our daily intentions!!

As a final note, to help protect your teeth and the more sensitive tissues of your mouth and esophagus, you may want to dilute your ACV or lemon juice in a good amount of water if you can, and/or brush your teeth after 30 minutes of drinking.

4. While following the Livy Method, we are aiming to consume at least six meals and snacks a day, with a good mix of carbs, protein, and healthy fat at each meal. The Livy Method also focuses on eating to satisfaction and not overeating during these meals. This ensures that the digestive system is not overloaded and can handle the amount of food we give it! This helps to prevent heartburn from the stomach acids going back from the stomach into the esophagus, and may also prevent any subsequent gas, nausea, or vomiting. This also maximizes nutrient absorption! Even though you will reach a point where you won't necessarily be eating this often, the principles will be the same, eating what makes you feel good, eating to satisfaction and nurturing your body!

5. The Livy Method also recommends eating earlier in the evening and not too late at night! As discussed, eating before dark or up to two hours after sunset promotes better digestion. This allows your body to focus on rest and repair as opposed to digestion when our natural levels of melatonin are at their highest! This also allows more time for our food to travel from our stomach to our small intestine, reducing the risk of reflux. Sleeping on our left side is the most optimal position for digestion as it applies the least amount of pressure on our LES, and promotes better flow in the digestion pathway. Lying on our right side causes increased pressure on our LES, and is the least favoured position for digestion.

6. Because many of us come into this process with digestive issues, we are less able to absorb and process nutrients, vitamins, and minerals from our food. This is why supplementation is recommended as a companion to the food plan. It can help our bodies function the most optimally and can also help heal our bodies, eventually allowing us to process our nutrients better on our own. As discussed in The Basics of Digestion, adding in prebiotics and probiotics also aids in the production and absorption of B vitamins and vitamin K in the colon, and also improves the colonization of helpful bacteria in our digestive system, which is vital to the digestive process!

Check out this video on the importance of the microbiome of our digestive system!

https://www.youtube.com/watch?v=B9RruLkAUm8&t=329s

7. Canadian digestive bitters can also be very helpful for the digestive process as recommended in the supplements post. Digestive bitters are groups of herbs that have very bitter qualities and stimulate the bitter receptors that are found in the mouth, gut, and pancreas (contrary to popular belief that they are just found in the tongue). As a result, they stimulate the production of saliva and they can help to naturally stimulate gastric juices and bile flow, which results in enhanced digestion!

8. Maintaining a journal that includes a food diary is a great add when following The Livy Method. Journaling how certain foods make you feel can really give insights into what foods cause digestive discomforts or issues, and help you identify potential intolerances!

9. Stress management is imperative to the weight loss process and also helps manage the brain-gut connection! Using stress management techniques and the other methods recommended on plan decreases external stimulation that can literally "stress" our digestive system, promoting the body to function as best it can!

10. Finally, following the Livy Method ensures that you are adequately hydrated! Water as we all know here is vital to life and can maximize our success! It is involved in almost every chemical reaction in the body, particularly in the processing of our nutrients and the absorption of vitamins and minerals in the body. It can be particularly helpful in preventing constipation because water helps soften your stools! So… sip, sip, sip that water and get in just enough!

REFERENCES

AllHealthGo. (2018, August 30). *Living without a gallbladder* [Video]. Youtube. https://www.youtube.com/watch?v=l2eb7mSIvuk

Bernstein, S., & Khatri, M. (2020, December 7). *What is H. pylori?* WebMD. https://www.webmd.com/digestive-disorders/h-pylori-helicobacter-pylori

Bhargava, H.D. (2020, September 11). *Gerd.* WebMD. https://www.webmd.com/heartburn-gerd/guide/reflux-disease-gerd-1#:~:text=Gastroesophageal%20reflux%20disease%2C%20or%20GERD,get%20heartburn%20or%20acid%20indigestion.

Bolen, B., & Hall, M. (2020, December 7). *Keep a food diary to identify food triggers.* Verywell Health. https://www.verywellhealth.com/how-to-keep-a-food-diary-1945006

Brennan, D. (2021, November 15). *What is hypochlorhydria?* WebMD. https://www.webmd.com/digestive-disorders/what-is-hypochlorhydria

Cuenca, L. (2013, May 30). The bittersweet truth of sweet and bitter taste receptors. *Harvard University: The Graduate School of Arts and Sciences.* https://sitn.hms.harvard.edu/flash/2013/the-bittersweet-truth-of-sweet-and-bitter-taste-receptors/

Dunne, C., Dolan, B., & Clyne, M. (2014). Factors that mediate colonization of the human stomach by helicobacter pylori. *World Journal of Gastroenterology, 20*(19), 5610–5624. https://doi.org/10.3748/wjg.v20.i19.5610

Granger, N.D., Morris, J. D., Kvietys, P. R., & Granger, J. P. (2018). *Physiology and Pathophysiology of Digestion.* Morgan & Claypool Life Science Publishers.

Guy-Evans, O., & McLeod, S. (2021, May 18). *Parasympathetic nervous system functions.* SimplyPsychology. https://www.simplypsychology.org/parasympathetic-nervous-system.html#:~:text=The%20parasympathetic%20nervous%20system%20is,voluntary%20control%2C%20therefore%20being%20automatic.&text=The%20parasympathetic%20nervous%20system%20leads%20to%20decreased%20arousal.

Healthwise Staff. (2020, April 25). *GERD: Controlling heartburn by changing your habits.* C.S. Mott Children's Hospital: University of Michigan Health. https://www.mottchildren.org/health-library/ut1339

Harvard Health Publishing. (2020, July 6). *Understanding the stress response: Chronic activation of this survival mechanism impairs health.* Harvard Medical School. https://www.health.harvard.edu/staying-healthy/understanding-the-stress-response

Heda, R., Toro, F., & Tombazzi, C.R. (2021, May 9). *Physiology, pepsin.* StatPearls Publishing. https://www.ncbi.nlm.nih.gov/books/NBK537005/#:~:text=Parietal%20cells%20within%20the%20stomach,hydrogen%20ions%20and%20decrease%20pH.

How to manage acid reflux after bariatric surgery. (n.d.). Southern Nevada Bariatrics. Retrieved March 30, 2022, from https://www.southernnevadabariatrics.com/blog/how-to-manage-acid-reflux-after-bariatric-surgery

Intrinsic factor. (2022, March 21). MedlinePlus. Retrieved March 30, 2022, from https://medlineplus.gov/ency/article/002381.htm#:~:text=Intrinsic%20factor%20is%20a%20protein,cells%20in%20the%20stomach%20lining.

Irritable bowel syndrome (IBS). (2020, September 24). Cleveland Clinic. Retrieved March 30, 2022, from https://my.clevelandclinic.org/health/diseases/4342-irritable-bowel-syndrome-ibs

Mayo Clinic Staff. (2021, July 8). *Chronic stress puts your health at risk: Chronic stress can wreak havoc on your mind and body. Take steps to control your stress.* Mayo Clinic. https://www.mayoclinic.org/healthy-lifestyle/stress-management/in-depth/stress/art-20046037#:~:text=Cortisol%20also%20curbs%20functions%20that,reproductive%20system%20and%20growth%20processes.

Mayo Clinic Staff. (2021, May 18). *Helicobacter pylori (H. pylori) infection.* Mayo Clinic. https://www.mayoclinic.org/diseases-conditions/h-pylori/symptoms-causes/syc-20356171

Mayo Clinic. (2010, April 22). *Heartburn, acid reflux, GERD* [Video]. Youtube. https://www.youtube.com/watch?v=TdK0jRFpWPQ

Mayo Clinic Staff. (2020, October 10). *Gastroparesis.* Mayo Clinic. https://www.mayoclinic.org/diseases-conditions/gastroparesis/symptoms-causes/syc-20355787#:~:text=Gastroparesis%20is%20a%20condition%20that,food%20through%20your%20digestive%20tract

Morris, J.D., Granger, D. N., Granger, J. P., & Kvietys, P. R. (2018). *Physiology and Pathophysiology of Digestion: Part 2.* Biota Publishing.

Nambudripad, R. (2021, February 28). *SIBO: A doctor's guide to the root cause of bloating and IBS* [Video]. Youtube. https://www.youtube.com/watch?v=1WPv2FijZ5s

Nelson, D. (2020, March 3). *What does pH stand for and mean?* Science Trends. https://sciencetrends. com/what-does-ph-stand-for-and-mean/

Overview: Gallbladder removal. (2021, December 8). NHS. Retrieved March 30, 2022, from https://www.nhs.uk/conditions/gallbladder-removal/#:~:text=Living%20without%20a%20 gallbladder,continuously%20into%20your%20digestive%20system

Sethi, S., & Anthony, K. (2019, March 7). *How to increase stomach acid at home. Healthline.* https:// www.healthline.com/health/how-to-increase-stomach-acid#outlook

Stomach. (n.d.). National Cancer Institute. https://training.seer.cancer.gov/anatomy/digestive/regions/ stomach.html#:~:text=Four%20different%20types%20of%20cells,Chief%20cells

The brain-gut connection. (n.d). Johns Hopkins Medicine. Retrieved March 30, 2022, from https:// www.hopkinsmedicine.org/health/wellness-and-prevention/the-brain-gut-connection

Water Science School. (2019, June 19). *pH scale.* United States Geological Survey. https://www. usgs.gov/media/images/ph-scale-0#:~:text=pH%20is%20a%20measure%20of,hydroxyl%20 ions%20in%20the%20water

Warwick, K.W., & Eske, J. (2020, July 29). *How can you naturally increase stomach acid?* Medical News Today. https://www.medicalnewstoday.com/articles/how-to-increase-stomach-acid

Your digestive system: 5 ways to support gut health. (n.d.). Johns Hopkins Medicine. Retrieved March 30, 2022, from https://www.hopkinsmedicine.org/health/wellness-and-prevention/ your-digestive-system-5-ways-to-support-gut-health

HORMONES IMPORTANT TO WEIGHT LOSS & DIGESTION PART 2: HORMONES OF HUNGER AND SATIETY AND TIMING OF DIGESTION

In this post we are continuing the conversation of the hormones that are involved in digestion and are important to weight loss. The goal of these posts is to help provide some foundational information and create an understanding of how our bodies function. We will also discuss how implementing The Livy Method optimizes our health, wellness, and mindfulness, by providing an environment where our bodies no longer feel the need to store fat!

We will be focusing on the hormones that are imperative to regulating our hunger and feelings of satiety, or what we at Weight Loss By Gina like to call, eating to satisfaction! We will also be looking at the concept of breakfast and how making it high in protein sets up our day for success. Finally, we will conclude our discussion on digestion by looking at how long it takes our bodies to process and digest the foods that we eat. All of these topics can give us more insight into the "rhyme and reason" behind the different tweaks and the organization of The Livy Method Food Plan, and how it promotes weight loss.

HUNGER

In the science post The Migrating Motor Complex (MMC) and Hunger, we discussed how the feeling of "hunger" is a fairly complex concept that can be influenced by many things including physical/physiological, emotional, social, economic, and mental factors. In fact, many of us have lost touch with gauging hunger signals, or never really become in tune with them in the first place.

We discussed strategies for reconnecting with these signals such as journaling, using a hunger scale, revisiting the four mindfulness questions at every meal and snack. We also discussed the importance of being in the moment when you are eating, minimizing distractions, to really tune into your food and how it is making you feel!

Let's dive in a bit deeper and look closer at the physiological processes that occur in our bodies that drive our feelings of hunger, but also lead to our feelings of satisfaction when we have eaten enough.

WHAT ARE HORMONES?

Hormones are defined as a special substance produced in the body that contains "chemical messengers" that control and regulate the activity of certain cells or organs (Davis, C.P., 2021, March 29). They are secreted into the blood or extracellular fluid by one cell and in turn, alter the functioning of other "targeted" cells. These target cells may be in glands, tissues, and other cells. The target cells recognize the hormone circulating that is specific to it, and become a "receptor" allowing the hormone to activate it! In fact, many hormones are active in more than one physical process and may have multiple functions!

Many hormones are secreted by special **glands** and are essential for every activity of life, including the processes of digestion, metabolism, growth, reproduction, and our mood.

There are two types of glands. **Endocrine glands,** which are ductless glands that release the hormones they make directly into the bloodstream. These glands form part of what we know as the **endocrine system**. The other type of gland that is present in the body is called an **exocrine gland** (for example sweat glands and lymph nodes). These are not considered part of the endocrine system as they do not produce hormones, and they release their product through a duct.

Neurotransmitters, although not specifically hormones, are also special chemical messengers that help carry, promote, and balance signals between neurons (also known as nerve cells) and target cells throughout the body. Neurotransmitters are more specific to the central nervous system.

Neurotransmitters can have strong influences on our hunger and satiety cues and signals!

Here is a great video that briefly talks about hormones and how they work in the body.

https://www.youtube.com/watch?v=-SPRPkLoKp8

This video explains the endocrine system for those that want to learn a little more about how it works!

https://www.youtube.com/watch?v=ER49EweKwW8

This video talks about how neurotransmitters travel across neurons in the body.

https://www.youtube.com/watch?v=WhowH0kb7n0&t=5s

Now that we understand a little more about how hormones and neurotransmitters work in our body, let's talk about how these chemical messengers influence our hunger, satiety, and can influence weight loss!

INSULIN

As we discussed in the Science Post <u>Hormones Important to Weight Loss & Digestion Part 1-Insulin,</u> the pancreas has a major role in digestion by producing and secreting digestive enzymes. However, it also produces the hormone insulin, which is responsible for regulating and storing glucose (a simple sugar that is broken down from food) in the muscles, liver, and fat cells, for later use when needed.

To recap, the beta cells in your pancreas monitor your blood sugar level every few seconds. When your blood glucose rises after you eat, the beta cells release insulin into your bloodstream. Insulin acts like a key, unlocking muscle, fat, and liver cells, so that glucose can penetrate them. Once inside, the cells convert glucose into energy to use right then, or store it to use later.

As glucose moves from the bloodstream into the cells, blood sugar levels start to drop. The beta cells in the pancreas can tell this is happening, so they slow down the amount of insulin they are making. At the same time, the pancreas slows down the amount of insulin that it's releasing into the bloodstream. When this happens, the amount of glucose going into the cells also slows down.

After you haven't eaten for a few hours, your blood glucose level drops, and your pancreas stops producing insulin. Alpha cells in the pancreas begin to produce glucagon, signaling the liver to break down stored glycogen and turn it back into glucose. This glucose then travels to your bloodstream to replenish your supply until you are able to eat again.

Insulin resistance has become an increasingly common condition in current society and causes the cells in the body to stop responding to insulin. This results in the body producing even more insulin, in an effort to increase the possibility of glucose absorption. This condition eventually may result in high blood sugar, because the insulin cannot move glucose into your cells, and is linked to obesity, inflammation, type 2 diabetes and heart disease. Although more research is needed, insulin resistance may be linked to carrying excess weight and to a lack of exercise.

Insulin sensitivity can be thought of as the opposite of insulin resistance. It means that your cells are having a healthy response to the insulin being produced in the body. By following The Livy Method, you are already actively focusing on habits that will help improve insulin sensitivity, such as:

REGULAR EXERCISE AND MOVING YOUR BODY

Research supports that exercise, at both high and moderate intensities, that increases your heart rate and breathing, results in your muscles using more glucose from the body (Landes, E., & Jones, J., 2022, January 26). Over time, this can lower your blood sugar levels and also makes the insulin in your body work better. You will also receive these benefits for hours after your activity or workout.

However, strenuous exercise can sometimes increase blood sugar temporarily after you stop exercising, and very intense exercise can cause the body to make more stress hormones which can lead to an increase in blood sugar, as well as stress on the body. This can also help explain one of the reasons why over exercise is not a good weight loss tool! We will be discussing this further down when we discuss the hormone cortisol.

IMPROVE YOUR SLEEP HABITS

Not getting enough sleep, or not getting quality sleep, is linked to obesity and insulin resistance.

According to the Sleep Foundation, sleep can both raise and lower glucose levels. Our bodies experience a cycle of changes every day, called a circadian rhythm, which naturally raises blood sugar levels at night and when a person sleeps. These natural blood sugar elevations are not a cause for concern.

Restorative sleep however, may lower elevated blood sugar levels by promoting healthy systems. Decreased sleep is a risk factor for increased blood sugar levels. Even partial sleep deprivation of only 1 to 2 hours in a night, increases risk of insulin resistance, which can in turn increase blood sugar levels. As a result, a lack of sleep has been associated with diabetes.

More research is needed to better understand the connection between sleep and blood sugar. However, the following factors have been found to influence the relationship between sleep and blood sugar levels (Sleep Foundation. Retrieved 2022, March):

- The amount of time a person sleeps (7-8 hours has been discussed as ideal).

- The stages of sleep a person experiences.

- The time of day of a person sleeps (considerations for shift workers).

- Age (as people age, they often have more difficulty sleeping).

- Eating habits (for example eating before sleep and poor nutrition, which overlaps with nutrition and sleep)

Why Does Sleep Affect Blood Sugar? Researchers are beginning to uncover why sleep affects blood sugar and which underlying mechanisms are involved. So far, they've learned that the following physiological factors play a role in the relationship between sleep and blood sugar:

- Cortisol (the stress hormone) is increased by sleep deprivation and increases glucose.

- Insulin sensitivity is reduced by sleep deprivation and impacts glucose.

- The time of day a person sleeps impacts insulin and cortisol levels, both of which affect glucose.

- Increases in growth hormone accompany glucose increases during sleep.

- Oxidative stress and inflammation are increased by sleep deprivation and impact glucose.

- **C-reactive protein (CRP)** and other inflammatory markers are increased by sleep deprivation and can impact glucose.

FOLLOWING THE LIVY METHOD FOOD PLAN HELPS REGULATE INSULIN!

Eating a diet which includes protein, as well as healthy fats from nuts, avocados and good oils like extra-virgin olive oil, and eating a diet rich in carbohydrates that are known to keep blood sugars stable and are high in fiber, such as whole grains, fruits, legumes, and includes many vegetables, may help reduce insulin resistance. Decreasing your intake of saturated and trans fats may also help.

MAINTAIN A MODERATE WEIGHT

In people that are overweight, healthy weight loss and weight management may improve insulin sensitivity.

LEPTIN

Leptin is a hormone made by the fat cells that creates the feeling of "fullness" that works by telling your **hypothalamus**, the portion of your brain that regulates appetite, that you're full. It works in conjunction with the hormone **ghrelin** that increases appetite, and also plays a role in body weight.

Of the two hormones, leptin appears to have a greater influence in our body's energy balance. Some researchers even think that leptin helps regulate ghrelin.

In general, the more fat you have, the more leptin is in your blood. However, the level varies depending on many factors, including when you last ate and your sleep patterns.

However, people with obesity may experience **leptin resistance**. This means the message to stop eating doesn't reach your brain, eventually causing you to overeat. In turn, your body may produce even more leptin until your levels become elevated. The concept of this is very similar to that of insulin resistance.

The direct cause of leptin resistance is unclear, but it may be due to inflammation, gene mutations, and/or excessive leptin production, which can occur with obesity.

Inflammation is a big component of this phenomenon, according to endocrinologist Scott Isaacs, MD (McCulloch, M., 2015). "Leptin resistance (as well as insulin resistance) is caused by fat cells, especially in visceral or belly fat, producing large numbers of inflammatory chemicals or cytokines, which block the effects of leptin," Isaacs explains. He adds that eating healthful foods, including ones rich in anti-inflammatory antioxidants and omega-3 fats, can improve leptin resistance.

Although no known treatment exists for leptin resistance, a few lifestyle changes may help lower leptin levels. Here are a few tips that may help and all recommended by The Livy Method. As you will notice reading through the discussion of all the hormones and neurotransmitters, the tips will all come to be quite repetitive!

MAINTAIN A HEALTHY WEIGHT

Because leptin resistance is associated with obesity, it's important to maintain a healthy weight. Additionally, research suggests that a decrease in body fat may help reduce leptin levels. Like insulin resistance, and recommended above, reducing abdominal/visceral fat can greatly help reduce the inflammation that may contribute to leptin resistance.

IMPROVE YOUR SLEEP QUALITY

Leptin levels may be related to sleep quality in people with obesity. Although this association may not exist in people without obesity, there are numerous other reasons to get better sleep.

EXERCISE REGULARLY

Research links regular, consistent exercise to a decrease in leptin levels.

GHRELIN

The hormone ghrelin, is essentially the opposite of leptin. It's one of the primary and most powerful hunger-stimulating hormones involved in regulating hunger. It is produced and secreted from the stomach lining, that sends a message to your hypothalamus indicating that your body needs food. The main function of ghrelin appears to be to stimulate an increase in appetite. But some researchers believe that ghrelin is not as important in determining appetite as once thought (Magee, E., & Nazario, B., n.d.). They think that its role in regulating body weight may actually be a more complex process.

Normally, ghrelin levels are highest before eating and lowest after a meal, and appear to cycle through about every 4 hours. German researchers have suggested that ghrelin levels play a big role in determining how quickly hunger comes back after we eat. Normally, ghrelin levels go up dramatically before you eat, which signals hunger. They then go down for about three hours after the meal.

Eating at regular intervals is in sync with this cycle, but after overnight fasting, ghrelin levels are increased. Ghrelin levels rise approximately two times immediately before a meal, and then decrease to their lowest levels about one hour after a meal.

Ghrelin is a short-acting hormone, and it appears that there is not a limiting level, that just builds until you eat. Importantly, it doesn't seem to be affected by what you ate yesterday! Thus, it is important to eat when you are hungry, and not let these levels build too high, which may reinforce overeating as recommended by The Livy Method!

Although one might think that ghrelin levels are higher in an obese person, thus driving more hunger, the opposite is true. Human studies have found that ghrelin levels actually are lower in the obese, but they're more sensitive to its appetite-stimulating effects. This increased sensitivity may lead to overeating.

TIPS TO MANAGE GHRELIN LEVELS

One reason weight loss can be difficult is that restricting calories often leads to increased ghrelin levels, leaving you hungry. Additionally, metabolism tends to slow down and leptin levels decrease. The Livy Method reinforces feeding into these hunger cues thus preventing ghrelin levels from getting too high, and also giving your body what it needs! This is why it is important to eat when you are hungry!

MAINTAIN A MODERATE BODY WEIGHT

Obesity may increase your sensitivity to ghrelin, ultimately increasing your appetite.

TRY TO GET GOOD QUALITY SLEEP

Poor sleep may lead to increases in ghrelin, overeating, and weight gain.

EAT REGULARLY

Because ghrelin levels are highest before a meal, listen to your body and eat when you're hungry and then just eat to satisfaction! These are all fundamental principles of The Livy Method!

CORTISOL

Cortisol is known as the stress hormone and is produced by your adrenal glands, as discussed previously in the science post Issues With Digestion.

To recap, during times of stress, the release of cortisol, alongside the hormone epinephrine (also known as adrenaline) engages our sympathetic nervous system, which is commonly called the "fight or flight" response. This is so our bodies can fight the emergency!

While it's important for your body to release cortisol in dangerous situations, chronic high levels may lead to many health issues, including heart disease, diabetes, low energy levels, high blood pressure, sleep disturbances, and weight gain.

Certain lifestyle factors, which include inadequate or poor sleep habits, chronic stress, and an unhealthy diet, may contribute to high cortisol levels.

Importantly, obesity appears to raise cortisol levels, but high levels may also cause weight gain, creating a negative feedback loop, reinforcing the body's need to store fat!

Here are how strategies recommended by The Livy Method may help manage cortisol levels:

OPTIMIZE SLEEP

Chronic sleep issues, including insomnia, sleep apnea, and irregular sleep habits (like those of shift workers), may contribute to high cortisol levels. Focus on developing a regular bedtime and sleep schedule may help with lowering cortisol levels!

EXERCISE REGULARLY

Cortisol levels temporarily increase after high intensity exercise, but regular exercise generally helps decrease levels by improving overall health and lowering stress levels. However, stressing the body with strenuous exercise or over exercising may have the opposite effect, and in fact increase cortisol levels.

PRACTICE MINDFULNESS

Research suggests that regularly practicing mindfulness lowers cortisol levels (Landes, E., & Jones, J., 2022, January 26). Try adding meditation and other relaxation techniques to your daily routine. Epsom salt baths are also a great way to relax as the warmth and the magnesium in the Epsom salts, relaxes muscles, helping to decrease stress, and ultimately cortisol levels!

MAINTAIN A MODERATE BODY WEIGHT

Because obesity may increase cortisol levels and high cortisol levels can cause weight gain, maintaining a moderate weight may help keep levels in check.

EAT A BALANCED DIET

Research has shown that diets high in added sugars, refined grains, and saturated fat may lead to higher cortisol levels. Following a plan like The Livy Method may help lower cortisol levels.

ESTROGEN

Estrogen is a sex hormone responsible for regulating the female reproductive system, as well as the immune, skeletal, and vascular systems. Although estrogen is also present and is an important hormone for males as well!

Levels of this hormone change during life stages such as pregnancy, nursing, and menopause, as well as throughout the menstrual cycle. For men as testosterone declines with age, estrogen levels increase.

High levels of estrogen, which are often seen in people with obesity, are associated with an increased risk of certain cancers and other chronic diseases.

Conversely, low levels, typically seen in women with aging, perimenopause, and menopause, may affect body weight and body fat, therefore also increasing risk of chronic diseases.

Individuals with low estrogen levels often experience an accumulation of weight around the abdomen, which should now be a familiar concept. This metabolic visceral fat, can lead to other health problems which should also sound familiar, such as high blood sugar, high blood pressure, and heart disease.

By following The Livy Method, you will naturally keep estrogen levels stable by doing the following:

TRY TO MANAGE YOUR WEIGHT

Weight loss or maintenance may reduce the risk of heart disease due to low estrogen levels in women ages 55–75. Research also supports healthy weight maintenance for reducing chronic diseases in general.

EXERCISE REGULARLY

Low estrogen levels may decrease levels of energy that may affect your motivation for exercising. However, regular exercise is still an important aspect of maintaining health.

FOLLOW A HEALTHY DIET LIKE THE LIVY METHOD

Diets high in processed foods, sugar, and refined grains have been shown to increase estrogen levels, which may raise the risk of chronic disease. Limiting these foods increases the likelihood of reversing some of these health issues.

NEUROPEPTIDE Y

Neuropeptide Y (NPY) is a hormone produced by cells in your brain and nervous system that stimulates appetite and decreases energy expenditure in response to prolonged fasting or stress.

Because it may stimulate eating, NPY is associated with obesity and weight gain.

NPY production is activated in fat tissue and may increase fat storage and lead to abdominal/visceral weight gain and metabolic syndrome, a condition that can increase the risk of chronic diseases.

Research has shown that NPY's mechanisms that lead to obesity may also increase inflammation in the body, further worsening health conditions.

Here are some tips for maintaining healthy levels of NPY:

EXERCISE

Some studies suggest that regular exercise that increases your heart rate and rate of breathing may help decrease NPY levels, though research is mixed.

EAT A NUTRITIOUS DIET, LIKE THE LIVY METHOD

Although more research is needed, a diet high in fat, processed foods, and added sugars may increase NPY levels. Following a nutrition food plan like The Livy Method may help lower NPY levels!

GLUCAGON-LIKE PEPTIDE-1

Glucagon-like peptide-1 (GLP-1) is a hormone produced in the digestive system when nutrients enter the intestines. This hormone also plays a major role in keeping blood sugar levels stable and making you feel full.

Research suggests that people that struggle with obesity may have issues with GLP-1 signaling.

Here are some tips to help maintain healthy levels of GLP-1:

EAT PLENTY OF PROTEIN

Adding in protein rich foods have been shown to increase GLP-1 levels. The good news is that protein is an important part of The Livy Method, as it is highlighted in breakfast and dinner, but also an important component in almost all meals and snacks!

CONSIDER TAKING PROBIOTICS

Preliminary research suggests that probiotics may increase GLP-1 levels, though more human research is needed. These are recommended along with prebiotics (to feed these good gut bacteria!) as part of The Livy Method supplements list!

CHOLECYSTOKININ

Like GLP-1, cholecystokinin (CCK) is a satiety hormone produced by cells in your digestive system after a meal. It has an important role in energy production, protein synthesis, digestion, and other bodily functions. It also increases the release of the fullness hormone leptin which we discussed earlier.

People that struggle with obesity may have a reduced sensitivity to CCK's effects, which may lead to chronic overeating, similar to the hormone ghrelin. In turn, this may further reduce CCK sensitivity, creating a negative feedback loop, and a cycle of overeating, worsening the likelihood of increased weight gain.

Here are some tips for maintaining healthy levels of CCK:

EAT PLENTY OF PROTEIN

Some research suggests a diet high in protein may help increase CCK levels, and therefore help increase feelings of fullness.

EXERCISE

While research is limited, some evidence supports regular exercise for increasing CCK levels.

PEPTIDE YY

Peptide YY (PYY) is another gut hormone that has a role in decreasing the appetite, leading to increased feelings of satiety. PYY levels may be lower in those that struggle with obesity, and may lead to an increase in appetite and overeating. Maintaining sufficient levels are believed to play a major role in reducing food intake and decreasing the risk of obesity.

Here are some ways to promote healthy levels of PPY in your body:

FOLLOWING A WELL-BALANCED DIET LIKE THE LIVY METHOD

Eating a well-balanced diet that includes protein, fruits and vegetables may promote healthy PYY levels and fullness. Although more research is needed.

EXERCISE

While research on exercise and PYY levels is conflicting, staying active and moving your body is generally beneficial for health, well-being and stress management!

DOPAMINE

Interconnected with the hormones involved in satiety and hunger are neurotransmitters, one of which includes dopamine. Dopamine has a direct effect in activating the reward and pleasure centers in the brain, which can affect both mood and food intake.

Those that struggle with obesity often have a blunted dopamine pathway because of chronic exposure to highly palatable foods, such as foods that are high in added sugar and fats. This over-exposure, which leads to a blunted response when eating, has been suggested to contribute to increased reward-seeking behavior, including overeating.

EAT A BREAKFAST THAT IS HIGH IN PROTEIN

WHAT IS BREAKFAST?

Breakfast is unique because it breaks a time of fasting (after a night of sleep). You are considered a breakfast eater if you eat your first meal of the day following your longest period of sleep, within 2 to 3 hours of waking and if your meal contains food or beverage from at least one food group. This is why The Livy Method recommends eating within 2.5 hours of waking if you are active once awake.

Eating a breakfast that is high in protein has been shown to be one of the best methods of reducing post meal cravings and increasing dopamine levels, but also decreasing a blunted response to it. Protein contains amino acids, several of which are the building blocks of dopamine. Thus, increasing protein consumption has been suggested to increase the production of dopamine in the body!

In addition, getting enough of one amino acid, tyrosine, is an important component in the production of dopamine. Top tyrosine sources include meat, poultry, eggs, fish, cheese, soybeans, and peanuts.

There is also compelling data that shows improved satiety and reduced appetite with the consumption of a high-protein breakfast in normal-weight individuals!!!

SHOULD YOU EAT BREAKFAST?

In the past, skipping breakfast has been associated with weight gain.

However, there is evidence showing that recommendations to eat or skip breakfast have no effect on weight gain or loss (Bjarnadottir, A, 2017, June 3).

That being said, eating breakfast may be a good idea for other reasons. It may improve mental performance in school children, teenagers and certain patient groups. Although, this may also depend on the quality of the breakfast, and as discussed, a high protein breakfast can prove to be very beneficial!

Protein activates the body's signals that curb appetite, which reduces cravings and overeating, mostly due to a decrease in the hunger hormone ghrelin and a rise in the fullness hormones peptide YY, GLP-1 and cholecystokinin. Interestingly, several studies have now demonstrated that eating a high-protein breakfast changes these hormones throughout the day!

BREAKFAST EATERS TEND TO HAVE HEALTHIER HABITS

Many observational studies show that breakfast eaters tend to be healthier, and are less likely to be overweight/obese, and have a lower risk of several chronic diseases. This is mostly likely because those that put the time and energy into having breakfast, also tend to place importance on prioritizing their health in other ways.

A high protein breakfast has been shown to benefit muscle health and to support weight loss by increasing muscle mass, energy expenditure (calories burned), satiety hormones, glucose regulation and by decreasing the desire to snack at night .

Eating a high protein breakfast, has also been shown to improve the body's response to foods high in carbohydrate, up to 4-hours after the breakfast meal. A study looked at the effect of a high protein breakfast compared to a high fat or high carbohydrate breakfast on the body's ability to control glucose and insulin, following the consumption of white bread, four hours after the breakfast meal. Participants consuming a high protein breakfast had improved blood sugar control and insulin levels after consuming the white bread!

This all further reinforces that starting your day with a breakfast making protein the star of the show, not only helps to reduce cravings, improve the feelings of satiety, but also may help boost your mood at the start of the day!

SEEK PLEASURE FROM OTHER ACTIVITIES

The classic approach of finding an alternate activity to get your mind off a craving has benefits beyond distraction. Activities such as listening to music and doing yoga also increase dopamine levels, and can also feed into feeling good!

CONSUME OMEGA-3 FATS

Omega-3 fats, by supplementation and included from foods rich in Omega 3 fats such as salmon and other fatty fishes, can increase the number of dopamine receptors and dopamine levels. Omega-3 fats also are anti-inflammatory and may help improve leptin sensitivity. Because of all the benefits they have, Omega 3 supplementation is also recommended as part of The Livy Method basic supplements list!

Now that we've discussed some of the important hormones and neurotransmitters involved in our hunger and feelings of satisfaction, let's complete our discussion of digestion with a short synopsis of how long it takes the average person to actually process, digest, and move food through their body.

BREAKING DOWN DIGESTION SPEED

Why is it that after eating certain foods, you can feel full for hours, but after others, you're looking for a snack within minutes?

HOW LONG DOES FOOD TAKE TO DIGEST?

The entire digestive process can take several hours. Food generally stays in your stomach between about 40 to 120-plus minutes. Then add another 40 to 120 minutes for time spent in the small bowel. The denser the food, composed with protein and/or fat, the longer it takes to digest. It can take about 24-36 hours for digested food to be eliminated from the body. Longer in those that have digestive issues.

Simple carbohydrates, such as plain rice, pasta or simple sugars, average between 30 and 60 minutes in the stomach, but with added proteins and fats, can take upwards of between two to four hours to leave your stomach.

HOW LONG DOES IT TAKE WATER TO DIGEST?

Liquids leave the stomach faster because there is less to break down:

Plain water: 10 to 20 minutes.

Simple liquids (clear juices, tea, sodas): 20 to 40 minutes.

Complex liquids (smoothies, protein shakes, bone broths): 40 to 60 minutes.

Please note that these times are estimates and how long it takes to digest food varies on factors depending on body type, metabolism, medications, the types of food you eat, level of physical activity overall exercise fitness, if you are living a sedentary versus physically active lifestyle, past surgeries you've endured, and stress level.

Is it possible to tell when your stomach is empty?

Just because you feel hungry doesn't mean your stomach is empty. Our hunger cues, as discussed, can be hormonally regulated, so if you have a high level of hunger hormones circulating, you may feel hungry, even if your stomach is full. Your perception of these sensations is also highly individual, but as discussed before, journaling, using a hunger scale, asking yourself the 4 questions, and following the Livy Method as designed, will help you become more in tune with your hunger and feelings of satisfaction when eating just enough.

REFERENCES

About us. (n.d.). Sleep Foundation. Retrieved March 30, 2022, from https://www.sleepfoundation.org/about-us

Biggers, A., & Jewell, T. (2019, October 22). *Risk factors of having high or low estrogen levels in males.* Healthline. https://www.healthline.com/health/estrogen-in-men

Bjarnadottir, A. (2017, June 3). *Is Skipping Breakfast Bad for You? The Surprising Truth.* Healthline. https://www.healthline.com/nutrition/is-skipping-breakfast-bad

Brown, G. (2019, June 24). *Difference between hormones and neurotransmitters.* Difference Between. http://www.differencebetween.net/science/health/difference-between-hormones-and-neurotransmitters/#:~:text=Hormones%20are%20chemical%20signals%20secreted,the%20brain%20and%20the%20body.

Cherry, K., & Lakhan, S. (2021, July 8). *The role of neurotransmitters.* Verywell Mind. https://www.verywellmind.com/what-is-a-neurotransmitter-2795394

Davis, C.P. (2021, March 29). *Medical definition of hormone.* MedicineNet. https://www.medicinenet.com/hormone/definition.htm

Digestion and absorption of carbohydrates. (2018, October 12). Lane Community College. Retrieved March 30, 2022, from https://media.lanecc.edu/users/powellt/FN225OER/Carbohydrates/FN225Carbohydrates4.html

Gao, C., Liu, Y., Gan, Y., Bao, W., Peng, X., Xing, Q., Gao, H., Lai, J., Liu, L., Wang, Z., & Yang, Y. (2020). Effects of fish oil supplementation on glucose control and lipid levels among patients with type 2 diabetes mellitus: a meta-analysis of randomized controlled trials. *Lipids in Health and Disease, 19,* 87 (2020). https://doi.org/10.1186/s12944-020-01214-w

Glands. (n.d.). You and Your Hormones. Retrieved March 30, 2022, from https://www.yourhor-mones.info/glands/#:~:text=is%20a%20gland%3F-,A%20gland%20is%20an%20organ%20 which%20produces%20and%20releases%20substances,hormones)%20directly%20 into%20the%20bloodstream.

Hawley, A. (2018, December 17). *Protein, its what's for breakfast.* American Society for Nutrition. https://nutrition.org/protein-its-whats-for-breakfast/#:~:text=A%20high%20protein%20 breakfast%20has,desire%20to%20snack%20at%20night%20.

Hjalmarsdottir, F. (2017, June 22). *How protein at breakfast can help you lose weight.* Healthline.https://www.healthline.com/nutrition/ protein-at-breakfast-and-weight-loss#5-Healthy-Snacks-That-Can-Help-You-Lose-Weight

Hormones, receptors and target cells (n.d.). Vivo Pathophysiology. Retrieved March 30, 2022, from http://www.vivo.colostate.edu/hbooks/pathphys/endocrine/basics/hormones.html

How long does it take to digest food: Breaking down digestion speed. (2021, April 19). Cleve-land Clinic. Retrieved March 30, 2022, from https://health.clevelandclinic.org/ how-long-does-it-take-to-digest-food/

Hunger and fullness signals. (2021, March). Alberta Health Services. Retrieved March 30, 2022, from https://www.albertahealthservices.ca/assets/info/nutrition/if-nfs-hunger-and-fullness-signals.pd

Khanacademymedicine. (2015, April 16). *Hormone control of hunger* [Video]. Youtube. https://www. youtube.com/watch?v=EVkFPeP5sFI

Landes, E., & Jones, J. (2022, January 26). *9 hormones that affect your weight and how to improve them.* Healthline. https://www.healthline.com/nutrition/9-fixes-for-weight-hormones

Magee, E., & Nazario, B. (n.d.). *Your 'hunger hormones': How they affect your appetite and your weight.* WebMD. https://www.webmd.com/diet/features/your-hunger-hormones

Mawer, R., & Feller, M. (2021, October 8). *What is ghrelin? All you need to know about this hormone.* Healthline. https://www.healthline.com/nutrition/ghrelin

McCulloch, M. (2015). Appetite hormones. *Today's Dietitian, 17*(7), 26. https://www.todaysdietitian. com/newarchives/070115p26.shtml

Narayan, R. [Khanacademymedicine]. (2014, May 15). *Control of the GI tract: Gastrointestinal system physiology* [Video]. Youtube. https://www.youtube.com/watch?v=_kfB2qKjdgM

Pradhan, G., Samson, S. L., & Sun, Y. (2013). Ghrelin: much more than a hunger hormone. *Current Opinion In Clinical Nutrition and Metabolic Care, 16*(6), 619–624. https://doi.org/10.1097/ MCO.0b013e328365b9be

Purves, D., Augustine, G.J., Fitzpatrick, D., Katz, L.C., LaMantina, A., McNamara, J.O., & Williams, S.M. (2001). Neuroscience (2nd Edition). Sinauer Associates. https://www.ncbi.nlm.nih.gov/books/NBK10957/

Shaikh, J., & Uttekar, P.S. (2021, September 1). *Does it take 30 minutes to digest food?* MedicineNet. https://www.medicinenet.com/does_it_take_30_minutes_to_digest_food/article.htm

van Galen, K.A., ter Horst, K.W., & Serlie, M.J. (2021). Serotonin, food intake, and obesity. *Obesity Reviews, 22*(7), e2210. https://doi.org/10.1111/obr.13210

Wurtman, J.J., & Schrader, J. (2010, August 5). *Serotonin: What it is and why it's important for weight loss: Serotonin is nature's own appetite suppressant.* Psychology Today. https://www.psychologytoday.com/us/blog/the-antidepressant-diet/201008/serotonin-what-it-is-and-why-its-important-weight-loss

Yeung, A.Y., & Tadi, P. (2021, November 14). *Physiology, obesity neurohormonal appetite and satiety control.* StatPearls Publishing. https://www.ncbi.nlm.nih.gov/books/NBK555906/

THE SCIENCE OF FAT AND FAT LOSS

Welcome back to the science posts, where we are providing some foundational information and understanding of how our bodies function, and how implementing The Livy Method optimizes our health, wellness, and mindfulness, by providing an environment where our bodies no longer feel the need to store fat!

In this science post we are following up the conversation about the concept of detoxification, with how the body utilizes and releases fat in the weight loss process. So, to better understand what fat loss really is and what happens in the body to make this process happen, let's take a deeper dive into fat and fat metabolism!

WHAT ARE FATS?

Fats which are also called "fatty acids" or "lipids", are an essential component of the homeostatic function of the human body. They also contribute to some of the body's most vital processes.

Fats and oils are categorized in chemistry as a chemical compound called an ester, which is described as any class of organic compounds that react with water to produce alcohols, and organic or inorganic acids.

Fats are fatty, waxy, or oily compounds that are soluble in organic solvents (dissolve in a substance that contains carbon and nonpolar, for example paint thinner) and insoluble in polar solvents such as water.

These include:

- Fats and oils (triglycerides)
- Phospholipids
- Waxes
- Steroids

The human body is composed of two main types of fat tissue. White fat is important in energy metabolism, heat insulation, and cushioning. Brown fat, also called brown adipose tissue, is a special type of body fat that is turned on (activated) when you get cold. Brown fat produces heat to help maintain your body temperature in cold conditions. Brown fat is found mostly in newborn babies, between the shoulders, and is important for thermogenesis (making heat without shivering). Scientists used to believe that only babies had brown fat. They also thought this fat disappeared by the time most people reached adulthood. However, researchers now know that even adults have small reserves of brown fat (Marcin, A., Hodgson, L. 2022, January 24) It's typically stored in small deposits around the shoulders and neck.

A third type of fat called beige (or brite) fat has been identified in humans, and is a relatively new area of research. These fat cells function along the spectrum between brown and white fat cells. Similarly to brown fat, beige cells can help utilize fat rather than store it. It is thought that certain hormones and enzymes are released when you are stressed, cold, or during exercise, which can help convert white fat into beige fat. This is an exciting area of research to possibly help prevent obesity and maximize healthy body fat levels.

When you are first born, your body does not have much white fat to help insulate and retain body heat; although there are white fat cells, there is not much fat stored in them.

Brown fat cells are somewhat smaller than white, are composed of several smaller fat droplets, are iron rich (hence the brown colour), and are loaded with mitochondria which can generate heat. A new-born baby produces heat primarily by breaking down fat molecules into fatty acids in brown fat cells. Instead of those fatty acids leaving the brown fat cell, as happens in white fat cells, they get further broken down in the mitochondria and their energy is released directly as heat. Brown fat contains more mitochondria than white fat, and has generated interest among researchers because it appears to be able to use regular body fat as fuel. In addition, exercise and the exposure to cold may stimulate hormones that activate brown fat.

All people have some "constitutive" brown fat, which is the kind you're born with. There's also another form that's "recruitable." This means it can change to brown fat under the right circumstances. This recruitable type is found in muscles and white fat throughout your body.

RECAP OF THE DIGESTION OF FAT

When you eat food that contains fat, mostly triglycerides, it is digested through the stomach and intestines.

In the intestines, the following happens: large fat droplets get mixed with bile salts from the gallbladder in a process called emulsification. The mixture breaks up the large droplets into several smaller droplets called micelles, increasing the fat's surface area. The pancreas secretes enzymes called lipases that attack the surface of each micelle and break the fats down into their components of glycerol and fatty acids. These components get absorbed into the cells lining the intestine. Once in the intestinal cell, the parts are reassembled into fat molecules (triglycerides) with a protein coating called chylomicrons. This protein coating makes the fat dissolve more easily in water. The chylomicrons are then released into the lymphatic system. They do not go directly into the bloodstream because they are too big to pass through the wall of the capillaries (which are a tiny network of blood vessels). The lymphatic system eventually merges with the veins, at which point the chylomicrons are able to pass into the bloodstream. Fat molecules get broken down into glycerol and fatty acids and are then reassembled because fat molecules are too big to easily cross cell membranes. So, when passing from the intestine through the intestinal cells into the lymph, or when crossing any cell barrier, the fats must first be broken down. However, when fats are being transported in the lymph or blood, it is better to have a few large fat molecules than many smaller fatty acids, because the larger fats do not "attract" as many excess water molecules by osmosis as many smaller molecules would.

The fat that we store in our body is also stored as triglycerides. When you eat, your body converts any energy it does not need to use right away into triglycerides. The triglycerides are then stored in your fat cells. Later, hormones release triglycerides for energy between meals if you need them. Triglycerides also provide insulation to cells, and aid in the absorption of fat-soluble vitamins.

A triglyceride is made up of glycerol (a 3-carbon sugar alcohol/polyol) and 3 fatty acids. Fatty acids are chains of hydrogen and carbon. They are composed of differing lengths and various degrees of saturation. The molecule ends with something called a carboxylic acid group. How they are "bonded" allows for the creation of many different types of fatty acids. Fatty acids in biological systems usually contain an even number of carbon atoms and are typically 14 carbons to 24 carbons long.

Check out this video for more information on the molecular structure of triglycerides!

https://www.khanacademy.org/science/ap-biology/chemistry-of-life/properties-structure-and-function-of-biological-macromolecules/v/molecular-structure-of-triglycerides-fats

Fats are also an essential component of the cell membrane in our body's cells. In the cell membrane, phospholipids are arranged in a bilayer, providing cell protection and serving as a barrier to certain molecules. The structure is typically made of a glycerol backbone, 2 fatty acid tails (which are hydrophobic, meaning the structure tries to avoid water molecules), and a phosphate group (which are hydrophilic, meaning that group is attracted to water molecules). These molecules are called phospholipids, and are amphipathic (having parts that are both hydrophobic and hydrophilic). The hydrophilic part faces outward and the hydrophobic part faces inward. This physical arrangement of the cell membrane helps to monitor and act as a gatekeeper, as to which molecules can enter and exit the cell. For example, nonpolar molecules and small polar molecules, such as oxygen and water, can easily diffuse in and out of the cell. Large polar molecules, for example, glucose, cannot pass freely so they need the help of transport proteins.

Another type of lipid is wax. Waxes are esters made of a long-chain alcohol and a fatty acid. Waxes provide protection. Cerumen (also known as earwax) helps protect the skin of the ear canal.

Another class of lipids includes steroids, which have a structure of four fused rings. One important type of steroid is cholesterol. Cholesterol is produced in the liver and is the most common steroid. Cholesterol is the precursor to many steroid hormones such as estrogen, testosterone, and cortisol. It is also the precursor to vitamin D as well as bile salts, which help in the emulsification of fats and their subsequent absorption by cells. Cholesterol is also an important part in the composition of the cell membrane. Cholesterol is inserted in the bilayer of the cell membrane and has a big influence on the fluidity of the membrane.

WHY IS DIETARY FAT IMPORTANT?

Most of the fat that we need can be made by our bodies, however, there are certain fats that our bodies cannot manufacture but are essential for our health and bodily functions.

These fats, are called "essential" fats, essential fatty acids (EFAs), or polyunsaturated fats. Essential fats include Omega-3 fats (found in foods such as fish and flax seed) and Omega-6 fats (found in foods such as nuts, seeds, and corn oil).

Other components of omega-3 fatty acid that are found in fatty fish and shellfish are called eicosapentaenoic acid (EPA) and docosahexaenoic acid (DHA). Fish can contain the metal mercury which acts as a toxin in the body, so choosing a good quality Omega-3 supplement, or fish lower in mercury like salmon, anchovies, herring, sardines, Pacific oysters, trout, Atlantic mackerel, and Pacific mackerel will help provide the EPA and DHA that your body needs.

Fat is an important component in our diet because:

- Fat helps the body absorb and process fat soluble vitamins like vitamins A, D, E, and K

- Fat helps to keep our skin healthy

- Essential fats like Omega-3 are important for heart health and brain health. Omega-3 fatty acids may reduce inflammation throughout the body. Inflammation can cause damage to your blood vessels, leading to heart disease and stroke. Omega-3 fatty acids may benefit heart health by: decreasing triglycerides levels, slightly lowering blood pressure, reducing blood clotting that could lead to clots therefore decreasing your risk of stroke and heart attack, decreasing heart failure risk and reducing arrhythmias (Mayo Clinic 2019, September).

The omega-3 fatty acids EPA and DHA are critical for normal brain function and development throughout all stages of life. EPA and DHA seem to have important roles in the developing baby's brain, and are also vital for the maintenance of normal brain function throughout life. They are abundant in the cell membranes of brain cells, preserving cell membrane health and facilitating communication between brain cells. In older adults, lower levels of DHA in the blood have been associated with smaller brain size, which is a sign of accelerated brain aging. It is also thought that Omega-3 fatty acids also reduce inflammation in the brain.

- Healthy unsaturated fats, like monounsaturated fats and polyunsaturated fats, can help lower levels of LDL cholesterol. Monounsaturated fats are found in avocados, peanut butter, nuts like almonds, hazelnuts, cashews, and pecans, and seeds, such as pumpkin, sesame, and sunflower seeds. They are also found in plant oils such as olive, peanut, safflower, sesame, and canola oils. A study from Harvard researchers (Harvard Health Publishing *2021, April 19)* found that consuming monounsaturated fats, especially from nuts and olive oil, can lower a person's risk of heart disease — especially if the healthy fat replaces saturated fat and refined carbs (which can also raise LDL low density lipoprotein levels, the type of cholesterol that causes plaque build-up in the arteries). Unsaturated fats help to raise the HDL high density lipoprotein (good) cholesterol levels. HDL picks up excess LDL in the blood and moves it to the liver, where it is broken down and discarded. The goal is to have a high HDL-to-LDL ratio for a healthy blood lipid profile. The researchers added that any benefit from consuming monounsaturated fats may be negated if a person continues to consume too much saturated fat.

- Fat adds flavour to food by making food taste better.

- Fat keeps you feeling satisfied longer after a meal as it helps to regulate blood sugar levels and the hormones involved in hunger and satiety. Fat also takes the digestive system longer to process and digest, thus also making you feel fuller longer.

Although fats are a healthy part of our diet, it is still important to acknowledge that only up to 10% of our fat intake should come from saturated fats. Saturated fat includes foods like meat, dairy and coconut oil. Those monitoring their cholesterol should be mindful of their saturated fat intake.

Fats are generally recommended to account for about 30% of our diet, with the majority of fat intake coming from the healthy unsaturated fats listed above. Trans fat (partially hydrogenated fats) found in processed food can be detrimental to our health, so avoid these as much as possible.

Check out this video for more details discussing the differences between these kinds of fats.

https://www.youtube.com/watch?v=mvvx2yQRbzQ

Now that we discussed the fundamentals of fat, let's talk about how our bodies use it for stored energy, and how it is released from the body!

RECAP ON THE PROCESS OF METABOLISM

When you are not eating, whether active or at rest, your body must draw on its internal energy stores of complex carbohydrates, fat, and proteins to provide your body with the energy it needs to do all the things it needs to do to keep you alive! Important activities like breathing, keep your heart pumping, digesting, or providing energy for that run you enjoy.

Most of the cells in your body use glucose along with amino acids (the building blocks of protein) and fats for energy. However, glucose is the main source of fuel for your brain. Nerve cells and chemical messengers located there need it to help them process information, and having access to glucose is very important for overall brain function. Your brain uses about 60% of the glucose that our bodies use. However, glucose does not always have to come immediately from foods and beverages. Glucose is also generated by the body to ensure that we always have the amount that is needed. One way that this is achieved, is by breaking down something called glycogen, in order to free up the glucose it contains.

Glycogen is released by an important hormone called glucagon. When the body doesn't need to use glucose for energy, it is stored in the liver and muscles by insulin. Glycogen is this stored form of connected glucose molecules. When the body needs a quick boost of energy or is not getting glucose from food, glycogen is broken down to release glucose into the bloodstream to be used as fuel by the cells. Your body can store enough glycogen in order to keep you fueled for about a day. This process is called glycogenolysis.

The body can also produce glucose through a process called gluconeogenesis. This process occurs when the body (mainly the liver, then kidneys and to a less extent the small intestine) makes glucose from non-carbohydrate sources which include lactate (what our bodies produce during exercise), glycerol (is produced when fats are digested, can be used for energy or stored in adipose tissue) and amino acids. Gluconeogenesis occurs when glycogen stores become low and glucose consumption is too low or nonexistent, such as during periods of starvation or prolonged fasting. Although the body has enough glycogen stored in the muscles and liver to last about a day, after approximately 14 hours in a fasted state it will begin to increase its percentage of gluconeogenesis, generating energy in increased ratios as time goes on. In this stage, energy that is stored in adipose tissue all around your body in the form of triglycerides will be liberalized. In the fat cell, other types of lipases (enzymes that break down fats) work to break down fats into fatty acids and glycerol in a process called lipolysis. These lipases are activated by various hormones, such as glucagon, epinephrine, and growth hormone. The resulting glycerol and fatty acids are released into the blood and travel to the liver through the bloodstream. Once in the liver, the glycerol and fatty acids can be either further broken down directly to get energy, or used to make glucose.

One very important consideration though, is that skeletal muscle (composed of amino acids) can be used as a source when generating glucose through the pathway of gluconeogenesis. This can lead to muscle wasting and loss over time which can have a major impact on the body!

An additional alternative form of energy that can be generated if needed, is the formation of ketone bodies from our fat reserves. Ketone bodies can serve as a fuel source if glucose levels are too low in the body. Ketones serve as fuel in times of prolonged starvation, carbohydrate deprivation, or when patients suffer from uncontrolled diabetes and cannot utilize most of the circulating glucose. In these scenarios, fat stores are liberated, generating ketone bodies to the body and brain for energy.

So, in losing weight, what happens to the fat we use for energy?

The body disposes of fat through a series of very complex metabolic pathways. For those of you that are interested in the biochemistry behind each of these processes, these videos are a great way to understand the different pathways of fat metabolism described simply above:

https://www.youtube.com/watch?v=9lElznAeI48

https://www.youtube.com/watch?v=Qep3wooEw5M

https://www.ninjanerd.org/lecture/mobilization-of-triglycerides

https://www.ninjanerd.org/lecture/fatty-acid-synthesis-part-1

https://www.ninjanerd.org/lecture/fatty-acid-oxidation-part-2

https://www.ninjanerd.org/lecture/the-metabolic-map-lipids

https://www.ninjanerd.org/lecture/lipoprotein-metabolism-chylomicrons-vldl-idl-ldl-hdl

This is where things become very interesting!!

As the body begins to draw on our fat stores for energy, although the number of fat cells remains the same, each fat cell simply gets smaller.

The by-products of the metabolism of fat are processed by the body in the following ways:

As water, through your skin (when you sweat) and your kidneys (when you urinate), and as carbon dioxide (CO_2) through your lungs (when you breathe out). Exercise also increases your respiratory rate, so more CO_2 (and the by-products of fat) leaves your body when you work out. Being well hydrated is well documented in supporting the body in fat loss (also allowing for the release of fat by-products through urine). Fat breakdown also generates heat, which keeps body temperatures normal.

What happens to body fat when you exercise?

Your muscles first utilize stored glycogen for energy. After about 30 to 60 minutes of aerobic exercise, your body starts utilizing mainly fat stores depending on the intensity of the activity. If you are exercising moderately, this takes about an hour.

Building your muscle mass will raise your basal metabolic rate, and the amount of energy your body uses at rest.

This leads us to the most interesting theory about how most of our fat leaves our body.

A study conducted by a team of Australian researchers Meerman and Brown (2014), calculated exactly what happens to our fat when we drop weight, and revealed that we don't convert our missing mass into heat or energy. We actually breathe it out.

Their results reveal that 22 pounds (10 kg) of fat turns into 18.5 pounds (8.4 kg) of carbon dioxide, which is exhaled when we breathe, and 3.5 pounds (1.6 kg) of water, which we then excrete through our urine, tears, sweat and other bodily fluids.

Lead author of the paper Ruben Meerman, a physicist, first became interested in the biochemistry of weight loss when he dropped 33 pounds (15 kg). However, when he asked his doctors where this weight went, he was surprised by the fact no one could tell him.

After surveying 150 doctors, dieticians, and personal trainers, he discovered that more than half thought that fat was converted into heat or energy as we break it down.

But, as a physicist, Meerman knew that this would violate the **law of conservation of mass**. This law states that in a closed or isolated system, matter cannot be created or destroyed. It can change forms but is conserved. This law also helped scientists understand that substances did not disappear as result of a reaction (as they may appear to do), rather they transform into another substance of equal mass.

We put on weight in the form of fat when excess stores of energy are converted into triglycerides (compounds made up of carbon, hydrogen, and oxygen), and are then stored in lipid droplets inside fat cells. To lose weight, you need to break down those triglycerides to access their carbon.

The results of this study showed that in order to completely break down 22 pounds (10 kg) of human fat, we need to inhale 64 pounds (29 kg) of oxygen (and somewhere along the way, burn 94,000 calories). This reaction produces 62 pounds (28 kg) of CO_2 and 24 pounds (11 kg) of water. Their calculations show that the lungs are the primary excretory organ for fat!

However, they couldn't work out exactly what was happening to the fat cells in this reaction. After months of research, Meerman discovered a formula from a paper published in 1949 that solved the problem. It showed that oxygen atoms are shared between the carbon and hydrogen in fat at a ratio of 2:1 (forming carbon dioxide and water). This allowed them to come up with the final figure of 84 percent of a fat molecule's atoms being exhaled as carbon dioxide, and the remaining 16 percent ending up as water.

However, this doesn't mean that simply breathing deeply will help us lose weight, energy is still required to unlock the carbon and break down the fat in the first place.

Meerman stated that "You can only breathe so many times a day; on a day of rest, you breathe around 12 times a minute so 17,280 times you'll breathe in a day and each one takes 10 milligrams of carbon with it, roughly."

Hopefully you found this interesting!

Check out this video for more details!

https://www.youtube.com/watch?v=C8ialLlcdcw

REFERENCES

Ahmed, S., Shah, P. & Ahmed, O. (2021, May 9). *Biochemistry, lipids*. StatPearls Publishing. https://www.ncbi.nlm.nih.gov/books/NBK525952/

Betts, G.J., Young, K.A., Wise, J.A., Johnson, E., Poe, B., Kruse, D.H., Korol, O., Johnson, J.E., Womble, M., & DeSaix, P. (2019, May 29). *Anatomy and physiology*. Openstax. https://open-textbc.ca/anatomyandphysiologyopenstax/chapter/lipid-metabolism/

Cannon, B., Nedergaard, J. (2008). Neither fat nor flesh. *Nature, 454*, 947–948. https://doi.org/10.1038/454947a

Cleveland Clinic. (2019, January 17). *Where does body fat go when you lose weight?* https://health.cleve-landclinic.org/where-does-body-fat-go-when-you-lose-weight/#:~:text=Your%20body%20must%20dispose%20of,(when%20you%20breathe%20out)

Constant, F., Popkin, B.M. & Gardner, C.D (2012). Drinking water is associated with weight loss in overweight dieting women independent of diet and activity. *Obesity, 16(11), 2481-2488.* https://doi.org/10.1038/oby.2008.409

El-Zayat, S.R., Sibaii, H. & El-Shamy, K.A. (2019). Physiological process of fat loss. *Bulletin of the National Research Centre*, 43. https://doi.org/10.1186/s42269-019-0238-z

Feingold, K. R. (2021). Introduction to lipids and lipoproteins. In K. R. Feingold (Eds.) et. al., Endotext. Mdtext.com, Inc. https://pubmed.ncbi.nlm.nih.gov/26247089/

Freudenrich, C. (n.d.). How fat cells work. How Stuff Works. https://science.howstuffworks.com/life/cellular-microscopic/fat-cell3.htm

Harvard Health Publishing. (2021, April 19). *Know the facts about fats.* Harvard Medical School. https://www.health.harvard.edu/staying-healthy/know-the-facts-about-fats#:~:text=%-22Fat%20helps%20give%20your%20body,your%20body%20absorb%20vital%20nutrients.

Health e-University. (n.d.) *What are fats?* https://www.healtheuniversity.ca/EN/CardiacCollege/Eating/Fats/

Hensrud, D. (2020, November 5). *What is brown fat? How is it different from other body fat?* Mayo Clinic. https://www.mayoclinic.org/healthy-lifestyle/weight-loss/expert-answers/brown-fat/faq-20058388#:~:text=Brown%20fat%2C%20also%20called%20brown,mitochondria%20than%20does%20white%20fat.

Khan Academy. (2015, July 14). *Molecular structure of triglycerides (fats) | Biology* [Video]. Youtube. https://www.youtube.com/watch?v=OpyTJbzA7Fk

Laskowski, E. R. (2020, April 21). *When you lose weight, where does the lost body fat go?* Mayo Clinic. https://www.mayoclinic.org/healthy-lifestyle/weight-loss/expert-answers/body-fat/faq-20058251

LCR Staff Writer. (2019, November 6). *Weight loss info: What does fat in urine look like?* LCR Health. https://lcrhealth.com/fat-loss-urine-color/

Link, R., Chin, K. (2021, February 18). *Can peeing cause lasting weight loss?* Healthline. https://www.healthline.com/nutrition/do-you-lose-weight-when-you-pee

Marcin, A., Hodgson, L. (2022, January 24). *Brown fat: What you should know.* Healthline. https://www.healthline.com/health/brown-fat#purpose

Mayo Clinic Staff. (2020, September 29). *Triglycerides: Why do they matter?* Mayo Clinic. https://www.mayoclinic.org/diseases-conditions/high-blood-cholesterol/in-depth/triglycerides/art-20048186#:~:text=Triglycerides%20are%20a%20type%20of,triglycerides%20for%20energy%20between%20meals.

Mayo Clinic Staff. (2019, September 28). *Omega-3 in fish: How eating fish helps your heart.* Mayo Clinic. https://www.mayoclinic.org/diseases-conditions/heart-disease/in-depth/omega-3/art-20045614#:~:text=Omega%2D3%20fatty%20acids%20are,Decreasing%20triglycerides

Meerman, R., Brown, A. J. (2014). When somebody loses weight, where does the fat go? *BMJ, 349(7257).* https://doi.org/10.1038/oby.2008.409

Ninja Nerd. (2018, January 6). *Metabolism | Lipoprotein metabolism | Chylomicrons, vldl, idl, ldl, & hdl* [Video]. Youtube. https://www.youtube.com/watch?v=wQY0xpwqPfQ

Ninja Nerd. (2017, June 19). *Metabolism | Fatty acid oxidation: Part 2* [Video].Youtube. https://www.youtube.com/watch?v=jxylGoJP9jY

Ninja Nerd. (2017, June 14). *Metabolism | The metabolic map: Lipids* [Video]. Youtube. https://www.youtube.com/watch?v=Wm7UR0zCQzM

Ninja Nerd. (2017, June 7). *Metabolism | Mobilization of triglycerides* [Video]. Youtube. https://www.youtube.com/watch?v=lD62q1hUae4&t=1s

Ninja Nerd. (2017, May 29). *Metabolism | Fatty acid synthesis: Part 1* [Video]. Youtube. https://www.youtube.com/watch?v=nBFSz63T1c0

Oregon State University. (2019, June). *Essential fatty acids.* https://lpi.oregonstate.edu/mic/other-nutrients/essential-fatty-acids

Pearson, K. (2017, December 5). *How omega-3 fish oil affects your brain and mental health.* Healthline. https://www.healthline.com/nutrition/omega-3-fish-oil-for-brain-health#TOC_TITLE_HDR_3

https://www.thoughtco.com/definition-of-conservation-of-mass-law-604412

SciShow. (2015, December 21). *The deal with fat* [Video]. Youtube. https://www.youtube.com/watch?v=mvvx2yQRbzQ

SciShow. (2015, January 13). *When you burn fat, where does it go?* [Video]. Youtube. https://www.youtube.com/watch?v=C8ialLlcdcw

The Editors of Encyclopedia Britannica. (2021, May 31.). *Ester.* Encyclopedia Britannica. https://www.britannica.com/science/ester-chemical-compound

Watson, H. (2015). Biological membranes. *Essays in Biochemistry, 59,* 43–69. https://doi.org/10.1042/bse0590043

Wondersofchemistry. (2019, March 4). *Fat metabolism introduction* [Video]. Youtube. https://www.youtube.com/watch?v=Qep3wooEw5M

Wondersofchemistry. (2018, March 31). *Lipolysis* [Video]. Youtube. https://www.youtube.com/watch?v=9lElznAeI48

SUGARS AND THE BRAIN

The goal of these posts is to help provide some foundational information and create an understanding of how our bodies function. We will also discuss how implementing The Livy Method optimises our health, wellness, and mindfulness, by providing an environment where our bodies no longer feel the need to store fat!

In this post, we are taking a closer look at sugar and non-nutritive sugars (NNS), alternatively known as artificial sweeteners. We already examined sugar quite closely, discussing all the reasons why it is beneficial to minimise the intake of it, especially if maximising the program. However, let's take a closer look at how sugar and NNS affect us, more specifically our brain, and how they may influence our bodies, and even the choices we make!

WHY DO WE LIKE SUGAR?

Sugar provides energy to our bodies in the form of calories, so humans, like most other creatures, have evolved to enjoy it. Our primitive ancestors were scavengers. Sugary foods are excellent sources of energy, so we have evolved to find sweet foods particularly palatable. Foods with unpleasant, bitter and sour tastes can be unripe, poisonous or rotting. These foods could cause sickness, so we are more likely to avoid those foods.

We need food to survive, and we need the amount that nature has provided for us in the perfect package, which is food in its whole form. This often includes fibre or other substances that allow for a slower digestion, and does not usually facilitate a fast rise in blood sugar, as well as it is more likely to create a feeling of satiety.

Therefore, to maximise our survival as a species, this innate brain system has us seeking out these foods.

Sugar comes in a variety of forms. To recap, glucose is the simplest form of carbohydrates and only has one sugar molecule, which is called a **monosaccharide**. Other monosaccharides that may sound familiar include fructose, galactose, and ribose, which the body also processes or may produce for energy.

We have discussed the importance of how our body breaks down our food into these simple sugars in order to provide energy to the body in the science post on Insulin. There was also discussion on how added sugar affects our bodies. But let's take a deeper dive into how added sugar affects our brain and nervous system, after a refresher on how our body processes these added sugars.

WHAT IS ADDED SUGAR OR FREE SUGARS?

The World Health Organization (WHO) has been cautioning people to reduce their intake of "free sugars" to less than 10 percent of daily calories since 1989. The organization says that doing so can lower the risk of becoming obese or overweight, or experiencing tooth decay. Free sugars include both the sugars naturally found in honey and fruit juice, and sugar added to food and drinks. On food labels, added sugars include words such as glucose, fructose, corn syrup, brown sugar, dextrose, maltose, and sucrose, as well as many others.

As we had discussed, the most significant sources of added sugar in today's diet consists primarily of the simple sugar fructose. Fructose is a fairly sweet, naturally occurring sugar. It comes from most fruits, and even some vegetables.

However, the majority of sources of fructose that people tend to consume are table sugar (which is called **sucrose**, made from sugar cane or beets, is composed of 50% glucose and 50% fructose), honey, agave nectar, fruit juices, palm sugar and (**HFCS**) high fructose corn syrup (HFCS is a highly processed and inexpensive substitute for cane sugar that was introduced in the 1970s, which is made from corn. It's used to sweeten a variety of processed foods, including soda, candy, baked goods, and cereals). Today's sugars are often refined and concentrated.

After we ingest food, the stomach and small intestine go right to work in breaking the food down into its simplest form of glucose, which is absorbed and then released into the bloodstream. Once in the bloodstream, glucose can be used immediately by the cells for energy, or stored in our bodies to be used later. However, glucose and fructose are metabolised very differently by the body. Before it can be used by the body, fructose needs to be converted into glucose, which is conducted by the liver. While every cell in the body can use glucose, the liver is the only organ that can metabolise fructose when ingested in significant amounts!

Before the mass production of refined sugar, humans rarely consumed fructose in high amounts. But as food science has developed over the years, our food has greatly changed from its very simple former self. When people eat a diet that is high in calories and high in fructose, the liver is thought to become overloaded and starts turning the fructose into fat. Many scientists believe that excess fructose consumption may be a key driver in many of the most serious diseases today. These include obesity, type 2 diabetes, insulin resistance, heart disease, and even cancer. However, more human evidence is needed. Although, researchers debate the extent to which fructose contributes to these disorders, there is a considerable mounting body of evidence justifying the concerns.

THE DATA BEHIND SUGAR

In 2015, the WHO further suggested reducing free sugar daily intake to less than 5 percent of calories, about 6 teaspoons, for optimising health. In the United States In 2017–2018, the average daily intake of added sugars was 17 teaspoons for children and young adults aged 2 to 19 years, as well as in adults over 20 years of age. Added sugar also accounts for 14 percent of the average person's daily calorie intake. Most of this comes from beverages, including energy drinks, alcoholic drinks, soda, fruit drinks, and sweetened coffee and teas.

Other common sources are snacks. These don't just include the obvious, like brownies, cookies, dough-nuts, and ice cream. You can also find large quantities of added sugar in bread, salad dressing, granola bars, cereals, and even fat-free yoghurts to name a few.

In Canada, a health report released on October 20, 2021 from Statistics Canada, found that in a 2015 Canadian Community Health Survey (CCHS), the total sugar intake in Canada per person was estimated at 105.6 g/day. While this was down from the 110.0 g/day reported in a CCHS conducted in 2004, it was concluded that the apparent reduction between 2004 and 2015 may actually be caused by misreporting as a result of changes in survey methodology. They also reported that total sugar consumption from foods actually increased between 2004 and 2015, while total sugar intake from beverages decreased.

The Office of Disease Prevention and Health Promotion in the Dietary Guidelines for Americans 2020-2025, suggest cutting the consumption of added sugars to less than 10 percent of calories per day. This is actually in line with WHO's older recommendations, that were stated earlier back in 1989!

However, to help consumers, the Food and Drug Administration (FDA) has developed a new food label that lists added sugars separately, which manufacturers are required to use (though some smaller manufacturers had until 2021 to comply).

https://www.fda.gov/food/food-labeling-nutrition/changes-nutrition-facts-label

Canada has also updated their food labels, which now identifies the total percentage of sugars in a product. This change was imposed by the Canadian Food Inspection Agency (CFIA), with compliance to be enforced by Dec 15, 2022.

https://www.canada.ca/en/health-canada/services/food-labelling-changes.html

Check out the video to see how sugar can be hidden in the foods we buy!

https://www.ted.com/talks/robert_lustig_sugar_hiding_in_plain_sight?language=en

HOW DOES SUGAR AFFECT OUR BRAIN?

There is an increasing body of research that tells us excess sugar could be as addictive as some street drugs and have similar effects on the brain. The concept of food addiction is a very controversial subject among scientists and clinicians. While it is true that you can become physically dependent on certain drugs, it is debated whether you can be addicted to food when you need it for basic survival. There are also those that caution us in our language when using words like addiction when describing things like food. The drug crisis is very serious, and those with addiction are physiologically driven to get more drugs. This can also be said for those with other addictions such as alcohol and sex. They may resort to crime and violence to do so, whereas those seeking out food wouldn't necessarily go to those lengths. However, our environment today is abundant with sweet, energy dense, processed foods, which we have easy access to. Our portion sizes have also increased to a much greater degree. What is clear, is these foods are having some effects on us, and our drive to have more of it.

Given the rise of obesity, one could argue towards the theory that sugar can in fact be addictive to some sort of degree. However, despite the differing opinions regarding this, researchers and nutritionists can agree that sugar has addictive properties and we need to be having less of it. Furthermore, in certain individuals with certain predispositions, this could manifest as having a compulsion towards sugary foods.

Check out this video on the effects of sugar and the brain!

https://www.ted.com/talks/nicole_avena_how_sugar_affects_the_brain?language=en

DOPAMINE

Sugar increases activity in certain parts of our brains, which means that those parts become excited due to the incoming nutrition. When we eat sweet foods the brain's reward system, called the mesolimbic dopamine system, gets activated. Brain activation happens because of electrical activity that occurs within cells called neurons. A neuron is a nerve cell that sends and receives electrical and chemical signals.

All brain activity occurs in the form of electricity that is sent down small "wires" or "tunnels" in the neurons called axons. The electrical signal through the axons then results in the release of brain chemicals called neurotransmitters, which are a chemical substance released by neurons in the brain that send messages to our bodies and muscles.

Interconnected with the hormones involved in satiety and hunger are neurotransmitters, one of which includes dopamine. Eating sugar releases opioids and dopamine in our bodies. This is the link between added sugar and compulsive behaviour. Dopamine has a direct effect in activating the reward and pleasure centres in the brain, which can affect both mood and food intake.

Those that struggle with obesity often have a blunted dopamine pathway because of chronic exposure to highly palatable foods, such as foods that are high in added sugar and fats. This over-exposure, which leads to a blunted response when eating, has been suggested to contribute to increased reward-seeking behaviour, including overeating.

When a certain behaviour causes an excessive release of dopamine, you experience sensations of pleasure that you are inclined to re-experience, and so repeat the behaviour. As you repeat that behaviour more and more, your brain adjusts to release less dopamine. The only way to feel the same amount of pleasure as before, is to repeat the behaviour in increasing amounts and frequency. This then leads to the blunted response that was described above, subsequently leading one to seek out more sugar which ultimately leads to substance (sugar) abuse and weight gain. Also, every time we have sugar, we reinforce neuropathways, causing the brain to become increasingly hardwired to crave sugar, from a habit formation perspective.

Check out these videos to learn more about the dopamine reward system and the mesolimbic dopamine pathway system!

https://www.youtube.com/watch?v=YzCYuKX6zp8&t=10s

https://www.youtube.com/watch?v=f7E0mTJQ2KM&t=36s

Check out this video about the potentially addictive effects of sugar on the brain!

https://www.youtube.com/watch?v=ShQYz8AwKJE

HYPOTHALAMUS

As discussed in the science post The Set Point Theory, the hypothalamus, a small region of the brain located at the base of the brain, near the pituitary gland, is involved in the integration of signals directed to it from hormones like leptin (from adipose or fat cells), ghrelin (from the digestive system), insulin (the pancreas), along with many other hormones that regulate our hunger and satiety. Your metabolism constantly adjusts up or down based on a variety of signals. The set point theory also suggests that your weight may go up or down temporarily but will ultimately return to its normal set range. The signalling system we have in place helps to maintain our weight.

Some researchers (Jung & Kim, 2013) believe that the reactive signal system stops working efficiently over time and leptin and insulin resistance develop, causing us to gain weight. As discussed, the thought is that foods that are high in fat and sugar, like many processed foods available today, lead to not only inflammation in the body, but also in the brain. Because the hypothalamus is so important in regulating, and interpreting the signals involved in hunger, satiety, and metabolism, inflammation can lead to a disruption in the pathway of these signals and even in how fat is stored. This can lead to weight gain. This further corroborates the negative impact that sugar and processed high fat foods have on our brain!

MANAGING CRAVINGS

Many people experience food cravings. Cravings can occur particularly when one is stressed, hungry, or their gastronomic senses are inundated with the sight, sound, and aroma of their favourite foods being prepared.

To overcome cravings, we need to inhibit our natural response to indulge in these tasty foods. A network of inhibitory neurons is critical for adjusting our behaviour. These neurons are concentrated in the prefrontal cortex, a key area of the brain involved in decision-making, impulse regulation and delaying gratification.

https://www.youtube.com/watch?v=i47_jiCsBMs&t=2s

Inhibitory neurons are like the brain's brakes and release the neurotransmitter GABA or Gamma Aminobutyric Acid. GABA is considered an inhibitory neurotransmitter because it blocks, or inhibits, certain brain signals and decreases activity in your nervous system. When GABA attaches to a protein in your brain known as a GABA receptor, it produces a calming effect. This can help with feelings of anxiety, stress, and fear. It may also help to prevent seizures.

Research in rats has shown that eating high sugar diets can alter inhibitory neurons. Rats that were fed a high sugar diet were also less able to regulate their behaviour and make decisions.

This shows that there is the potential that what we eat can influence our ability to make choices that are beneficial to us, and may underlie why diet changes can be so difficult for people.

A 2017 study asked people to rate how much they wanted to eat a high calorie snack when they were hungry versus when they had recently eaten. The people who regularly ate a high-fat, high-sugar diet rated their cravings for snack foods higher even when they were not hungry. This suggests that regularly eating high-sugar foods could heighten cravings, creating a negative feedback loop of wanting more and more of these foods.

However, there is good news! Our taste buds can adapt to accept less sugar in a fairly short period of time. Following a plan like The Livy Method that promotes eating nutrient dense, whole foods, which are naturally lower in sugar, is a great way to support the body in addressing cravings. By reducing sugar, especially concentrated sugars (as recommended by The Livy Method), not only limits the amount of sugar ingested, but also makes foods that are less sweet seem sweeter. This is a common finding by members when participating in the plan. In fact, members often comment on how they start to really enjoy the natural taste and flavours of the food they eat. They also describe how when they indulge in eating sweet or processed food, it doesn't taste as good as they remember, or they can taste the chemicals and additives in the food which they never noticed before.

SUGAR AND MEMORY

Another brain area that can be affected by high sugar diets is the hippocampus. The hippocampus is a part of the brain found in the inner folds of the bottom middle section of the brain, known as the temporal lobe. Its main functions involve human learning and memory.

The hippocampus is part of the limbic system, which is associated with the functions of feeling and reacting. The limbic system is situated on the edge of the cortex, and it includes the hypothalamus and the amygdala. These structures help control different bodily functions, such as the endocrine system and what is commonly known as the "fight or flight" response.

The hippocampus helps humans process and retrieve two kinds of memory, declarative memories and spatial relationships.

Declarative memories are those related to facts and events. Examples include learning how to memorise speeches or lines in a play.

Spatial relationship memories involve pathways or routes. For example, when a cab driver learns a route through a city, they use spatial memory. Spatial relationship memories appear to be stored in the right hippocampus.

The hippocampus is also where short-term memories are turned into long-term memories. These are then stored elsewhere in the brain. Research has shown that nerve cells continue to develop throughout adulthood, and that the hippocampus is one of the few places in the brain where new nerve cells are generated.

Similar to animal research, there is emerging evidence that a Western-style (WS) diet – high in saturated fat and added sugar – impairs human hippocampal functioning. However, the conditions under which this occurs are not fully understood.

According to a scientific systematic review (Taylor et al, 2021), regular consumption of a Western-style diet places individuals at higher risk for mild cognitive impairment and dementia. With progressive memory loss and hippocampal damage being an early feature and neurological sign of dementia, diet-induced hippocampal impairment may have significant ramifications by initiating or speeding-up the disease process. Furthermore, the same physiological changes associated with a Western-style diet, including increased hippocampal inflammation and reduced hippocampal neurogenesis (the formation of new neurons), are associated with the pathology of dementia.

There are also further consequences in having an impaired hippocampus resulting from the western-style diet. The hippocampus has a role in appetite regulation, by its involvement in recalling previously consumed food to assist with conscious adjustment of intake – such as recalling what you recently ate, and so moderating your intake accordingly. When satiated, the hippocampus may automatically inhibit retrieval of pleasant food-related memories. Thus, when looking at food when satiated, it will no longer lead to the recollection of how pleasant it is to eat, thereby dulling desire. It is suggested that impaired hippocampal inhibition leads to an increase in the intake of the very foods (highly palatable sweet and fatty foods) that caused the hippocampal damage in the first place, creating a "vicious cycle". This model is actually called the vicious cycle model and is likely to lead to slow, long term weight gain.

Finally, the hippocampus seems to be involved in appetitive interoception. Interoception is the perception of sensations from inside the body. This includes the perception of physical sensations related to internal organ function such as a heart beat, respiration, satiety, as well as the autonomic nervous system activities that are related to emotions. Hippocampal impairment has been linked to interoceptive insensitivity which can result in a disconnection with hunger/satiety and thirst cues. This may lead to overconsumption, resulting in weight gain and obesity over the long term.

Check out this video on the hippocampus and limbic system!

https://www.youtube.com/watch?v=2K3GAaC2SEI

Check out this video on the effects of sugar on the brain and hippocampus

https://www.youtube.com/watch?v=Dacv_OoM62s

NON-NUTRITIVE SWEETENERS (NNS)

From reviewing this information, it can be seen that a diet high in sugar, especially when paired with poor quality fats (often seen in processed foods), has detrimental effects on not only our bodies, but our brain!

This is why there is a market for non-nutritive sweeteners. The purpose of these products is to satisfy the desire for a sweet taste, but has few or negligible calories. The thought is people can continue to enjoy the taste of "sweet", while being able to manage weight/weight loss and health issues such as diabetes.

NNS are made by chemical alternatives, altering existing sugars or amino acids, or are made from the derivatives of plants. Some examples of NNS are aspartame (Equal, NutraSweet), cyclamate (Sucaryl, Sugar Twin, Sweet 'N Low), saccharin, sucralose (Splenda), sugar alcohols (mannitol, sorbitol, and xylitol. Note: if you eat too much of them, sugar alcohols can cause diarrhea and bloating), polydextrose, stevia, steviol glycosides, and erythritol, amongst many others. The regulation of NNS varies in different countries, allowing for different product availability depending on where you live. NNS are found in many different products, and may even be listed as an ingredient that is not identified as a low sugar product, or used as an additive.

THE SCIENCE BEHIND THE USE OF NNS

When going down the rabbit hole of research into this area, it is honestly difficult to navigate how NNS truly affects us. There have been many studies that do report the safety of these products, which does allow for wide scale use of them through regulatory bodies such as the FDA and Health Canada. However, it is identified that there is still a need for both further primary research, and high quality comprehensive systematic reviews including meta-analyses, to inform future recommendations about the health benefits and risks of NNS, to advise and support health care practice and public health decision-making. There are noted controversies of the existing evidence between different artificial sweeteners surrounding their use.

Although NNS maintains a similar palatability as natural sugars, the way the body processes them is different. Interestingly, the gut microbiota may play a major role in the physiological effects of artificial sweeteners on body weight regulation and glucose homeostasis. According to Pang, Goossens, & Blaak (2021) there is mechanistic evidence that artificial sweeteners may induce gut microbiota dysbiosis, by altering the gut microbiota composition and function.

The gut microbiota appears to react differently to NNS than to real sugar. These organisms become less able to break down real sugars the more that they are exposed to artificial sweeteners. Not being able to break down sugars is a concern, because this change in the microbiota can affect the ability of our bodies to digest and process the nutrients from the food we eat. This can potentially lead to deficiencies in vitamins and minerals!

Although different physiological processes are involved in the effect of NNS on metabolic health, meta-analyses of Randomised Control Trials (RCTs) or RCTs and prospective cohort studies, suggest that artificial sweeteners may have a neutral effect on body weight and glycemic control, respectively, or may have a beneficial effect on long-term body weight regulation. Even though the majority of human studies report no significant effects of artificial sweeteners on body weight and glycemic control, it should be emphasised that the study duration of most studies is limited. Furthermore, unlike rodent studies, long-term studies investigating the underlying physiological effects of body weight control and metabolic health of humans and NNS use are scarce and therefore warranted. This is important to consider when interpreting the results.

Notably, artificial sweeteners are metabolised differently and may not all elicit the same metabolic effect. For instance, components of NNS may affect the gut microbiota composition directly and others are easily digested and absorbed. It is also important to note, most NNS provide little to no energy, so should not affect your blood sugar. However, this is not true in the case of sugar alcohols. They are a carbohydrate, and a hybrid form of sugar and alcohol. These products can affect your blood sugar, so those with diabetes should still be mindful of them.

Not all studies investigating the effects of artificial sweeteners on body weight control and glucose homeostasis, take into account the different metabolic pathways of distinct artificial sweeteners. Therefore, human data on the effects of distinct artificial sweeteners are limited or lacking. The difference in metabolic fate of artificial sweeteners may underlie conflicting findings that have been reported related to their effects on body weight control, glucose homeostasis, and underlying biological mechanisms. Therefore, making conclusions of the metabolic effects of a single artificial sweetener to all artificial sweeteners is not appropriate.

An example of this is that there is growing evidence that indicates certain artificial sweeteners like sucralose reduce insulin sensitivity and affect the gut bacteria.

It is recommended that future studies should consider the metabolic pathways of different artificial sweeteners. Also, further (long-term) human research investigating the underlying physiological pathways of different artificial sweeteners on microbiota alterations and its related metabolic pathway is warranted to evaluate the potential impact of their use.

Finally, although Stevia in the purified form, called stevioside (known as stevia extract or Stevia rebaudiana), is considered safe to use, whole stevia leaves or crude stevia extracts are not recommended, as there is not enough information about their potential impact on your health. There's concern that raw stevia herb may harm your kidneys, reproductive system, and cardiovascular system. It may also drop blood pressure too low or interact with medications that lower blood sugar.

The WHO has released this 2022 systematic review and meta-analysis of the health effects of the use of non-sugar sweeteners.

https://ewgagdyvsuu.exactdn.com/wp-content/uploads/2022/04/Health-effects-of-the-use-of-non-sugar-sweeteners-a-systematic-review-and-meta-analysis.pdf

Currently, project SWEET, a European Commission Horizon 2020 funded project and human multicenter study is being conducted over 5 years. It is supported by a consortium of 29 pan-European research, consumer and industry partners, who will develop and review evidence on long term benefits and potential risks involved in switching over to sweeteners and sweetness enhancers (S&SEs) in the context of public health and safety, obesity, and sustainability. Check out their website to follow their findings!

https://sweetproject.eu/

Check out this excellent video synopsis on the complexity of reviewing the literature related to NNS.

https://www.youtube.com/watch?v=L6pJrxmDYEI

Check out this video on the microbiome that includes some discussion on the effects of NNS on the microbiome.

https://www.youtube.com/watch?v=IDqMB6C1uys

THE TAKEAWAY ON SUGAR AND NNS

After examining all the research on sugar and NNS, what is clear is that reducing both are beneficial to your health. The science is clear on the effect sugar has on the reward centre of the brain, and the impact of a diet high in sugar and fat, typical of today's processed diet, on the incidence of obesity and disease, also causing inflammation in the body and the brain.

An alternative has been presented to feed our sugar cravings in the form of NNS, which are presented as a safe alternative. However, the question is why do we need to feed into our need and want of sugar, with an alternative that is processed, chemically altered, made in a lab, and still needs more long term, rigorous human study? Other "sugar free" products often contain additives, dyes, colours, flavours and preservatives. These products are often marketed as "healthy"!

The Livy Method recommends eating whole, natural foods, that includes the option of adding in natural sugars on occasion if desired. This combined with proper hydration, and eating to satisfaction, allows one to experience and enjoy food as it was meant to be experienced.

Sweetness inundates our senses, dulling them over time. By reducing the amount of sweet we eat, our taste buds can actually "reset", and foods less sweet, actually taste sweeter. Therefore, we can actually enjoy eating foods in their natural state, while our bodies and brains reap all the nutritional benefits, becoming healthier because of it. Now that is truly sweet!

REFERENCES

Avena, N. (2017, September). *How sugar affects the brain* [Video]. TED. https://www.ted.com/talks/nicole_avena_how_sugar_affects_the_brain?language=en

Ahmed, S. H., Guillem, K., & Vandaele, Y. (2013). Sugar addiction: pushing the drug-sugar analogy to the limit. *Current opinion in clinical nutrition and metabolic care, 16*(4), 434–439. DOI: 10.1097/MCO.0b013e328361c8b8

BioBrainBuddies. (2020, May 8). *Memory and the hippocampus* [Video]. Youtube. https://www.youtube.com/watch?v=2K3GAaC2SEI

Changes to the nutrition facts label. (2022, March 7). U.S. Food and Drug Administration. https://www.fda.gov/food/food-labeling-nutrition/changes-nutrition-facts-label

Chong, C. P., Shahar, S., Haron, H., & Din, N. C. (2019). Habitual sugar intake and cognitive impairment among multi-ethnic Malaysian older adults. *Clinical Interventions in Aging, 14*, 1331–1342. https://doi.org/10.2147/CIA.S211534

Edwards, S. (2016). *Sugar and the brain.* Harvard Medical School. https://hms.harvard.edu/news-events/publications-archive/brain/sugar-brain

Government of Canada. (2008, April 30). *The safety of sugar substitutes.* https://www.canada.ca/en/health-canada/services/healthy-living/your-health/food-nutrition/safety-sugar-substitutes.html

Government of Canada. (2022, June 30). *Food labelling changes.* https://www.canada.ca/en/health-canada/services/food-labelling-changes.html

Guo, Y., Zhu, X., Zeng, M., Qi, L., Tang, X., Wang, D., Zhang, M., Xie, Y., Li, H., Yang, X., & Chen, D. (2021). A diet high in sugar and fat influences neurotransmitter metabolism and then affects brain function by altering the gut microbiota. *Translational Psychiatry, 11.* https://doi.org/10.1038/s41398-021-01443-2

Grech, A., Kam, C.O., Gemming, L., & Rangan, A. (2018). Diet-quality and socio-demographic factors associated with non-nutritive sweetener use in the Australian population. *Nutrients, 10*(7). doi: 10.3390/nu10070833

Healthline Medical Network. (2019, March 7). *What does gamma aminobutyric acid (GABA) do?* Healthline. https://www.healthline.com/health/gamma-aminobutyric-acid

How sweet it is: All about sugar substitutes. (2021, November 30). U.S. Food and Drug Administration. https://www.fda.gov/consumers/consumer-updates/how-sweet-it-all-about-sugar-substitutes

Hyman, M. (2018, January 15). *What's worse for you: Sugar or artificial sweetener?* Cleveland Clinic. https://health.clevelandclinic.org/whats-worse-sugar-or-artificial-sweetener/

Khanacademymedicine. (2014, June 25). *Reward pathway in the brain: Processing the environment* [Video]. Youtube. https://www.youtube.com/watch?v=YzCYuKX6zp8&t=10s

Kanwal, J.K. (2016, January 11). Brain tricks to make food taste sweeter: How to transform taste perception and why it matters. Science in the News. https://sitn.hms.harvard.edu/flash/2016/braintricks-to-make-food-taste-sweeter-how-to-transform-taste-perception-and-why-it-matters/

Jung, C. H., & Kim, M. S. (2013). Molecular mechanisms of central leptin resistance in obesity. Archives of Pharmacal Research, 36(2), 201–207. https://doi.org/10.1007/s12272-013-0020-y

Lee, A. A., & Owyang, C. (2017). Sugars, sweet taste receptors, and brain responses. Nutrients, 9(7). https://doi.org/10.3390/nu9070653

Leech, J., & Kubala, J. (2021, November 12). *What are sugar alcohols, and are they a healthy sugar swap?* Healthline. https://www.healthline.com/nutrition/sugar-alcohols-good-or-bad

Link, R. (2019, April 18). *Is stevia safe? Diabetes, pregnancy, kids, and more.* Healthline. https://www.healthline.com/nutrition/is-stevia-safe

Lohner, S., Toews, I. & Meerpohl, J.J. (2017). Health outcomes of non-nutritive sweeteners: Analysis of the research landscape. *Nutrition Journal, 16.* https://doi.org/10.1186/s12937-017-0278-x

Lustig, R. (2019, March.). *Sugar: Hiding in plain sight* [Video]. TED. https://www.ted.com/talks/robert_lustig_sugar_hiding_in_plain_sight?language=en

Mesolimbic pathway. (n.d.). Neuroscientifically Challenged. https://neuroscientificallychallenged.com/glossary/mesolimbic-pathway

Myüz, H., & Hout, M.C. (2019). Trick or treat? How artificial sweeteners affect the brain and body. *Frontiers for Young Minds, 7*(51). doi: 10.3389/frym.2019.00051

Neuroscientifically Challenged. (2015, February 13). *2-Minute neuroscience: Reward system* [Video]. Youtube. https://www.youtube.com/watch?v=f7E0mTJQ2KM&t=36s

Neuroscientifically Challenged. (2019, September 4). *2-Minute neuroscience: Prefrontal cortex* [Video]. Youtube. https://www.youtube.com/watch?v=i47_jiCsBMs&t=2s

Pang, M.D., Goossens, G.H., & Blaak, E.E. (2021). The impact of artificial sweeteners on body weight control and glucose homeostasis. *Frontiers in Nutrition, 7.* doi:10.3389/fnut.2020.598340

Petre, A. (2020, August 19). *Artificial sweeteners: Good or bad?* Healthline. https://www.healthline.com/nutrition/artificial-sweeteners-good-or-bad

Pugle, M. (2022, January 27). *How your body tries to prevent you from losing too much weight.* Healthline. https://www.healthline.com/health-news/how-your-body-tries-to-prevent-you-from-losing-too-much-weight

Price, C. J., & Hooven, C. (2018). Interoceptive awareness skills for emotion regulation: Theory and approach of mindful awareness in body-oriented therapy (MABT). *Frontiers in Psychology, 9.* https://doi.org/10.3389/fpsyg.2018.00798

Project overview. (n.d.). Sweet Project. https://sweetproject.eu/

REICHELT, A. (2019, December 26). *A neuroscientist explains what sugar really does to our brains.* Science Alert. https://www.sciencealert.com/research-shows-sugar-can-change-your-brain-here-s-how

Rios-Leyvraz, M., & Montez, J. (2022). *Health effects of the use of non-sugar sweeteners: A systematic review and meta-analysis.* Geneva: World Health Organization. https://ewgagdyvsuu.exactdn.com/wp-content/uploads/2022/04/Health-effects-of-the-use-of-non-sugar-sweeteners-a-systematic-review-and-meta-analysis.pdf

Rivera, L.S. (2020, January 15). *Effects of sugar on the brain: Cravings and inflammation.* UVAHealth. https://blog.uvahealth.com/2020/01/15/effects-sugar-brain/

Ruiz-Ojeda, F. J., Plaza-Díaz, J., Sáez-Lara, M. J., & Gil, A. (2019). Effects of sweeteners on the gut microbiota: A review of experimental studies and clinical trials. *Advances in Nutrition, 10*(Suppl.1), S31–S48. https://doi.org/10.1093/advances/nmy037

SciShow. (2019, January 14). *Are artificial sweeteners bad for you?* [Video]. Youtube. https://www.youtube.com/watch?v=L6pJrxmDYEI

Stevenson, R.J., Francis, H.M., Attuquayefio, T., & Ockert, C. (2017). Explicit wanting and liking for palatable snacks are differentially affected by change in physiological state, and differentially related to salivation and hunger. *Physiology & Behavior, 182,* 101-106. https://doi.org/10.1016/j.physbeh.2017.10.007

Taylor, Z.B., Stevenson, R.J., Ehrenfeld, L., Francis, H.M. (2021). The impact of saturated fat, added sugar and their combination on human hippocampal integrity and function: A systematic review and meta-analysis. *Neuroscience & Biobehavioral Reviews, 130,* 91-106. https://doi.org/10.1016/j.neubiorev.2021.08.008

TEDx Talks. (2016, June 27). *Microbiome: Gut bugs and you* [Video]. Youtube. https://www.youtube.com/watch?v=IDqMB6C1uys

TEDx Talks. (2016, June 29). *This is your brain on sugar* [Video]. Youtube. https://www.youtube.com/watch?v=xCXtcoUxJZc

TEDx Talks. (2017, March 1). *Society's sweet tooth... the brain's response to sugar* [Video]. Youtube. https://www.youtube.com/watch?v=ShQYz8AwKJE

TEDx Talks. (2018, September 25). *Misunderstanding dopamine: Why the language of addiction matters* [Video]. Youtube. https://www.youtube.com/watch?v=aqXmOb_fuN4

U.S. Department of Agriculture and U.S. Department of Health and Human Services. (2020, December). *Dietary guidelines for Americans 2020-2025 (9th ed).* https://www.dietaryguidelines.gov/sites/default/files/2020-12/Dietary_Guidelines_for_Americans_2020-2025.pdf

World Health Organization. (2015, March 4). *WHO calls on countries to reduce sugars intake among adults and children.* https://www.who.int/news/item/04-03-2015-who-calls-on-countries-to-reduce-sugars-intake-among-adults-and-children

Yang, Q. (2010). Gain weight by going diet? Artificial sweeteners and the neurobiology of sugar cravings: Neuroscience 2010. *The Yale Journal of Biology and Medicine, 83*(2), 101–108. https://www.ncbi.nlm.nih.gov/pmc/articles/PMC2892765/#!po=59.3750

Yeung, A.W.K., & Wong, N.S.M. (2020). How does our brain process sugars and non-nutritive sweeteners differently: A systematic review on functional magnetic resonance imaging studies. *Nutrients, 12.* https://doi.org/10.3390/nu12103010

MAINTENANCE AND THE MICROBIOME

This is the final science post, where the goal of these posts is to help provide some foundational information and create an understanding of how our bodies function. We will also discuss how implementing The Livy Method optimises our health, wellness, and mindfulness, by providing an environment where our bodies no longer feel the need to store fat!

We have talked about our microbiome in previous science posts, and how our health can be influenced by it. Just by following The Livy Method for these last 12 weeks, has had a major influence on our gut health and microbiome. In fact, as some of us head into maintenance, eating what makes us feel good, reinforces eating the foods that feed these good bacteria, continuing to keep us healthy. Let's review all that we have discussed about the microbiome and then take a deeper dive into it.

THE MICROBIOME- A REVIEW

According to the National Institute of Environmental Health Science (NIEHS) in the United States, the microbiome is defined as the collection of all microbes, such as bacteria, fungi, viruses, and their genes, that naturally live on our bodies and inside us.

Bacteria, viruses, fungi and other microscopic living things are referred to as microorganisms, or microbes, for short. Although microbes are so small that they require a microscope to see them, they contribute in big ways to human health and wellness. They protect us against pathogens, help our immune system develop, help to produce vitamins that our body needs, and enable us to digest food to produce energy.

Because the microbiome is a key connection between the body and the environment, these microbes can affect health in many ways and can even affect how we respond to certain environmental substances. Some microbes alter environmental substances in ways that make them more toxic, while others act as a buffer and make environmental substances less harmful.

HOW CAN THE MICROBIOME AFFECT HEALTH?

More than 2,000 years ago, Hippocrates, the Greek physician who many attribute to the foundation of modern medicine, suggested that all disease begins in the gut. It turns out he was onto something (Gunnars, K., 2019, February)!

Studies examining the diversity of the human microbiome started with Antonie van Leewenhoek, who, as early as the 1680s, had compared his oral and fecal microbiota (What is Biotechnology?). He noted the striking differences in microbes between these two habitats and also between samples from individuals in states of health and disease in both of these sites. Thus, studies of the profound differences in microbes at different body sites, and between health and disease, have existed since the science of microbiology itself. What is new today is the ability to use scientific techniques to gain insight into why these differences exist, and to understand how we can affect transformations from one state to another.

The human microbiome has a different community of microbes located in different areas in the body. Trillions of these microbes exist mainly inside your intestines and on your skin. Most of the microbes in your intestines are located in the large intestine in an area called the cecum, and they are referred to as the gut microbiome. They are also found in other areas of the body such as the oral and nasal cavities, and the conjunctiva of our eyes.

According to Healthline, although many different types of microbes live inside you, bacteria are the most studied. In fact, there are more bacterial cells in your body than human cells. It is estimated that there are roughly 40 trillion bacterial cells in your body and only 30 trillion human cells. That means you are more bacterial than human!

Altogether, these microbes may weigh as much as 2–5 pounds (1–2 kg), which is roughly the weight of your brain. Together, they function and are considered as an extra organ in your body, playing a huge role in your health.

THE MICROBIOME AND DIGESTION

Humans have evolved to live with microbes for millions of years. During this time, microbes have learned to play very important roles in the human body. In fact, without the gut microbiome, it would be very difficult to survive. Interestingly, the food you eat affects the diversity of your gut bacteria.

There are up to 1,000 species of bacteria in the human gut microbiome, and each of them plays a different role in your body. Most of them are extremely important for your health, while others may cause disease. Interestingly, on average a person carries about 160 species in their gut.

As discussed in the science post The Basics of Digestion, the gut flora in our colon help to ferment the indigestible food and produce vitamins such as Vitamin K and B vitamins that are reabsorbed by the colon. But that's not all, an estimated 80% of our immune system is found in our gut. Having a healthy digestive system, which includes a good balance of our healthy gut flora, ensures a healthier immune system and better nutrient absorption. This is why the Livy Method recommends taking a good quality probiotic, along with a prebiotic (if needed), to help feed those good microbes. Eating the high fibre, nutrient rich foods on plan not only gives our body what it needs, but is also vital in supporting our gut flora!

A person's core microbiome begins to develop from birth and is formed in the first years of life, but can change over time in response to different factors including diet, medications, and environmental exposures. You are first exposed to microbes when you pass through your mother's vaginal canal. However, new evidence suggests that babies may come in contact with some microbes while inside the womb.

Breastfeeding introduces beneficial bacteria to a baby's gut which also contributes to their microbiome.

As you grow, your gut microbiome begins to diversify, meaning it starts to contain many different types of microbial species. Higher microbiome diversity is considered good for your health.

Differences in the microbiome may lead to different health effects from environmental exposures and may also help determine individual susceptibility to certain illnesses. Environmental exposures can also disrupt a person's microbiome in ways that could increase the likelihood of developing conditions such as diabetes, obesity, cardiovascular and neurological diseases, allergies, and inflammatory bowel disease.

As your microbiome grows, it affects your body in a number of ways, including:

- **Digesting breast milk:** Some of the bacteria that first begin to grow inside babies' intestines are called ***Bifidobacteria***. They digest the healthy sugars in breast milk that are important for growth.

- **Influencing your immune system:** The gut microbiome also influences how your immune system works. By communicating with immune cells, the gut microbiome can influence how your body responds to infection.

- **Influencing your brain health:** Some research suggests that the gut microbiome may also affect the central nervous system, which controls brain function. See below for more details.

Digesting fibre: Certain bacteria digest fibre, producing short-chain fatty acids in the gut, which are important for gut health. Fibre may help prevent weight gain, diabetes, heart disease and the risk of cancer.

Short-chain fatty acids are fatty acids with fewer than 6 carbon atoms. They are produced when the friendly gut bacteria ferment fibre in your colon and are the main source of energy for the cells lining it.

Excess short-chain fatty acids are used for other functions in the body. For example, they may provide roughly 10% of your daily energy needs. Short-chain fatty acids are also involved in the metabolism of important nutrients like carbohydrates and fat.

About 95% of the short-chain fatty acids in your body are: acetate (C2), propionate (C3), and butyrate (C4). Propionate is mainly involved in producing glucose in the liver and small intestine, acetate is important for energy production and synthesis of lipids, and butyrate is the preferred energy source for cells that line the colon (Brown, M.J., 2021, October).

Many factors affect the amount of short-chain fatty acids in your colon, including how many microorganisms are present, the food source, and the time it takes food to travel through your digestive system.

Eating a lot of fibre-rich foods, such as fruits, vegetables, and legumes, is linked to an increase in short-chain fatty acids. However, the amount and type of fibre you eat affects the composition of bacteria in your gut, which affects what short-chain fatty acids are produced.

For example, studies have shown that eating more fibre increases butyrate production, while decreasing your fibre intake reduces production.

The following types of fibre are best for the production of short-chain fatty acids in the colon:

- **Inulin.** You can get inulin from artichokes, garlic, leeks, onions, wheat, rye, and asparagus.
- **Fructooligosaccharides (FOS).** FOS are found in various fruits and vegetables, including bananas, onions, garlic, and asparagus.
- **Resistant starch.** You can get resistant starch from grains, barley, rice, beans, green bananas, legumes, and potatoes that have been cooked and then cooled.
- **Pectin.** Good sources of pectin include apples, apricots, carrots, oranges, and others.
- **Arabinoxylan.** Arabinoxylan is the most common fibre in wheat bran, making up about 70% of the total fibre content.
- **Guar gum.** Guar gum can be extracted from guar beans, which are legumes.

Some types of cheese, butter, and cow's milk also contain small amounts of butyrate.

THE MICROBIOME AND WEIGHT GAIN

There are thousands of different types of bacteria in your intestines, most of which benefit your health. However, having too many unhealthy microbes can lead to disease. An imbalance of healthy and unhealthy microbes is sometimes called gut dysbiosis, and it may contribute to weight gain.

Some studies have shown that the gut microbiome differed completely between identical twins, one of whom was obese and one of whom was healthy. This demonstrated that differences in the microbiome were not genetic.

Interestingly, in one study, when the microbiome from the obese twin was transferred to mice, they gained more weight than those that had received the microbiome of the lean twin, despite both groups eating the same diet. These studies show that microbiome dysbiosis may play a role in weight gain.

Fortunately, probiotics are good for a healthy microbiome and can help with weight loss, by helping to strengthen our gut health which can fall in line with our weight loss goals. Nevertheless, some studies suggest that the effects of probiotics on weight loss on their own are probably quite small, with people losing less than 2.2 pounds (1 kg). However, probiotics are suggested with The Livy Method as they help with weight loss by improving digestion.

THE MICROBIOME AND IBS AND IBD

The microbiome can also affect gut health and may play a role in intestinal diseases like irritable bowel syndrome (IBS) and inflammatory bowel disease (IBD). The bloating, cramps and abdominal pain that people with IBS experience may be due to gut dysbiosis. This is because the microbes produce a lot of gas and other chemicals, which contribute to the symptoms of intestinal discomfort.

However, certain healthy bacteria in the microbiome can also improve gut health. Certain *Bifidobacteria* and **Lactobacilli**, which are found in probiotics and yoghurt, can help seal gaps between intestinal cells and help heal the intestines. These species can also prevent disease-causing bacteria from sticking to the intestinal wall. In fact, taking certain probiotics that contain *Bifidobacteria* and *Lactobacilli* can reduce symptoms of IBS.

Additionally, lower levels of short-chain fatty acids were linked to worsen ulcerative colitis.

Human studies also suggest that short-chain fatty acids, especially butyrate, can improve symptoms of ulcerative colitis and Crohn's disease. Furthermore, improvements in inflammation were associated with an increase in butyrate production due to its anti-inflammatory properties.

THE MICROBIOME AND THE HEART

Interestingly, the gut microbiome may even affect heart health. A recent study in 1,500 people found that the gut microbiome played an important role in promoting "good" HDL cholesterol and tri-glycerides. Certain unhealthy species in the gut microbiome may also contribute to heart disease by producing trimethylamine N-oxide (TMAO). TMAO is a chemical that contributes to blocked arteries, which may lead to heart attacks or stroke.

Certain bacteria within the microbiome convert choline and L-carnitine, both of which are nutrients found in red meat and other animal-based food sources, to TMAO, potentially increasing risk factors for heart disease. However, other bacteria within the gut microbiome, particularly *Lactobacilli*, may help reduce cholesterol when taken as a probiotic.

This is in-line with The Livy Method that encourages eating lots of vegetables, heavier carbs in the form of whole grains, darker rices, fruits, legumes, fermented foods, encouraging higher fibre content to feed the microbes in the gut, ultimately encouraging the growth of beneficial microbes. Many of the foods are also prebiotics which feed these flora. Eating foods like dandelion greens, garlic, onions, leeks, asparagus, bananas, barley, oats, apples, cocoa, flax seeds, wheat bran, and seaweed are great for feeding our beneficial bacteria. It is also recommended to go meat free occasionally or when you can, to help support the gut.

THE MICROBIOME AND BLOOD SUGAR

According to Barra et al. (2021), the gut microbiota can also influence blood glucose. Lower bacterial diversity correlates with insulin resistance and higher adiposity (having more fat).

Type 2 diabetes (T2D) is associated with an altered composition of the gut microbiota, where the lower relative abundance of **Firmicutes *Clostridia***, but higher ***Betaproteobacteria*** in diabetic humans was associated with higher blood glucose. There are many correlations between taxonomy (taxonomy is the science of naming, describing and classifying organisms and includes all plants, animals and micro-organisms of the world) and possible host functions. For example, the Firmicutes phylum consists predominantly of SCFA butyrate-producing bacteria; specifically, certain *Clostridia* which have anti-inflammatory properties and are less abundant in individuals with T2D.

Faecalibacterium prausnitzii is another butyrate-producing strain that is associated with improvements in glucose tolerance in patients who have undergone gastric bypass surgery, suggesting that bacterial metabolites can also affect glucose homeostasis. In addition, branched-chain amino acids produced by ***Bacteroides vulgatus*** species positively correlate with insulin resistance. Therefore, short-chain fatty acids seem to help regulate blood sugar levels and improve insulin resistance, especially in people with diabetes or insulin resistance.

Very interestingly, although there are fewer examples of microbes or microbial communities causing changes in blood glucose, the microbiota from obese mice can transmit higher blood glucose into germ-free mice independently of changes in adiposity.

THE MICROBIOME AND THE BRAIN

The gut microbiome may even benefit brain health in a number of ways! Certain species of bacteria can help produce chemicals in the brain called neurotransmitters. An example of this is serotonin. Serotonin is a neurotransmitter which sends signals between your nerve cells. Serotonin is found mostly in the digestive system (stomach and intestines), although it's also in blood platelets and throughout the central nervous system. Serotonin is most commonly known for helping to regulate our mood, but is also involved in digestion, clotting, sleeping, eating, bone health, and libido.

According to Caltech (2015, April), although serotonin is well known as a brain neurotransmitter, it is estimated that 90 percent of the body's serotonin is made in the digestive tract. In fact, altered levels of this peripheral serotonin have been linked to diseases such as irritable bowel syndrome, cardiovascular disease, and osteoporosis. Therefore, it can be seen that if our gut health can influence even this one neurotransmitter, it potentially can influence so many aspects of our health!

Furthermore, the gut is physically connected to the brain through millions of nerves. Thus, the gut microbiome may also affect brain health by helping to influence the messages that are sent to the brain through these nerves. Some studies have shown that people with various psychological disorders have different species of bacteria in their guts, compared to healthy people. This suggests that the gut microbiome may affect brain health. However, it's unclear if this is simply due to different dietary and lifestyle habits.

THE MICROBIOME AND PHASE III DETOXIFICATION

As discussed in the science post Detox, if phase I and II occur effectively, toxins can be eliminated by the kidneys and bowels via urine and stool. Although the liver is thought of as our primary detoxification organ, it requires a large variety of nutrients that must first be absorbed via the digestive system, in order to function optimally. Ironically though, the digestive system is also the initial site of exposure to ingested toxins. Due to these factors, it is recognized that there is an additional third phase of detoxification which occurs primarily in the digestive system.

The third phase of detoxification refers to a highly concentrated anti-porter (transport) system of proteins in the body. There are many anti-porters being researched, particularly P-glycoprotein, an anti-porter in the small intestine that moves toxins from cells into the gut. This transport system ensures the movement of harmful compounds out of the cell and into the detoxification organs.

A healthy diet and microbiome are key to the success of phase III, whereas digestive inflammation leads to the impairment of it. If phase III is compromised, an accumulation of toxins within the cell occurs. Errors in P-glycoprotein expression have been linked to Alzheimer's disease, and suspected to play a role in stress management and inflammatory bowel disease.

ORAL BACTERIA AND THE LINK TO HEALTH

Rheumatoid arthritis and pneumonia are just two diseases that have been linked to gum disease. According to Domini et al. (2019) bacteria normally present in the mouth can also release toxins that make their way into the brain. Once there, they may contribute to Alzheimer's disease. Maintaining good dental hygiene is not just important for oral health, but can be very important for our overall health, including our brain!

Over 6 billion bacteria, including 700 different species, reside inside your mouth. Some promote health, others provoke disease. It is thought that there are about 15 to 20 harmful strains, but that will continue to evolve over time, and we learn more about how these species interact with each other.

Your mouth, or what scientists refer to as the oral microbiome, is "a complex community with lots of communication between bacteria of the same species as well as across species,". When your teeth feel slimy and in need of a brushing, that is an indication of their presence.

Oral bacteria also thrive inside your cheeks and on your tongue, palate, tonsils, and gums. Your mouth is a great habitat for unicellular (one cell) microorganisms. It's constantly moist, has a fairly neutral pH, and a warm temperature. However, despite this perfect environment to sustain the bacteria, you do end up swallowing bacteria that end up in your gut. As discussed in the science posts on digestion, our acidic stomach acid is a protective mechanism that kills bacteria that may enter the stomach to protect us from getting sick! This is why a healthy digestive system is so important.

Furthermore, there is another portal of entry for bacteria to access our bodies via our mouths. Every time we chew, brush, or floss, these microbes can get pushed into the small vessels in our gums, which gives them access into the bloodstream.

In a healthy mouth, the immune system keeps microbes from entering the body and causing infection. However, when you have chronic gum disease or other oral infections, this system is compromised.

When oral bacteria access the bloodstream, they can travel to organs throughout the body, including the brain.

One known organism with the ability to cause harm in other parts of the body is *Porphyromonas gingivalis*, or Pg. Pg has been linked to a number of serious health issues, including pneumonia, rheumatoid arthritis, heart disease, hepatitis, and esophageal cancer.

Researchers now know it can sneak across the blood-brain barrier, a network of dense cells that protects the brain from harmful substances. Once there, Pg can cause pathological changes.

Researchers have observed Pg in the brains of deceased people with Alzheimer's disease. Surprisingly, Pg major proteins called gingipains, were found in the brains at a level much higher in those that had Alzheimer's disease, than in those with healthy brains of the same age. This supports that Pg may have a large influence on Alzheimer's disease. Currently there is an area of research looking into drugs and possible vaccines to eradicate and limit its spread.

Migration of bacteria from one part of the body to another is a natural process, which can't completely be prevented. However, the number of bacteria that can get into the bloodstream may be reduced by improved oral care. Here's how to do so:

BRUSH AND FLOSS

According to the Canadian Dental Association (CDA) you should brush your teeth for at least 2-3 minutes, ideally, brushing after every meal, because the bacterial attack on teeth begins minutes after eating. At the very least, brush once a day and always before you go to bed.

Flossing removes plaque and bacteria that you cannot reach with your toothbrush. It helps dislodge bits of food that would otherwise collect bacteria and contribute to inflammation and infection on the gums. If you don't floss, you are missing more than one-third of your tooth surface. Plaque is the main cause of gum disease. It is an invisible bacterial film that develops on your teeth every day. Within 24 to 36 hours, plaque hardens into tartar (also called calculus), which can only be removed by professional cleaning. Floss at least once a day, and plaque can be prevented from hardening into tartar.

See this link from the CDA on how to properly brush and floss your teeth.

https://www.cda-adc.ca/en/oral_health/cfyt/dental_care/flossing_brushing.asp

MOUTHWASH

Flossing and brushing are the two main recommendations for teeth care and health.

There is some discussion regarding whether or not mouthwash should be a part of the daily dental routine in a healthy person, and those without gum inflammation. There is some thought that mouthwash may disrupt the oral microbiome to allow for proper growth of good bacteria. It would be like comparing it to using antibiotics, which can wipe out the harmful bacteria that is making us sick, but also the beneficial bacteria. However, this is very individual and it would be important to speak to your dentist if you have any concerns related to your specific dental health, and health risks.

EAT MORE FRUITS AND VEGETABLES

Eating high-fibre foods, particularly fruits and vegetables, can reduce the progression of gum disease. Fibre creates more saliva in the mouth, which helps get rid of excess food and offsets harmful acids. Also, these foods keep us healthier in general which is important in preventing disease.

RINSE WITH WATER AFTER MEALS AND CHOOSE WATER AS THE BEVERAGE OF CHOICE

According to the CDA, sugar is one of the main causes of dental problems. Sugary drinks are also a major source of sugars in the diets of pre-teens and teens. As a result, consuming sugary drinks may lead to increased risk of cavities for children, and obesity and type 2 diabetes for the entire population.

Drinking water keeps you hydrated without the added sugars, sodium, and saturated fats, and it helps your body get rid of wastes.

Water also helps to buffer the collection of bacteria in your mouth until you can brush. Rinsing your mouth with water after meals and snacks, then brushing 30 to 45 minutes later, is a great addition to your mouth care.

BE VIGILANT IF YOU ALREADY HAVE A HEALTH ISSUE

People with certain diseases are more at risk for oral disease because they've already experienced a compromise in their immune system. Being vigilant in your oral health care may help lessen the impact.

IMPROVE YOUR GUT HEALTH AND MICROBIOME

There are many ways to improve your gut microbiome, all of which are a perfect compliment to The Livy Method including:

Eat a diverse range of foods: This can lead to a diverse microbiome, which is an indicator of good gut health. These include a source of healthy carbohydrates, good quality protein, and healthy fats.

In particular, legumes, beans and fruit contain lots of fibre and can promote the growth of healthy *Bifidobacteria*. Some high fibre foods that are good for your gut bacteria include:

- raspberries
- artichokes
- green peas
- broccoli

- chickpeas
- lentils
- beans
- whole grains
- bananas
- apples

Apples, artichokes, blueberries, almonds, and pistachios have also all been shown to increase *Bifidobacteria* in humans. *Bifidobacteria* are considered beneficial bacteria, as they can help prevent intestinal inflammation and enhance gut health.

Eat fermented foods and liquids: Fermented foods/liquids can reduce the amounts of disease-causing species in the gut. Fermented foods have undergone fermentation, a process in which the sugars they contain are broken down by yeast or bacteria.

Some examples of fermented foods/liquids are:

- yoghourt
- kimchi
- sauerkraut
- tempeh
- Fermented pickles
- kefir
- kombucha

Many of these foods are rich in *lactobacilli*, a type of bacteria that can benefit your health. Research shows that people who eat a lot of yoghourt appear to have more *lactobacilli* in their intestines. These people also have less *Enterobacteriaceae*, which is a type of bacteria associated with inflammation and a number of chronic conditions. Similarly, a number of studies have shown that yoghourt consumption can improve intestinal bacteria and decrease symptoms of lactose intolerance. What's more, yoghourt may also enhance the function and composition of the microbiome.

However, many yoghourts, especially flavoured yoghurt, contain high amounts of sugar. Therefore, it's best to opt for plain, unsweetened yoghurt or a flavoured yoghurt with minimal added sugar that is made only of milk and bacteria mixtures, also sometimes called "starter cultures." Additionally, to reap the gut health benefits, make sure the label reads "contains live active cultures."

Furthermore, fermented milk (kefir) may promote the growth of beneficial bacteria, such as *Bifidobacteria* and *lactobacilli*, while decreasing quantities of some other harmful strains of bacteria. Kimchi may also benefit the gut flora.

Limit your intake of artificial sweeteners: Some evidence has shown that artificial sweeteners like aspartame increase blood sugar by stimulating the growth of unhealthy bacteria like *Enterobacteriaceae* in the gut microbiome. Also, there is growing evidence that indicates certain artificial sweeteners like sucralose reduce insulin sensitivity and affect the gut bacteria. Check out the science post on Sugars and the Brain where this was discussed in more detail!

Eat prebiotic foods: As discussed above, prebiotics are a type of fibre that stimulates the growth of healthy bacteria. Taking a prebiotic along with your probiotic if needed as recommended in the Let's Talk Supplements Post can go a long way in building up the good bacteria in your digestive system, and help with the healing process.

Breastfeed for as long as possible: Breastfeeding is very important for the development of the gut microbiome. A baby's microbiome begins to properly develop at birth. However, studies suggest that babies may be exposed to some bacteria even before birth.

During the first 2 years of life, an infant's microbiome is continuously developing and is rich in beneficial *Bifidobacteria*, which can digest the sugars found in breast milk. What's more, breastfeeding is also associated with lower rates of allergies, obesity, and other health conditions that may be due to differences in the gut microbiota.

Eat whole grains: Whole grains contain lots of fibre and beneficial non-digestible carbohydrates like beta-glucan, which are digested by gut bacteria to benefit weight, cancer risk, diabetes and other issues. These carbohydrates are not absorbed in the small intestine and instead make their way to the large intestine to promote the growth of beneficial bacteria in the gut. Research suggests that whole grains can promote the growth of *Bifidobacteria*, *lactobacilli*, and *Bacteroidetes* in humans.

Whole grains can also increase feelings of fullness, reduce inflammation, and certain risk factors for heart disease. However, some people may have some issues with gluten and may have to limit or avoid the intake of it.

While this mostly applies to those with celiac disease or a sensitivity to gluten, more research is needed to determine whether eating grains that contain gluten may also alter the gut microbiome in healthy adults without these conditions.

Eat more plant-based meals: Vegetarian diets may help reduce levels of disease-causing bacteria such as *E. coli*, as well as inflammation and cholesterol. However, it is unclear if the benefits of a vegetarian diet on the gut microbiome are due to a lack of meat intake or if other factors may also play a role.

Eat foods rich in polyphenols: Polyphenols are plant compounds that have many health benefits, including reductions in blood pressure, inflammation, cholesterol levels, and oxidative stress. Human cells can't always digest polyphenols. Because they aren't absorbed efficiently, most polyphenols make their way to the colon, where they are digested by gut bacteria.

Some examples of foods rich in polyphenols are:

- cocoa and dark chocolate
- red wine
- grape skins
- green tea
- almonds
- onions
- blueberries
- broccoli

Polyphenols from cocoa can increase the amount of *Bifidobacteria* and *lactobacilli* in humans and reduce the quantity of *Clostridia*. Furthermore, these changes in the microbiome are associated with lower levels of triglycerides and C-reactive protein, which is a marker of inflammation.

The polyphenols in red wine have similar effects and have even been shown to increase levels of beneficial bacteria in people with metabolic syndrome. However, those that are mindful of supporting their liver may want to only have it on occasion as discussed in the science post Detox.

Take a probiotic supplement: Probiotics are live bacteria that can help restore the gut to a healthy state after dysbiosis. Probiotics may not permanently colonise the intestines; however, they may benefit your health by helping to change the overall composition of the microbiome and supporting your metabolism.

Probiotics may not have a big influence on the gut microbiome composition of healthy people, however, there is some evidence that probiotics may improve the gut microbiome in those with certain diseases.

Interestingly, a Spanish systematic by Álvarez-Arraño, V., & Martín-Peláez, S., (2021) reviewed 27 randomized control trials that met their criteria indicates that both probiotics and synbiotics (a combination of a probiotic and prebiotic), specifically certain strains of Lactobacillus gasseri, L. rhamnosus, L. plantarum, L. curvatus associated with other Lactobacillus species and/or with species from the Bifidobacterium genus, have the potential to aid in weight and fat loss in overweight and obese populations. There is still a need, though, for clinical trials, in order to state more accurate recommendations in terms of strains, doses and intervention times.

Take antibiotics only when necessary: Antibiotics kill many bad and good bacteria in the gut microbiome, possibly contributing to weight gain and antibiotic resistance. Thus, only take antibiotics when medically necessary. If taking Antibiotics, speak to your HCP about taking probiotics to help maintain your good bacterial flora.

As it can be seen, by following all the recommendations of The Livy Method, which facilitates strengthening the health of your microbiome, you may experience not only weight loss, but overall improvements in your health and wellness. Our bodies are not compartmentalised, separate systems. Our bodies are a unique symphony of so many different moving parts, living cells, organisms and systems, that all work together to keep us alive and functioning as best as we can. However, we choose how we fuel, maintain, and take care of it. The better we are able to invest in our health and selves, the more harmonious that symphony of our microbiome is.

Check out these great videos and resources to better understand our microbiome, they have been shared in other Science Posts but are worth watching:

https://www.youtube.com/watch?v=B9RruLkAUm8&t=329s

https://www.youtube.com/watch?v=IDqMB6C1uys

IMPACTT (Canada)

https://www.impactt-microbiome.ca/

link to the Human Microbiome Project

https://hmpdacc.org/ihmp/

https://hmpdacc.org/hmp/

https://hmpdacc.org/

EU Microbiome Support

https://www.microbiomesupport.eu/about/

European Commission food 2030

https://ec.europa.eu/info/research-and-innovation/research-area/environment/bioeconomy/food-systems/food-2030_en#:~:text=Food%202030%20is%20the%20EU's,is%20fit%20for%20the%20future.

Dr. Svetlana U. Perović has personally curated a list of microbiome events that are free and mostly virtual.

https://github.com/SvetlanaUP/Microbiome-conferences-c

https://whatisbiotechnology.org/index.php/science/summary/microbiome/the-human-microbiome-refers-to-the-complete-set-of-genes

And this concludes the science series for this round of The Livy Method Program. Hopefully you enjoyed this learning journey that we have embarked on together.

REFERENCES

About. (n.d.). Microbiome Support. https://www.microbiomesupport.eu/about/

Álvarez-Arraño V., Martín-Peláez, S. (2021) Effects of Probiotics and Synbiotics on Weight Loss in Subjects with Overweight or Obesity: A Systematic Review. *Nutrients*, 17;13(10):3627. doi: 10.3390/nu13103627. PMID: 34684633; PMCID: PMC8540110.

Baldi, S., Mundula, T., Nannini, G., & Amedei, A. (2021). Microbiota shaping - the effects of probiotics, prebiotics, and fecal microbiota transplant on cognitive functions: A systematic review. *World journal of Gastroenterology*, *27*(39), 6715–6732. https://doi.org/10.3748/wjg. v27.i39.6715

Barra, N. G., Anhê, F. F., Cavallari, J. F., Singh, A. M., Chan, D. Y., & Schertzer, J. D. (2021). Micronutrients impact the gut microbiota and blood glucose, *Journal of Endocrinology*, *250*(2), R1-R21.https://doi.org/10.1530/JOE-21-0081

Berg, G., Rybakova, D., Fischer, D., Cernava, T., Vergès, M. C., Charles, T., Chen, X., Cocolin, L., Eversole, K., Corral, G. H., Kazou, M., Kinkel, L., Lange, L., Lima, N., Loy, A., Macklin, J. A., Maguin, E., Mauchline, T., McClure, R., Mitter, B., … Schloter, M. (2020). Microbiome definition re-visited: Old concepts and new challenges. *Microbiome*, *8*(1). https://doi. org/10.1186/s40168-020-00875-0

Brown, M.J. (2021, October 11). *How short-chain fatty acids affect health and weight.* Healthline. https://www.healthline.com/nutrition/short-chain-fatty-acids-101

Claus, S. P., Guillou, H., & Ellero-Simatos, S. (2016). The gut microbiota: A major player in the toxicity of environmental pollutants? *NPJ biofilms and microbiomes*, *2*. https://doi.org/10.1038/npjbiofilms.2016.3

Deo, P. N., & Deshmukh, R. (2019). Oral microbiome: Unveiling the fundamentals. *Journal of Oral and Maxillofacial Pathology*, *23*(1), 122–128. https://doi.org/10.4103/jomfp.JOMFP_304_18

Dobell, C. (1920). The discovery of the intestinal protozoa of man. *Proceedings of the Royal Society of Medicine*, *13*(Sect Hist Med), 1–15. https://www.ncbi.nlm.nih.gov/pmc/articles/PMC2151982/

Dominy, S.S., Lynch, C., Ermini, F., Benedyk, M., Marczyk, A., Konradi, A., Nguyen, M., Haditsch, U., Raha, D., Griffin, C., Holsinger, L. J., Arastu-Kapur, S., Kaba, S., Lee, A., Ryder, M. I., Potempa, B., Mydel, P., Hellvard, A., Adamowicz, K., … Potempa, J. (2019). Porphyromonas gingivalis in Alzheimer's disease brains: Evidence for disease causation and treatment with small-molecule inhibitors. *Science Advances*, *5*(1). DOI: 10.1126/sciadv.aau3333

Flossing & brushing. (n.d.). Canadian Dental Association. https://www.cda-adc.ca/en/oral_health/cfyt/dental_care/flossing_brushing.asp

Food 2030. (n.d.). European Commision Research and Innovation. https://research-and-innovation.ec.europa.eu/research-area/environment/bioeconomy/food-systems/food-2030_en#:~:text=Food%202030%20is%20the%20EU's,is%20fit%20for%20the%20future.

Gunnars, K. (2019, February 27). *Does all disease begin in your gut? The surprising truth*. Healthline. https://www.healthline.com/nutrition/does-all-disease-begin-in-the-gut

Guo, Y., Zhu, X., Zeng, M., Qi, L., Tang, X., Wang, D., Zhang, M., Xie, Y., Li, H., Yang, X., & Chen, D. (2021). A diet high in sugar and fat influences neurotransmitter metabolism and then affects brain function by altering the gut microbiota. *Translational Psychiatry, 11*. https://doi.org/10.1038/s41398-021-01443-2

. Y., Song, K. P., & Chan, K. G. (2016). Porphyromonas gingivalis: An overview of periodontopathic pathogen below the gum line. *Frontiers in Microbiology, 7*. https://doi.org/10.3389/fmicb.2016.00053

Human microbiome project. (2020, August 20). National Institutes of Health. http://commonfund.nih.gov/hmp/

IMPACTT. (n.d.). Integrated Microbiome Platforms for Advancing Causation Testing and Translation. https://www.impactt-microbiome.ca/

Kristensen, N. B., Bryrup, T., Allin, K. H., Nielsen, T., Hansen, T. H., & Pedersen, O. (2016). Alterations in fecal microbiota composition by probiotic supplementation in healthy adults: A systematic review of randomized controlled trials. *Genome Medicine, 8*(1), 52. https://doi.org/10.1186/s13073-016-0300-5

Microbiome-conferences-etc. (n.d.). Github. https://github.com/SvetlanaUP/Microbiome-conferences-c

NIH human microbiome project. (n.d.). Human Microbiome Project. https://hmpdacc.org/

Scaccia, A. (2020, August 19). *Serotonin: What you need to know*. Healthline. https://www.healthline.com/health/mental-health/serotonin#functions

Sender, R., Fuchs, S., & Milo, R. (2016). Revised estimates for the number of human and bacteria cells in the body. *PLOS Biology, 14*(8). https://doi.org/10.1371/journal.pbio.1002533

Semeco, A., & Kelly, E. (2021, May 11). *The 19 best prebiotic foods you should eat*. Healthline. https://www.healthline.com/nutrition/19-best-prebiotic-foods

Shreiner, A. B., Kao, J. Y., & Young, V. B. (2015). The gut microbiome in health and in disease. *Current Opinion in Gastroenterology, 31*(1), 69–75. https://doi.org/10.1097/MOG.0000000000000139

Stoller-Conrad, J. (2015, April 9). *Microbes help produce serotonin in gut.* Caltech. https://www.caltech.edu/about/news/microbes-help-produce-serotonin-gut-46495

TEDx Talks. (2016, June 27). *Microbiome: Gut bugs and you | Warren Peters | TEDxLaSierraUniversity* [Video]. Youtube. https://www.youtube.com/watch?v=IDqMB6C1uys

TEDx Talks. (2019, December 12). *Your gut microbiome: The most important organ you've never heard of | Erika Ebbel Angle | TEDxFargo* [Video]. Youtube. https://www.youtube.com/watch?v=B9RruLkAUm8

Venegas, D. P., De la Fuente, M. K., Landskron, G., González, M. J., Quera, R., Dijkstra, G., Harmsen, H., Faber, K. N., & Hermoso, M. A. (2019). Short chain fatty acids (SCFAs)-mediated gut epithelial and immune regulation and its relevance for inflammatory bowel diseases. *Frontiers in Immunology, 10.* https://doi.org/10.3389/fimmu.2019.00277

Vijay, A., & Valdes, A.M. (2022). Role of the gut microbiome in chronic diseases: A narrative review. *European Journal of Clinical Nutrition, 76,* 489–501. https://doi.org/10.1038/s41430-021-00991-6

Welcome. (n.d.). Integrative Human Microbiome Project (iHMP). https://hmpdacc.org/ihmp/

What is taxonomy? (2010, April 6). Convention on Biological Diversity. https://www.cbd.int/gti/taxonomy.shtml#:~:text=Taxonomy%20is%20the%20science%20of,and%20microorganisms%20of%20the%20world.

Yano, J.M., Yu, K., Donaldson, G.P., Shastri, G.G., Ann, P., Ma, L., Nagler, C.R., Ismagilov, R.F., Mazmanian, S.K., & Hsiao, E.Y. (2015). Indigenous bacteria from the gut microbiota regulate host serotonin biosynthesis. *Cell, 161*(2), 264-276. DOI: 10.1016/j.cell.2015.02.047

Zheng, D., Liwinski, T., & Elinav, E. (2020). Interaction between microbiota and immunity in health and disease. *Cell Research, 30*(6), 492–506. https://doi.org/10.1038/s41422-020-0332-7

Zoe. (n.d.). https://joinzoe.com/

Fall 2022 Group: Tracking Sheet

Use the chart below to track your progress throughout the Fall 2022 Group. This chart can be used to help you pick up on patterns of behaviours and responses and give you a better idea of what weight loss looks like specifically to you. Feel free to fill in all or none of the columns or personalize what types of things you want to track in the notes section. Happy tracking!

September 2022										
			Meals and Snacks							
Date	**Weight**	**Water**	**B**	**S1**	**L**	**S2**	**S3**	**D**	**Supplements**	**Notes** (i.e., NSVs, BMs, Exercise, Sleep, Bonus snacks, etc.)
Sept 12			☐	☐	☐	☐	☐	☐	☐	
Sept 13			☐	☐	☐	☐	☐	☐	☐	
Sept 14			☐	☐	☐	☐	☐	☐	☐	
Sept 15			☐	☐	☐	☐	☐	☐	☐	
Sept 16			☐	☐	☐	☐	☐	☐	☐	
Sept 17			☐	☐	☐	☐	☐	☐	☐	
Sept 18			☐	☐	☐	☐	☐	☐	☐	
Sept 19			☐	☐	☐	☐	☐	☐	☐	
Sept 20			☐	☐	☐	☐	☐	☐	☐	
Sept 21			☐	☐	☐	☐	☐	☐	☐	
Sept 22			☐	☐	☐	☐	☐	☐	☐	
Sept 23			☐	☐	☐	☐	☐	☐	☐	
Sept 24			☐	☐	☐	☐	☐	☐	☐	

Fall 2022 Group: Tracking Sheet

Date	Weight	Water	Meals and Snacks B	S1	L	S2	S3	D	Supplements	Notes (i.e., NSVs, BMs, Exercise, Sleep, Bonus snacks, etc.)
Sept 25			☐	☐	☐	☐	☐	☐	☐	
Sept 26			☐	☐	☐	☐	☐	☐	☐	
Sept 27			☐	☐	☐	☐	☐	☐	☐	
Sept 28			☐	☐	☐	☐	☐	☐	☐	
Sept 29			☐	☐	☐	☐	☐	☐	☐	
Sept 30			☐	☐	☐	☐	☐	☐	☐	

September Notes:

_____

_____

_____

_____

_____

October 2022

Date	Weight	Water	Meals and Snacks B	S1	L	S2	S3	D	Supplements	Notes (BMs, Exercise, Period, Stress, Bonus snacks, etc.)
Oct 1			☐	☐	☐	☐	☐	☐	☐	
Oct 2			☐	☐	☐	☐	☐	☐	☐	
Oct 3			☐	☐	☐	☐	☐	☐	☐	

Fall 2022 Group: Tracking Sheet

Date	Weight	Water	Meals and Snacks						Supplements	Notes (i.e., NSVs, BMs, Exercise, Sleep, Bonus snacks, etc.)
			B	S1	L	S2	S3	D		
Oct 4			☐	☐	☐	☐	☐	☐	☐	
Oct 5			☐	☐	☐	☐	☐	☐	☐	
Oct 6			☐	☐	☐	☐	☐	☐	☐	
Oct 7			☐	☐	☐	☐	☐	☐	☐	
Oct 8			☐	☐	☐	☐	☐	☐	☐	
Oct 9			☐	☐	☐	☐	☐	☐	☐	
Oct 10			☐	☐	☐	☐	☐	☐	☐	
Oct 11			☐	☐	☐	☐	☐	☐	☐	
Oct 12			☐	☐	☐	☐	☐	☐	☐	
Oct 13			☐	☐	☐	☐	☐	☐	☐	
Oct 14			☐	☐	☐	☐	☐	☐	☐	
Oct 15			☐	☐	☐	☐	☐	☐	☐	
Oct 16			☐	☐	☐	☐	☐	☐	☐	
Oct 17			☐	☐	☐	☐	☐	☐	☐	
Oct 18			☐	☐	☐	☐	☐	☐	☐	
Oct 19			☐	☐	☐	☐	☐	☐	☐	

Fall 2022 Group: Tracking Sheet

Date	Weight	Water	Meals and Snacks						Supplements	Notes (i.e., NSVs, BMs, Exercise, Sleep, Bonus snacks, etc.)
			B	S1	L	S2	S3	D		
Oct 20			☐	☐	☐	☐	☐	☐	☐	
Oct 21			☐	☐	☐	☐	☐	☐	☐	
Oct 22			☐	☐	☐	☐	☐	☐	☐	
Oct 23			☐	☐	☐	☐	☐	☐	☐	
Oct 24			☐	☐	☐	☐	☐	☐	☐	
Oct 25			☐	☐	☐	☐	☐	☐	☐	
Oct 26			☐	☐	☐	☐	☐	☐	☐	
Oct 27			☐	☐	☐	☐	☐	☐	☐	
Oct 28			☐	☐	☐	☐	☐	☐	☐	
Oct 29			☐	☐	☐	☐	☐	☐	☐	
Oct 30			☐	☐	☐	☐	☐	☐	☐	
Oct 31			☐	☐	☐	☐	☐	☐	☐	

October Notes:

_____

_____

_____

_____

_____

Fall 2022 Group: Tracking Sheet

November 2022										
			Meals and Snacks							
Date	**Weight**	**Water**	**B**	**S1**	**L**	**S2**	**S3**	**D**	**Supplements**	**Notes** (BMs, Exercise, Period, Stress, Bonus snacks, etc.)
Nov 1			☐	☐	☐	☐	☐	☐	☐	
Nov 2			☐	☐	☐	☐	☐	☐	☐	
Nov 3			☐ ☐	☐ ☐	☐ ☐	☐ ☐	☐ ☐	☐ ☐	☐	
Nov 4			☐ ☐	☐ ☐	☐ ☐	☐ ☐	☐ ☐	☐ ☐	☐	
Nov 5			☐ ☐	☐ ☐	☐ ☐	☐ ☐	☐ ☐	☐ ☐	☐	
Nov 6			☐ ☐	☐ ☐	☐ ☐	☐ ☐	☐ ☐	☐ ☐	☐	
Nov 7			☐	☐	☐	☐	☐	☐	☐	
Nov 8			☐	☐	☐	☐	☐	☐	☐	
Nov 9			☐	☐	☐	☐	☐	☐	☐	
Nov 10			☐ ☐	☐ ☐	☐ ☐	☐ ☐	☐ ☐	☐ ☐	☐	
Nov 11			☐ ☐	☐ ☐	☐ ☐	☐ ☐	☐ ☐	☐ ☐	☐	
Nov 12			☐ ☐	☐ ☐	☐ ☐	☐ ☐	☐ ☐	☐ ☐	☐	
Nov 13			☐ ☐	☐ ☐	☐ ☐	☐ ☐	☐ ☐	☐ ☐	☐	
Nov 14			☐	☐	☐	☐	☐	☐	☐	

Fall 2022 Group: Tracking Sheet

Date	Weight	Water	Meals and Snacks						Supplements	Notes (i.e., NSVs, BMs, Exercise, Sleep, Bonus snacks, etc.)
			B	S1	L	S2	S3	D		
Nov 15			☐	☐	☐	☐	☐	☐	☐	
Nov 16			☐	☐	☐	☐	☐	☐	☐	
Nov 17			☐	☐	☐	☐	☐	☐	☐	
Nov 18			☐	☐	☐	☐	☐	☐	☐	
Nov 19			☐	☐	☐	☐	☐	☐	☐	
Nov 20			☐	☐	☐	☐	☐	☐	☐	
Nov 21			☐	☐	☐	☐	☐	☐	☐	
Nov 22			☐	☐	☐	☐	☐	☐	☐	
Nov 23			☐	☐	☐	☐	☐	☐	☐	
Nov 24			☐	☐	☐	☐	☐	☐	☐	
Nov 25			☐	☐	☐	☐	☐	☐	☐	
Nov 26			☐	☐	☐	☐	☐	☐	☐	
Nov 27			☐	☐	☐	☐	☐	☐	☐	
Nov 28			☐	☐	☐	☐	☐	☐	☐	
Nov 29			☐	☐	☐	☐	☐	☐	☐	

Fall 2022 Group: Tracking Sheet

Nov 30			☐	☐	☐	☐	☐	☐	☐	

November Notes:

_____

_____

_____

_____

_____

December 2022

Date	Weight	Water	B	S1	L	S2	S3	D	Supplements	Notes (BMs, Exercise, Period, Stress, Bonus snacks, etc.)
Dec 1			☐	☐	☐	☐	☐	☐	☐	
Dec 2			☐	☐	☐	☐	☐	☐	☐	
Dec 3			☐	☐	☐	☐	☐	☐	☐	
Dec 4			☐	☐	☐	☐	☐	☐	☐	
Dec 5			☐	☐	☐	☐	☐	☐	☐	
Dec 6			☐	☐	☐	☐	☐	☐	☐	
Dec 7			☐	☐	☐	☐	☐	☐	☐	
Dec 8			☐	☐	☐	☐	☐	☐	☐	
Dec 9			☐	☐	☐	☐	☐	☐	☐	
Dec 10			☐	☐	☐	☐	☐	☐	☐	

Fall 2022 Group: Tracking Sheet

Dec 11			☐	☐	☐	☐	☐	☐	☐	

			Meals and Snacks							
Date	**Weight**	**Water**	**B**	**S1**	**L**	**S2**	**S3**	**D**	**Supplements**	**Notes** (i.e., NSVs, BMs, Exercise, Sleep, Bonus snacks, etc.)
Dec 12			☐	☐	☐	☐	☐	☐	☐	
Dec 13			☐	☐	☐	☐	☐	☐	☐	

December Notes:

_____

_____

_____

_____

_____

Manufactured by Amazon.ca
Bolton, ON